"Today's AIDS sufferers represent, in many ways, the lepers of the '90s, and Christians should be the first to offer the same type of compassionate response that Jesus himself exemplified to the needy and suffering. Drs. Wood and Dietrich have put together a well-reasoned, conscientious treatise on the personal and social ramifications of this modern-day plague. I recommend their thoughtful analysis."—**Charles W. Colson**, Prison Fellowship

"Dr. Glenn Wood and Dr. John Dietrich are compassionate realists about AIDS. They give us accurate information about the illness, and call us to be loving truth-speakers who show mercy to its suffering victims." —**Dr. John White**, author of *Eros Defiled*

"The authors have shown themselves to be competent spokesmen for the medical and Christian communities. They have a dedication for scientific and biblical truth which causes the book to have an important impact on head and heart. Christians who are willing to submit to godly guidance to find their way through the complex issues of the AIDS crisis should read this book and put its principles into practice." —**Richard W. Goodgame, M.D.**, Assistant Professor of Medicine, Baylor College of Medicine, and recent medical missionary to Central Africa

"*The AIDS Epidemic* is a biblically solid and scientifically sound discussion of this tragic and complex problem. It offers unique insights into the whole sexual revolution. It will especially help pastors and lay leaders. I recommend it highly as the best Christian book I know of on the subject. —**Bill Counts**, senior pastor, Fellowship Bible Church (Texas)

"This is one of the finest books in print about the subject of AIDS. John Dietrich and Glenn Wood are deeply in love with Jesus Christ and with his lost and saved sheep. Because of their love for God and his people and because of their exceptional training and insight, I highly recommend this important book." —**Joe S. McIlhaney, Jr., M.D.**, author, *1250 Health-Care Questions Women Ask*

"This book, by two compassionate and skilled Christian doctors, will answer the questions many Christians are increasingly facing today in coming in contact with AIDS victims. It could well serve as a textbook for church seminars to help members deal with the AIDS phenomenon. It is accurate in its information, widely informed in its knowledge, and thorough in its discussion. As a California pastor, surrounded by the problem, I recommend it highly as a safe yet compassionate guide to the AIDS crisis." —**Ray C. Stedman**, Peninsula Bible Church (California)

Books in the Critical Concern Series:

- *Abortion: Toward an Evangelical Consensus*
- *Beyond Hunger: A Biblical Mandate for Social Responsibility*
- *Birthright: Christian, Do You Know Who You Are?*
- *Christian Countermoves in a Decadent Culture*
- *The Christian Mindset in a Secular Society*
- *The Christian, the Arts, and Truth*
- *Christians in the Wake of the Sexual Revolution*
- *The Controversy: Roots of the Creation-Evolution Conflict*
- *Decision Making and the Will of God*
- *Depression: Finding Hope and Meaning in Life's Darkest Shadow*
- *Euthanasia: Spiritual, Medical and Legal Issues in Terminal Health Care*
- *A Just Defense: The Use of Force, Nuclear Weapons and Our Conscience*
- *Life-Style Evangelism*
- *The Majesty of Man: The Dignity of Being Human*
- *The Trauma of Transparency: A Biblical Approach to Interpersonal Communication*
- *Worship: Rediscovering the Missing Jewel*

• A CRITICAL CONCERN BOOK •

The AIDS Epidemic
Balancing
Compassion & Justice

GLENN G. WOOD, M.D.
JOHN E. DIETRICH, M.D.

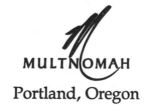

MULTNOMAH
Portland, Oregon

Unless otherwise indicated, all Scripture references are from the Holy Bible: New International Version, copyright 1973, 1978, 1984 by the International Bible Society. Used by permission of Zondervan Bible Publishers.

Scripture References marked KJV are from the Holy Bible: Authorized King James Version.

Scripture references marked NASB are from the New American Standard Bible, copyright The Lockman Foundation 1960, 1962, 1963, 1968, 1971, 1972, 1973, 1975, 1977. Used by permission.

Cover design by Durand Demlow
Cover illustration by Myles Pinkney
Edited by Rodney L. Morris

THE AIDS EPIDEMIC
©1990 by Glenn G. Wood and John E. Dietrich
Published by Multnomah Press
Portland, Oregon 97266

Multnomah Press is a ministry of Multnomah School of the Bible, 8435 N.E. Glisan Street, Portland, Oregon 97220

Printed in the United States of America

Library of Congress Cataloging-in-Publication Data

Wood, Glenn G.
    The AIDS epidemic : balancing compassion and justice / Glenn G. Wood, John E. Dietrich.
        p.   cm.
    Includes bibliographical references.
    ISBN 0-88070-309-1
    1. AIDS (Disease) 2. AIDS (Disease)—Religious aspects—Christianity. I. Dietrich, John E., 1950-   . II. Title.
RC607.A26W66 1990
362.1'969792—dc20   90-5554
                                                          CIP

92 93 94 - 5 4 3

To the people with AIDS,
of all ages, colors, and beliefs.
May this book help alleviate your
suffering in a small way,
and point you to the Lord of compassion.

He has showed you, O man , what is good.
And what does the LORD require of you?
To act justly and to love mercy
and to walk humbly with your God.
Micah 6:8

The authors have chosen to donate their profits from this book to Christian ministries to AIDS patients.

Contents

Acknowledgments   11

Part 1: Introduction
   1. The Earth Unchained from Its Sun   15
   2. The AIDS Epidemic Affects Everyone   23
   3. The Faces of AIDS   35
   4. The Shattered Dreams of the Sexual
      Revolution   51
   5. In the Beginning: The History of the
      AIDS Epidemic   83

Part 2: The Medical Description of AIDS
   6. The Spread of AIDS   113
   7. The Course, Diagnosis, and Treatment
      of AIDS   137
   8. The Prevention of AIDS   163
   9. The Air-tight Case against Casual
      Contagiousness   185

Part 3: The Church and AIDS
   10. The Need for a New Direction   211
   11. Homosexuality and Sins against
      the Body   229
   12. Christians and Sexuality   251
   13. Is AIDS the Judgment of God?   267
   14. A Biblically Based Model for
      Application   287
   15. Ministry Arenas   299

Part 4: Society and AIDS

    16. Civil Rights versus Social Responsibility   317

    17. Economics and AIDS   335

    18. Education and AIDS   353

    19. AIDS, Plagues, and Death   371

    20. Warnings and Opportunities   391

Glossary   405

Bibliography   413

Scripture Index   421

Subject Index   425

Acknowledgments

We first thank our wives (Nancy Wood and Merrilee Dietrich) and families (Kim, Rebecca, Justin, and Rachel Wood; Andrew, Timothy, and Abby Dietrich) for being so patient during this project, which turned out to be larger than any of us had anticipated. Biff Bivens and John Barnes were instrumental in providing early editing and guidance for two novice writers. This book would be much poorer without their valuable help. Rod Morris, our longsuffering editor at Multnomah, went through many trials inflicted by us, yet with nary a word of complaint. New writers could not have asked for a better friend and encourager.

Glenn thanks the professors at the Center for Advanced Biblical Studies, especially Bill Counts, Hud McWilliams, and Mark Arrington, for teaching him to think clearly, and University of Texas philosopher Robert Kane, who walks to a different drummer, but who realizes what the important questions are. Don Sunukjian brought his enormous talents in communications to bear on two of the more difficult chapters of the book. Gary McKnight, Gary Mason, and Ian Rogers provided books, clear thinking, and steadfast friendship throughout this project. Don and Debbie Vasser were gracious enough to give Glenn time off from the medical practice to do some of the writing.

John thanks his medical partner, Steven W. Parker, M.D., for reviewing several parts of the book and for being patient and supportive in this project, and his professors at Baylor for providing the opportunity to learn the discipline of infectious disease. His patients have willingly shared parts of their lives, teaching resiliency and tenderness sometimes even in the midst of dying. John also expresses deep gratitude to the men and women who have escaped from sexual and drug addiction; they confirm that victory is still available through prayer, conviction, and obedience.

Most of all, we praise our Lord who provided the example in his life of what true light is. Let no one be deceived by our exhortations within this work that we are good examples of what we call for in others. We too have been convicted by the truth of God's Word that we are unworthy vessels who by God's grace are continuing to be molded into his image.

PART 1

INTRODUCTION

For all have sinned and fall short of the glory of God, and are justified freely by his grace through the redemption that came by Christ Jesus (Romans 3:23-24).

If I speak in the tongues of men and of angels, but have not love, I am only a resounding gong or a clanging cymbal. If I have the gift of prophecy and can fathom all mysteries and all knowledge, and if I have a faith that can move mountains, but have not love, I o.n nothing (1 Corinthians 13:1-2).

The LORD is good to all;
   he has compassion on all he has made
(Psalm 145:9).

"Do I take any pleasure in the death of the wicked? declares the Sovereign LORD. Rather, am I not pleased when they turn from their ways and live?" (Ezekiel 18:23).

Chapter One

The Earth Unchained from Its Sun

*H*ave you not heard of that madman who lit a lantern in the bright morning hours, ran to the marketplace, and cried incessantly: "I seek God! I seek God!"—As many of those who did not believe in God were standing around just then, he provoked much laughter. "Has he got lost?" asked one. "Did he lose his way like a child?" asked another. "Or is he hiding? Is he afraid of us? Has he gone on a voyage? emigrated?"— Thus they yelled and laughed.

The madman jumped into their midst and pierced them with his eyes. "Whither is God?" he cried; "I will tell you. We have killed him—you and I. All of us are his murderers. But how did we do this? How could we drink up the sea? Who gave us the sponge to wipe away the entire horizon? What were we doing when we unchained this earth from its sun?"[1]

Friedrich Nietzsche, 1882

Friday, June 5, 1981, represents a watershed in modern life. On that day, the Centers for Disease Control published the first report of the disease now known as Acquired Immunodeficiency Syndrome or AIDS.[2]

No one during that pivotal summer realized the coming impact of this new crisis. However, it is now clear that AIDS is one of the most important illnesses of our day and that it will remain significant well into the next century. In the nineties, over one million people in the United States and several million more across the world will die from this frightening malady. The social, economic, and moral trauma of AIDS on all people will be considerable regardless of culture, gender, geographic location, or religious beliefs.

Many mistakes early in the epidemic have resulted in an increased loss of life. And even today, many secular groups have shortsighted goals that will result in further unnecessary death. This tragedy cries out for clarification and compassion from the followers of Christ. Unfortunately, the books for Christians about AIDS have been uneven at best, manipulative and mistake-ridden at worst. These works have tended to be medically inaccurate and biblically unbalanced, often searching for conspiracies that do not exist. They are narrow in scope and fail to give a complete account of how AIDS fits into the rest of our culture. The resulting books are half-truths that fail to present Christlike solutions.

The AIDS epidemic is a critical issue facing the body of Christ. Therefore, it is important that the complexities of this issue be explained so that Christians can act appropriately both individually and corporately. We should not under- or over-emphasize the severity of the calamity. We should not merely react to moves by political groups, but should be informed by the Word of God and inspired directly by the life of Christ. Only by integrating biblical truth with the best medical knowledge can there be hope for a reasoned response.

This is a comprehensive volume on the AIDS epidemic. Our desire is to see this book used as a reference by local congregations to assist in the difficult decisions every church will face. Consequently, there are several general goals we hope to accomplish.

GOAL ONE: GIVE ACCURATE MEDICAL INFORMATION

We will present the most accurate medical information available. Where the experts agree on medical aspects of the illness, we will reveal why that is the case. As you will discover, a surprising amount of what is known about AIDS was understood early in the epidemic. Moreover, the evidence for this is logical and easy to understand. By the use of clear models, we hope to show why some of the more inflammatory accusations of some writers, both secular and religious, are untrue and harmful.

On the other hand, we will alter the faulty advice of medical authorities that is unsupported scientifically or morally. As one social critic put it, "There is no value-free expertise."[3] Supposedly objective scientists evaluate information through their personal convictions, with their inherent strengths and weaknesses. Dr. Robert Redfield, one of the finest investigators of AIDS in the nation, has appropriately stated that "in the case of AIDS, medicine and morality teach us the same lesson."[4] Abstinence before marriage and monogamy within marriage are the simple answers to stopping the epidemic through sexual transmission. Yet, because of biased values, many medical experts and so-called ethicists refuse to acknowledge this.

In medical areas that are incompletely understood, such as the origin of the AIDS virus, we will not assert theories that have not been confirmed scientifically, although we will present some of the conflicting positions. In sobering circumstances it is vital to separate fact from fantasy. Thereby, we avoid hysteria and can take appropriate measures.

GOAL TWO: HUMANIZE THE ILLNESS

We will give actual case histories of people with AIDS in order to make it a more familiar illness for the church called to minister to all who suffer. In our youth-oriented culture intent on concealing aging, illness, and disability, it is natural for nonmedical Christians to be reluctant to

approach people with such a debilitating disease. But affliction never occurs apart from the patient, so it will be important to see the complete picture of people with AIDS. In
some cases this may include sins that have led to the illness,
but it will also include the loneliness of the outcast, estrangement of spouses and family members, and economic devastation of the patients. By the grace of God, for some it also
includes triumph over tragedy. We must never lose sight of
the truth that the disease called AIDS is as varied as the individuals who have it. By combining men, women, and children into a disease category, we run the risk of not
celebrating the individual as one created in the image of
God.

GOAL THREE: EXPLAIN THE CONTEXT OF AIDS IN OUR SOCIETY

We will examine the historical, political, religious, and
social circumstances that have allowed the rapid spread of
the disease. Contrary to the information given in the national
media, AIDS is not a self-sustaining epidemic. As we will
show, the moral climate of North America allowed the crisis
in the Western world to occur, and the political and social
milieu have sustained it. The enormity of the AIDS epidemic
is the result of our society's refusal to follow God's edicts on
sexuality. No epidemiologist can reasonably dispute this. Yet
seldom does the secular press express remorse about the
changes in sexual attitudes that will cost over a million lives
in the U.S. alone. This blindness will be easier to understand
as we examine the social history of the last several decades.

This is a complicated area to probe, and no secular or
Christian writer has described the complexities involved.
Our world of knowledge and experience is fragmented in
the twentieth century. Immense amounts of information are
coming to light yearly so that no one can process it all. More
significantly, given the supposed demise of God and the
resultant loss of absolute moral imperatives, the secular
world has no single way of ordering data and ideas. The loss
of belief in absolute truth has set society adrift from its

moorings—"the earth is unchained from the sun." The process of being set adrift from God is called secularization, but that only connotes the negative movement. The human soul, which longs for meaning and purpose, must then turn to something, an idol, to replace an absent God.[5] Dostoyevsky's aphorism that "if God does not exist everything is permitted" is prophetic; it is the theme of the twentieth century.[6] The idol adopted can be a political cause, material possessions, illegal drugs, personal power, sexual conquests, intellectual glory, deification of the individual, or a combination. Seen in this context, the AIDS epidemic and society's reluctance to change are much more understandable.

The secularist mood was euphoric at the beginning of this century, similar to the levity of the atheists in Nietzsche's parable.[7] But Nietzsche's madman understood the cataclysms to come far better than they. The actual fools are the ones who think so lightly of ousting God and making man the measure of all things. The terrible results were inevitable.

GOAL FOUR: EXPLAIN HOW AIDS HAS TRANSFORMED OUR SOCIETY

Society is never static. It is like a large organism constantly reacting and reforming itself depending on external and internal stresses. The AIDS epidemic has caused enormous changes in thinking in our culture that are going to become more pronounced as the death count escalates. Few areas of Western society will be unaffected. Therefore, we will investigate the impact on the economy, the media, communications, politics, law, entertainment, morals, and religion.

It is important for evangelical Christians, who have God's truth, to be involved in the coming deliberations as the global community changes. However, in the process of expressing the truth of Scripture we should not disgrace our opponents. The imagery of Christ as the Great Physician is particularly appropriate here. As his followers, we are to help heal people, not scold them like schoolmasters. When the church chastises the world, we appear as another political faction after its own ends. But as fallen creatures, we cannot adequately be healers without personal prayer and the power of the Holy Spirit.

GOAL FIVE: PRESENT OUR PERFECT MODEL

We will look at the life and teaching of Christ to see how he responded under similar circumstances. Although AIDS is a fresh challenge for the church, the principles Jesus set forth two millennia ago are just as applicable today as then. As we look through church history, we see mistakes made because of the tendency to depend upon the mind of man instead of the life of Christ. Once we understand the many medical and social manifestations of the AIDS epidemic, the proper answers become straightforward. We simply act as Christ did. He also lived in a world of relative values within the Roman empire and came into contact with many people with different worldviews.

Some of the particulars of AIDS will change, but the principles in Jesus' life and teaching will transcend all specifics of this tragedy or any other illness. As the AIDS epidemic unfolds, many current medical details will become outdated, but the needed response of the church will remain essentially the same.

The time for action is now to avoid an even greater tragedy than death from AIDS. That greater tragedy is to have the non-Christian world observe an uncaring church unworthy of the name of God and avoid turning to the only One who has taken the finality out of death. However, if the church will respond properly, a suffering world will be drawn powerfully to Christ. Then we can stand in triumph with him and announce to humanity:

"Where, O death, is your victory?
Where, O death, is your sting?"

Chapter 1, Notes

1. Friedrich Nietzsche, *The Gay Science*, trans. Walter Kaufmann (New York: Vintage Books, 1974), 181.

2. Centers for Disease Control, "*Pneumocystis* pneumonia—Los Angeles," *Morbidity and Mortality Weekly Report* 30 (1981):250-52.

3. Herbert Schlossberg, *Idols for Destruction* (Nashville: Thomas Nelson Publishers, 1983), 194.

4. Robert Redfield and Wanda Franz, *AIDS and Young People* (Washington, D.C.: Regnery Gateway, Inc., 1987), 25.

5. Schlossberg, *Idols*, 6.

6. Fydor Dostoyevsky, *Brothers Karamazov*, part 1, book 1, chapter 6.

7. Klaus Bockmuehl, "Secularisation and Secularism," in *The Best in Theology*, vol. 1 (Carol Stream, Ill.: Christianity Today Publishers, 1987), 177.

"'The LORD is slow to anger, abounding in love and forgiving sin and rebellion. Yet he does not leave the guilty unpunished; he punishes the children for the sin of the fathers to the third and fourth generation.' In accordance with your great love, forgive the sin of these people . . ." (Numbers 14:18-19).

Jesus said, "Father, forgive them, for they do not know what they are doing" (Luke 23:34).

Then [Stephen] fell on his knees and cried out, "Lord, do not hold this sin against them." When he had said this, he fell asleep (Acts 7:60).

Do not repay evil with evil or insult with insult, but with blessing, because to this you were called so that you may inherit a blessing (1 Peter 3:9).

Chapter Two

The AIDS Epidemic Affects Everyone

O ne year ago I was teaching a Bible study to a group of hospital workers. A pastor's wife in the group knew I was writing a book on AIDS and asked me to call her husband. They had a special problem in their church and needed advice.

I called her husband the next day. He was a young pastor of a growing storefront church. Like many growing churches, they had a Spirit-given excitement as they were seeing many confess Christ as Savior and others rededicate their lives to God. A young man named Frank had joined the church about two months before. He had become interested in a young woman in the congregation and came to talk to the pastor because he had an exceptional problem. Frank revealed to the pastor that he had just left the homosexual life-style but was infected with the AIDS virus. He was perfectly healthy otherwise, but he had not told his potential girlfriend about his exposure to AIDS. The pastor kept this conversation to himself initially, but felt an obligation to discuss this with the board of elders.

Some of the elders had heard the conflicting information about AIDS. They were worried Frank might transmit the illness to others by coughing or by close contact. They were concerned about the small Sunday school classrooms; should he be allowed in there? Only one toilet was available for this new group of believers, and the elders wondered about needed precautions. What should they do about communion? How should a basin be cleaned after an HIV-infected man has been baptized? The pastor was particularly anxious about the young woman Frank wanted to date. The pastor was aware that the homosexual life-style included a high level of impersonal sexual activity. Would Frank carry that level of promiscuity into his newfound heterosexuality and commit sin as well as transmit the disease?

Conversations like this are occurring in other parts of the country, and as the epidemic enlarges, pastors will increasingly be called upon to teach their flocks about this disease and how Christians are to respond to it. AIDS will become as commonplace in some congregations as cancer or car accidents. But where will pastors get their information? And will it be the correct information or falsehoods founded on fear?

To their credit, the pastor and board counseled and prayed with Frank with a loving desire to have the best for him. They never considered asking him to leave as long as he was repentant of his past sins and trying to avoid further immorality. They anointed him with oil and laid hands on him to pray for a cure. Frank stayed with the church another month. However, the pull of the homosexual subculture was too much for him. The pastor asked Frank to confess when he fell into sin. Frank refused, having decided his homosexuality was inborn. Frank left the church and refused to return the pastor's calls. Later, his phone was disconnected.

A small church had just had its first encounter with this new disease. It is unlikely it will be their last. Churches throughout the United States will have comparable experiences. I know of several men in our city who are infected with the virus and who attend evangelical churches where no one knows they have a time bomb ticking in their bodies. We are going down a dark tunnel with this disease, and there is a light at the end of the tunnel. Unfortunately, the light is an oncoming train about to have an impact on almost everyone in America.

Most people not directly affected by AIDS think it will have negligible influence on their lives. At the opposite extreme, a small, diverse group of authors, politicians, homosexual activists, and Christians think this epidemic will be the most devastating illness of all time. Both extremes are misleading and hinder proper responses to the epidemic. We desire to present a reasonable third position in which Christians do not underestimate the significance of the AIDS epidemic nor act as if the world were coming to an end. Christians are the most likely people to combine the compassion, fair-mindedness, and the *possibility* of unbiased responses that could make a major difference in this highly politicized disease.

What Is AIDS?

Acquired Immunodeficiency Syndrome is caused by a viral infection first described in the early 1980s. It is primarily a sexually transmitted disease, although an enlarging portion of AIDS victims have contracted the disease through blood exposure by sharing needles and syringes during intravenous drug abuse. It can also be passed from an infected woman to her baby during childbirth. The AIDS virus has had several different names but is now called Human Immunodeficiency Virus (HIV). (The acronym AIDS is used frequently in this book because of its familiarity. However, the most accurate terminology for this infection is HIV disease, which will be used interchangeably with the AIDS acronym.)

The virus has a long incubation period during which the infected individual appears healthy but is capable of transmitting the infection. This period without symptoms has made AIDS particularly dangerous. Thousands were infected with the virus before anyone knew the disease existed. These individuals then spread the HIV unknowingly to others.

The virus slowly destroys a critical portion of the immune system. Some people develop a milder form of the disease called AIDS Related Complex (ARC). These patients have less severe symptoms than those with complete AIDS, including chronic diarrhea, lymph node enlargement, high fevers, neurological problems, and weight loss. The patients may die at this stage, may have the debilitating symptoms for months or years, or may go on to develop full-blown AIDS as the immune destruction continues. Since HIV disease is now seen by scientists as a continuum ranging from no symptoms to severe secondary infections, the term ARC, which implies a distinct syndrome, is less frequently used.

In fully developed AIDS, the immune decay is complete, and the individual is susceptible to cancers and infections that rarely affect people with normal health. Although antibiotics and chemotherapy may help to prolong life, the vast majority of persons infected with HIV eventually die. (A more extensive development of the medical information will occur in Part 2.)

THE WORLD SITUATION

Silently, the spread of the HIV grew to epidemic proportions on several continents before AIDS was first described in 1981. By January 1989, 142 out of 177 countries reporting to the World Health Organization (WHO) had diagnosed cases of AIDS within their borders.[1] Between five and ten million people are infected with the virus worldwide.[2] Although AIDS has been reported in most countries, only a few regions are greatly affected. The primary areas are Africa, the Americas, and Europe. In these places dwell over 95 percent of the AIDS patients diagnosed thus far, although the WHO expects a slow spread into other regions.

The developing countries with large numbers of cases in Africa, the Caribbean, and South America have been especially hard hit. These regions already deal with severe health problems such as malnutrition, high infant mortality, and debilitating tropical diseases. Tourism, especially in Africa and Haiti, has decreased because of fear of AIDS, further limiting resources. Africans and Haitians have been discriminated against when they have gone outside their countries because of people's unwarranted fears of catching AIDS.

AIDS IN THE U.S.

HIV disease in the United States is primarily a disease of homosexual men, intravenous drug users, hemophiliacs, and other transfusion victims. These groups constitute over 90 percent of all AIDS patients. Because of the United States' large male homosexual population, the vast majority of its patients are men[3], unlike Africa where men and women are equally affected.[4] In the U.S., one to two million individuals may be infected with the virus,[5] many of these seemingly healthy young men. The exact number of people infected is unknown because of legal restrictions and the prohibitive costs of mass testing. Most of these people—perhaps all of them—will come down with full-blown AIDS.[6] Some sectors of greater New York City, San Francisco, and Los Angeles are being annihilated by a biological explosion. Roughly half of the male homosexuals in San Francisco are infected with HIV.[7]

HIV disease has also ravaged intravenous drug users, who represent over one-quarter of all AIDS patients. Infected drug users are concentrated in certain geographic clusters, such as the Northeast corridor, Atlanta, Miami, Detroit, San Francisco, and Denver.[8] Often in poor health to begin with, these people develop full-blown AIDS more rapidly and die sooner than any other group. Moreover, they are an important source of transmission to their sexual partners and to their newborn infants. One-half of all women with AIDS in the U.S. have histories of IV drug use and another 20 percent have had sexual partners who used IV drugs.[9] Many of the women support their drug habit by prostitution, thus potentially propagating the virus to many others. The infants of infected mothers have a 30 percent chance of contracting the disease before or during childbirth[10] and usually die within months of having their first symptoms.[11]

Nine out of ten severe hemophiliacs are now infected with HIV, acquired through frequent transfusions of Factor VIII, a blood product given to prevent their bleeding problems. Since they require fewer transfusions, about half of the males with a milder form of hemophilia are infected.[12] Hemophiliacs uninfected by 1985 have a very low chance of acquiring the infection because of blood donor screening and a special heat treatment of Factor VIII which destroys the virus.

AIDS has been diagnosed in every U.S. state, although some states have only a few cases. As in Africa, the epidemic is more urban than rural since IV drug abuse, homosexuality, and promiscuity occur more frequently there. Anonymity, high population density, and the uninhibited life-style common in big cities are all conducive to the spread of AIDS. However, just as the disease has spread from the epicenters of New York and California to other regions, so epidemiologists expect it to spread slowly to rural areas. The spread into the heterosexual, non-IV drug using populations has been slower than some experts expected, but will likely increase over time.

Even for those with little risk of infection, there is cause for concern. Economic consequences will occur, such as increasing insurance premiums, higher costs for hospitalization, and perhaps tax increases for government support of HIV-infected people. Homosexuals and people with AIDS are pressing for legal protection and the right to express alternate life-styles. A new openness has emerged in discussing previously forbidden topics such as condoms, homosexual practices, and prostitution. Many have suggested mandatory sex education for all school children.

Although these issues are significant, the AIDS epidemic will affect people in many more personal ways. With one to two million people in the U.S. infected with HIV, almost all of us will see a family member, a friend, a business associate, or a member of the church stricken by the infection. Here are some of the scenarios we may come across.

* * * * * *

You discover that Bill, a friend with whom you have worked for five years, is in the hospital with a rare form of pneumonia. Another employee knows that this type of pneumonia is never seen in people with healthy immune systems and concludes that Bill has AIDS. Having known Bill for a long time, you struggle with the idea that he is a homosexual or an IV drug abuser. Your work station is right next to Bill's. You have shared soft drinks and sampled his lunch and he yours. You worry about your chances of getting the illness, particularly since you have had more colds this year. You feel an obligation to visit Bill, but you're not sure what to say. As a Christian you think IV drug abuse and homosexuality are sins, but you also know that as an ambassador for Christ you are called to minister to the needy.

* * * * * *

A new family moves into your school district, and you discover that one of their children has already died of AIDS. The two remaining children are healthy but infected with the AIDS virus. One of the children will be in your child's class. You consider yourself open-minded and realize the experts say that AIDS is not casually transmitted. However, this is your child and you are reluctant to accept the experts' testimony. You take your child to school and recognize the infected child from his picture in the newspaper. Only about half of the children who are supposed to be in the class have actually come. As you seat your daughter in a chair some distance from the controversial child, he sneezes violently twice, and you notice he has a runny nose.

* * * * * *

You realize that tragedies such as AIDS make people reevaluate their life and beliefs; redeemed homosexuals are beginning to come to church in your community. Many have changed their life-styles and have accepted the beliefs of Christianity. Some are still effeminate, and you wonder if they have completely broken with their past life. Jason, the first redeemed homosexual you meet in your church, has no AIDS virus in his body by the grace of God. However, he is so excited about his life as a Christian that he starts bringing several of his homosexual friends to church, who confess their sins and ask for forgiveness. One of these men is very thin and has lumps around his neck, and you wonder if these are signs of AIDS. Another man asks for prayer because he is infected with HIV. You have already decided to accept these men because it is the Christian thing to do. However, others are concerned, and over several months church attendance drops noticeably. You are close to the pastor, who confides that collections have also fallen; if they go down much further the church will become insolvent. What do you and the pastor do?

* * * * * *

One of your best friends confides in a prayer group that she has just received terrible news. Her twenty-four-year-old son is in the hospital with severe diarrhea and has admitted to her that he is a homosexual and has AIDS. She goes to the hospital and meets her son's lover and two other homosexual buddies. She has never knowingly been around homosexual men and does not know what to say. She has no reservation about hugging her sick son but does not want to shake hands with his close friends. She is angry at these friends and fears they have effectively murdered her son by passing the virus on to him. How do you counsel her?

* * * * * *

A family joins the church in which you are the director of the children's education program. The parents confide to you that their two boys are hemophiliacs and are infected with HIV, but they reassure you that they cannot infect others. Both boys appear and act perfectly normal. The mother has asked you not to reveal this to anyone because of the controversy it would cause. You realize that sooner or later it will come out. Should you worry about placing her toddler in the same class with ten others of the same age? Do you respect her wishes to keep the secret? What about the rights of your best friend who has a child in the same class?

* * * * * *

A friend at church has just experienced the joy of her first baby. The baby seems normal for the first six months, but then fails to gain weight. Finally, the child gets severely ill with pneumonia and comes down with meningitis six weeks later. A children's infectious disease expert reveals that the child has AIDS. Your friend's husband tearfully confesses to her that about twice a month since their marriage he has been visiting prostitutes during business trips to the West Coast. He wants to kill himself because he realizes his sin has caused him, his wife, and their innocent child to come down with the disease. How do you minister to your friend?

* * * * * *

Your wife works as a registered nurse at the local hospital. She is asked to draw blood from a young male with an unknown illness. As she withdraws the needle the patient flinches, and she sticks her finger. She immediately washes her finger with soap and water. The patient's doctor desires to perform the antibody test to rule out HIV infection in the young man. Appropriate forms asking permission to test the blood are drawn up according to the law. He refuses. Brokenhearted, you and your wife realize that nothing can be done legally. The young man's physician confides that AIDS is a real possibility. You and your wife must wait two to three months before she can be tested for the AIDS virus. Then, assuming the first test is negative, she must wait again. For months. Only after the second test is drawn can she and you rest easily and resume normal marital relations, interrupted for fear of an HIV infection in her.

CONCLUSION

Those who become severely ill in Western countries are usually elderly and sick with cancer or heart disease. AIDS affects the young and healthy and causes much ambivalence, since sin is often involved. The story of AIDS is depressing, but not as ominous as some have said.

It is important that the church be well-informed. To bury our heads in the sand or to claim the sky is falling when it is not does no one any good. Once we have the proper information, the church must then respond appropriately based on the reality of Jesus Christ. Christians throughout history have formed hospitals, assisted the poor, and cared for lepers and others when no one else would. And Christians will be the ones caring for the AIDS patients as well (see Part 3: The Church and AIDS).

But to be adequately informed, to have a full understanding of AIDS's impact on people, we must turn from how AIDS affects us to see the perspective of the victims and the faces of AIDS.

Chapter 2, Notes

1. *Update: AIDS Cases Reported to the Global Programme on AIDS* (Geneva, Switzerland: World Health Organization, 1989).

2. J. M. Mann and J. Chin, "AIDS: A Global Perspective," *New England Journal of Medicine* 319 (1988):302-3.

3. Centers for Disease Control, "HIV/AIDS Surveillance," December 1989.

4. T. C. Quinn et al., "AIDS in Africa: An Epidemiologic Paradigm," *Science* 234 (1986):955-63.

5. Centers for Disease Control, "Quarterly Report to the Domestic Policy Council on the Prevalence and Rate of Spread of HIV and AIDS—United States," *Morbidity and Mortality Weekly Report* 37 (1989):551-59.

6. K-J Lui et al., "A Model-based Estimate of the Mean Incubation Period for AIDS in Homosexual Men," *Science* 240 (1988): 1333-35.

7. See Table 3-5 in J. J. Goedert and W. A. Blattner, "The Epidemiology and Natural History of Human Immunodeficiency Virus," in *AIDS: Etiology, Diagnosis, Treatment, and Prevention,* 2d

ed., ed. V. T. Devita, S. Hellman, and S. A. Rosenberg (New York: J.B. Lippincott, 1988), 43.

8. Centers for Disease Control, "Update: Acquired Immunodeficiency Syndrome Associated with Intravenous Drug Use—United States, 1988," *Morbidity and Mortality Weekly Report* 38 (1989):165-70; R. A. Hahn et al., "Prevalence of HIV Infection among Intravenous Drug Users in the United States," *Journal of the American Medical Association* 261 (1989):2677-84.

9. Centers for Disease Control, "Update: Acquired Immunodeficiency Syndrome—United States, 1981-1988," *Morbidity and Mortality Weekly Report* 38 (1989):229-35.

10. S. Blanche et al., "A Prospective Study of Infants Born to Women Seropositive for Human Immunodeficiency Virus Type 1," *New England Journal of Medicine* 320 (1989): 1643-48; M.F. Rogers et al., "Use of the Polymerase Chain Reaction for Early Detection of the Proviral Sequences of Human Immunodeficiency Virus in Infants Born to Seropositive Mothers," *New England Journal of Medicine* 320 (1989): 1649-54.

11. G.B. Scott et al., "Survival in Children with Perinatally Aquired Human Immunodeficiency Virus Type 1 Infection," *New England Journal of Medicine* 321 (1989): 1791-96.

12. Goedert and Blattner, "Epidemiology and Natural History," Table 3-6, 45.

The Lord is not slow in keeping his promise, as some understand slowness. He is patient with you, not wanting anyone to perish, but everyone to come to repentance (2 Peter 3:9).

"But if a wicked man turns away from all the sins he has committed and keeps all my decrees and does what is just and right, he will surely live; he will not die. None of the offenses he has committed will be remembered against him. Because of the righteous things he has done, he will live" (Ezekiel 18:21-22).

To some who were confident of their own righteousness and looked down on everybody else, Jesus told this parable: "Two men went up to the temple to pray, one a Pharisee and the other a tax collector. The Pharisee stood up and prayed about himself: 'God, I thank you that I am not like other men—robbers, evildoers, adulterers—or even like this tax collector. I fast twice a week and give a tenth of all I get.'

"But the tax collector stood at a distance. He would not even look up to heaven, but beat his breast and said, 'God, have mercy on me, a sinner.'

"I tell you that this man, rather than the other, went home justified before God. For everyone who exalts himself will be humbled, and he who humbles himself will be exalted" (Luke 18:9-14).

Chapter Three

The Faces of AIDS

*T*he most of our brethren were unsparing in their exceeding love and brotherly kindness. They held fast to each other and visited the sick fearlessly, and ministered to them continually, serving them in Christ. And they died with them most joyfully, taking the affliction of others, and drawing the sickness from their neighbors to themselves and willingly receiving their pains. And many who cared for the sick and gave strength to others died themselves, having transferred to themselves their deaths. . . .

Truly the best of our brethren departed from life in this manner, including some presbyters and deacons and those of the people who had the highest reputation; so that this form of death, through the great piety and strong faith it exhibited, seemed to lack nothing of martyrdom. . . .

But with the heathen everything was quite otherwise. They deserted those who began to be sick, and fled from their dearest friends. And they cast them out into the streets when they were half dead, and left the dead like refuse, unburied. They shunned any participation or fellowship with death; which yet, with all their precautions, it was not easy for them to escape.

Dionysius of Alexandria, A.D. 263

The following true stories are not unusual; they are representative of the trials people with AIDS routinely face. The signs and symptoms of AIDS vary for each person. The people, their circumstances, and their responses to adversity are unique. John has personally cared for each of these patients. Their case histories give a partial glimpse into what it means to have AIDS.

* * * * * *

Peter loved to skate. It gave him a sense of vitality like no other activity. The combination of speed, strength, and gracefulness that he brought to his sport allowed him to be a professional teacher. To all appearances, Peter had a full life. His colleagues and friends thought of him as likable, outgoing, and cheerful. He was always on the go, participating in professional figure skating competitions and teaching beginning lessons on the side. Peter worked well with kids; he was patient with them and quick to praise their slightest improvement.

However, the first time I met him, Peter appeared quite different. When I was called in as a consultant, he was already in the hospital, being treated by another physician. It was difficult to get his medical history because of his labored breathing. His struggle to breathe provided a sharp contrast to the athletic body I saw before me. It made me uneasy to see him in this state, not only because of his discomfort but also because a young man of thirty-five is not supposed to be so ill.

When the AIDS antibody test came back positive, Peter was devastated. Being in one of the high risk groups, Peter had a reason to fear AIDS, but he was still young enough to believe the lie that tragedy always happens to someone else. It would not take long for that myth of youth to leave him. Peter also thought he could overcome anything, given enough effort. It would take longer for this belief to disappear, since he still had strength left in his body. But as his strength faded over the next eighteen months, so did Peter's hope for a complete recovery.

That first episode of pneumonia was relatively easy to treat, and although it confirmed the diagnosis of AIDS, it seemed only a temporary setback in Peter's life. As a gifted figure skater, he was eager to get back to work and training. He was careful to do exactly as I asked to make the best of his therapy. Those several months after full recovery from the pneumonia found him back in the ice rink again and skating competitively. No one could have recognized that he had AIDS and that his immune system was slowly being destroyed.

Peter reveled in those nine months of health. Every time he practiced long and hard, it gave him the feeling that everything would be all right. The doctors must be wrong to say he had this illness. He was going to lick this thing. This phase of denial is understandable. It doesn't make sense that a healthy young man is going to die because a lab test says he has some virus. But the time of apparent health always comes to an end; then the struggle begins.

Fever and a twenty-pound weight loss brought him back to my office. A minor fungal infection that he had caught as a child, and then easily suppressed, had reactivated and was now spreading quickly throughout his body. Skating was no longer a possibility. Sadly, he would never skate again. The weakness and fatigue were frustrating. Peter lost teeth as his gums deteriorated, and he couldn't gain weight no matter how much he ate. At times he couldn't care less about food. I told Peter he had to eat even when he didn't feel hungry because he would need to keep his weight up. Then the wasting, unrelenting diarrhea began, making the weight loss worse. Going to the bathroom six, eight, ten times a day added to his discomfort; it was difficult for him to leave home because of it. I tried to find out what was causing the diarrhea, but all the diagnostic tests came back normal. Therefore, we had no reliable treatment for it. Blindness suddenly struck in his left eye, caused by another reactivated infection from his youth.

The last two months of his life were difficult because of his frailty. I was sorry to see Peter in this state, so weakened now and unable to work. The original fear was back. No one is ready to die in his thirties. His hopes for the future began to diminish as the reality of the disease became apparent. Skating was a subject we avoided. We both realized that the great love of his life was a fading memory. At this point, Peter only wanted to feel better.

Peter was always meticulously clean, even as he approached the end of his life. It was important to him to be well-groomed even though, due to his weakness, it took a lot of time to prepare to go out. His mother, who lived in the same town, usually came with him to my office in the latter stages of his disease. She was not a doting mother, but Peter needed her assistance and comfort over the last months. It was disheartening to him to have to depend on someone, even his mother, since he had always prided himself on his physical capabilities. He eventually moved back in with his parents, entirely dependent on them once again.

AIDS was not kind to Peter. He did not slowly, painlessly slip into oblivion. The illness pummeled his body into submission and then gave temporary reprieves before attacking again. Because of his training, Peter was stronger than most, but that simply made his deterioration more evident and prolonged. I treated each new attack with the best therapies, but I knew my efforts would soon be futile. I sometimes questioned why we continued, but Peter still had fading hopes. He had heard about this drug or that diet. He would bring in articles from newspapers about promising new therapies. But the hopes would shrivel under the relentless, exhausting attacks of the unseen enemy.

Finally, debilitated and tired, blind in one eye and emaciated, he arrived at the hospital for the last time with a new fever, cough, and pneumonia. We both knew it would soon be over. Peter's last few months of life had been miserable, and the physical and emotional strength he needed to continue fighting for his life had vanished. It was not easy to watch his body fail; it was more difficult to watch his spirit fade. I realized, as I observed his exuberance disappear, that the essence of the man was going as well.

His former homosexual life-style was a distant echo in his struggle for life. He had stopped all risky behavior from the time he understood how his infection was spread. I admired that about him, since many of my other patients ignored my advice and continued to engage in practices that threatened others. His parents were loving and supportive of him. Though he was a homosexual, this did not affect their interaction with him; they were concerned now with loving their son, helping him through his illness. Somehow I needed to keep Peter comfortable and be supportive to his mother and father at the same time.

Peter and I became friends during his final year, since I had seen him frequently. As his lungs became heavier with fluid and his breathing more labored, he sensed he had little time left. A few days before he died, he asked me to stay a minute to talk to him. He lay in bed, pale and gaunt, with oxygen tubes in his nose, holding an oxygen mask over his face. He struggled to speak. Peter looked me in the eye and asked me how much time he had left. It was not comfortable looking at those alert eyes when we were speaking of his death, and I turned away. After composing myself, I admitted that he would be alive only a short time more. We talked of spiritual matters as we had before, and this gave him some comfort. He believed in God, but I was unsure of Peter's standing in eternity.

Peter was rapidly deteriorating and getting increasingly short of breath. The end was near, and he knew it. He was trying to appear brave, yet fear was in his eyes. Speech had become all but impossible now, for it took all his energy just to breathe. He was not responding to the medicines available for this rare pneumonia. Into the evening, there was little his parents and I could do but watch him struggle. By morning he was becoming incoherent and losing consciousness. His parents asked me how long. I told them Peter would not survive another day and that nothing else could be done except to make him comfortable. I hugged his dad and mom, and they thanked me. Tears welled up in my eyes; they wept. They experienced severe emotional pain knowing they would have to bury their child. He should have buried them.

A few hours later Peter died, his body finally surrendering. Mercifully, in the end he was unconscious and not suffering. And importantly, he was not alone. His parents were there at his bedside, grieving silently as they watched their only son die.

* * * * * *

Stephen was twenty-three years old, married to Melanie, an attractive woman two years younger than himself. They had a one-year-old daughter. They had married young and were having some marital problems. But they both loved their little girl boundlessly. Since they were Christians, Stephen and his wife were trying to resolve their differences and strengthen their commitment to one another.

Stephen worked for a small hotel in town doing most everything that needed to be done, from maintenance work to greeting guests. He was a hard worker and consequently was reasonably paid. To add some exhilaration to his life, Stephen had bought a motorcycle a few years before. Melanie was not thrilled, but consoled herself knowing that her husband was a sensible man who wouldn't take needless risks.

But Stephen's common sense did not protect him completely. One day his motorcycle skidded on a rain-soaked street, pinning him underneath. Stephen's right thigh bone was broken in two places, and he tore the major artery to the leg. The surgeon was able to repair the leg without much problem, but due to large amounts of blood loss, Stephen was given two pints of blood.

Two and a half years had passed since that surgery and transfusion. Three days before I met him, Stephen began to experience a dry, hacking cough that quickly worsened. He went to a family doctor who diagnosed pneumonia and placed him in a community hospital. Despite strong intravenous antibiotics, Stephen's respiratory problems became worse. His doctor called me in to examine his patient. I was not sure why he was so sick, but it was clear that Stephen needed to be in an intensive care unit at a bigger hospital. He was transferred to a medical center and diagnostic tests were done to discover what was happening inside his lungs.

According to my exam and the history of Stephen's illness, he seemed to have *Pneumocystis carinii* pneumonia, the most common opportunistic infection occurring in AIDS patients. Yet Stephen told me he was married and had never had any homosexual affairs. He also denied the use of intravenous drugs. If he was telling the truth, then the only way he could have acquired HIV was through the blood transfusion two years before. That possibility frightened me, because all of the blood transfused in our area was from local donors. Most of the AIDS-contaminated blood in the nation had been taken from the east and west coasts. We had never seen a case of AIDS caused by a transfusion and were not expecting to see any this early in the epidemic.

Transferring Stephen to our intensive care unit and beginning new antibiotics did not prevent a steady downhill course. In a surgical procedure, a small piece of his lung was obtained to establish a diagnosis. It came back from the pathologist as positive for *Pneumocystis* organisms. Stephen had AIDS. The sinking feeling I immediately felt was more than just sadness for Stephen. I now had to worry about his wife and baby who likely had been exposed. I also was concerned about all the local patients who had received transfusions in the last two years. I knew that Stephen would be only the first of many transfusion-transmitted cases of AIDS in our city.

Shortly after Stephen was diagnosed, I had the painful

task of explaining to his wife that she and her daughter might be infected. Since her husband had the transfusion over two years before and they were having normal marital relations, her chance of being infected was high. Her daughter could have become infected during childbirth. Melanie sat stoically as I explained how the virus is spread, but her emotions and tears flowed as I explained that her seemingly healthy, happy one-year-old might also be infected. It was one of the most difficult conversations I have ever had.

Now the waiting began. To determine if she was infected with HIV, Melanie would have to wait until a test for the virus was developed or until she acquired an opportunistic infection like the one her husband had. In 1984, prior to the availability of accurate tests, those were the realities the family members of AIDS victims had to face.

Stephen continued to get worse. By this time he was unable to get sufficient oxygen into his blood because the pneumonia was so extensive, and we had to place him on a ventilator. Although Stephen was alert, it was impossible for him to talk with the tube inside his throat. Stephen had told me before he was placed on the ventilator that he feared death primarily because it would leave his family alone and without financial support. His hotel job had a small life insurance policy that would do little more than help bury him.

I did not know Stephen or his family long. The time between his diagnosis and death was only three weeks. But it was an especially difficult period for me to see this man ten years my junior spiral downward to inevitable death. Stephen had broken no ancient injunctions against adultery. He had not destroyed his body with drugs injected into his veins. He was a victim of the sin of someone else who had desired to give life through donating blood but instead had given death.

The nurses and respiratory therapists also suffered with me as we watched this tragedy. Stephen's wife and daughter came to see him every day. He continued to be alert, though unable to speak while on the ventilator. We could read in his eyes the various emotions that were washing over him. His eyes, always intelligent, showed fear, sadness, pain, and fatigue. They also expressed joy the moment his family came. Two days before Stephen died, I watched one of these visits with a broken heart. Stephen was playing peekaboo with his daughter, who was sitting in his lap. Her giggles intermingled with the sounds of the ventilator. Most of the nurses had to retreat quietly to wipe away their tears. It affected me deeply as I, too, had a one-year-old.

Soon the ventilator could not keep Stephen alive, and the room became silent. But while we could not give him new lungs or a strengthened immune system, God in his grace had already made him a new creature in Christ. The realization that soon he would be with his Lord gave Stephen a peace that was remarkable to see. His parents were also strong Christians and ministered to me in my grief much more than I did to them. Their gentle hugs soothed the anguish of my failure and his death. Although they were grieving also, they harbored no bitterness; they had already committed their son to their Lord. The peace of God enveloped us that day in a small intensive care waiting room. And I will never be the same.

Stephen and his wife had grown much closer during his illness; their minor differences were unimportant compared to this tragedy. Stephen died, but his wife had to go on living, waiting to find out whether she and her daughter were also infected. The blood test for HIV infection was available one year later, and Melanie was one of the first people I contacted to have the test done. By God's protection, both Melanie and her daughter were normal.

They would go on living, but with the deep scars of having watched an innocent man die a painful death. I discovered later that Stephen had not died in vain. In the last days of his life, he was writing to his friends to tell them about the joy of knowing the Lord and the serenity that he felt, knowing he would be with him soon.

* * * * * *

Tom had just graduated from a suburban high school and was faced with a problem most teenagers don't have—his father was dying of cancer. As difficult as that was, Tom was about to encounter another crisis.

Tom had started smoking pot two years before. When that high lost its appeal, he went on to harder drugs, shooting up occasionally under pressure from his friends. It was a choice he would later regret. Tom had also been arrested for selling small amounts of cocaine to close friends. He was not a hard-core drug user, just a confused kid who thought life was for partying and that his days would never end. He had never been in trouble before.

Tom now had a new problem, which was the reason I had originally met him. His occasional drug use had put him at risk for several infections, including HIV. He had never thought about those possibilities when he had tried the drugs. Although he had no symptoms at the time, his family doctor asked me to examine him for the viral infections IV drug users frequently acquire. When the test for AIDS came back positive, I was saddened and somewhat surprised. Even in 1986, we did not think of AIDS as infiltrating suburban high schools.

Tom, his mother, and I sat together in the exam room, and I explained what the positive test result meant. These types of meetings are always painful for me, and this one especially so since it involved such a young person. I told Tom that he was infected with the virus that causes AIDS and that he would probably have it for the rest of his life. Though he did not have full-blown AIDS now, he might come down with it at any time or he might never come down with it; nobody was sure of his chances. As I spoke, he fidgeted in his chair and grimaced at various points. I knew it would be difficult for anyone to understand or accept such a vague, unknown prognosis, much more so for a teenager. His mother was quiet while I spoke. In addition to facing the loss of her husband in the coming months, she now must consider the possible death of her son in the next few years. As I finished the session, she said they would do what they had to do.

I next talked to Tom privately to get a complete social history. I already knew he had shared needles with some of his friends, but I needed to find out how many and how often. He was embarrassed when I next asked about girlfriends and sexual contacts. He admitted that he had a steady girl and that he was sexually active with her. After all, it's just part of the party scene. He was beside himself with worry over how he would tell her. A month later, he returned and admitted he had not told her. I was not surprised, since most teenagers are not equipped emotionally to talk about life-and-death issues. The denial in the young is even stronger than the denial in the more mature men with whom I had similar discussions.

At the end of our trying conversation, I ordered another blood test to determine how much damage had already been done to Tom's immune system. The test measures the number of T-helper cells, a type of white blood cell that helps to organize the immune system. When the number falls to low levels, secondary infections or cancers are likely to occur. When Tom returned the next week, I had further bad news—his T-helper cells were already low. I recommended that he begin on an experimental drug called AZT, which slows the destruction of the T-helper cells. I explained that the drug is related to cancer chemotherapy and has significant side effects. Tom was depressed and burdened with decisions few teenagers are capable of making. He said he would think about it. I have not seen him since.

Now in prison and barely twenty years old, Tom must wait and alter his life plans because of a virus contracted while sharing a needle. Tom must wait for his prison release. He must wait as his father is dying and as his own immune system fails. Will he respond with maturity and not have sex with his girlfriend when he gets out? Will he stop using drugs? Will he tell the people he shared needles with to get tested for HIV infection? I have no way of knowing. All I can do is pray that he follows my advice, and that his family holds together under such tremendous burdens.

* * * * * *

The colors of the Christmas decorations throughout the

city contrasted with the drab gray-green of the emergency room walls. My thoughts of family and of the significance of the manger faded upon walking through the emergency room doors. I was there to see one of my AIDS patients, now sicker than ever with recurrent fever and chills. I stared, startled and saddened, at Gary. The physical and emotional hurt from the fresh black eye could easily be read on his lonely face.

I had first heard about Gary two months earlier when he had what probably was *Pneumocystis* pneumonia. A precise diagnosis couldn't be made in the little country town where he was treated. However, he had the classic symptoms of fever, dry and nonproductive cough, and slowly advancing shortness of breath. I spoke to his family doctor and told him what needed to be done. His symptoms disappeared and his chest X-ray cleared after his treatment—but only for a week. His fever and cough returned, but this time the chest X-ray did not look like a *Pneumocystis* pneumonia. He needed more sophisticated specialists and diagnostic tools, so he left his small town sixty miles away and came to Austin, a place that provided better medical care but where he had no friends.

Gary was in a sad state. At the time of his AIDS diagnosis, he had lost almost everything. No family came with him to the hospital. They had rejected both him and his homosexuality the month before. They told him to get out, that they didn't want to have anything to do with him. A friend accompanied Gary from his small town. Jeff seemed to be his big brother and guardian. He certainly seemed to care for Gary, helping him with the hospital paperwork, encouraging him, and setting up an apartment for him. Neither had much money and both, being without work, had no medical insurance.

After many tests, a widespread fungal infection common with AIDS was finally diagnosed. Appropriate medical therapy was initiated, and Gary had a gratifying response. Three weeks of hospitalization and thirty thousand dollars later, he was stable and well enough to go home—wherever that was going to be. But Gary had insufficient funds to buy the needed medication, at a cost of fifty dollars a week, that would control his infection. Finally money became available through private help, and Gary was discharged with Jeff.

Now in crisis again, Gary's black eye betrayed recent events. The blind fellow with him was not Jeff. Gary had been beaten up by Jeff on Christmas Day, in the midst of an argument, and suddenly was left alone without food or a place to live. Jeff "just couldn't handle it any more" and had taken off. Gary didn't have the money to pay for the apartment, so he was evicted. He went to the AIDS Services of Austin who put him in touch with his new companion, another person with AIDS, who had an apartment and food but needed someone to drive and do chores for him. Mutual need drove them to one another; their togetherness was gratifying to see.

I was amazed that Gary was not angry about the beating or his parents' rejection, but then he had grown used to rejection over the years. Gary had a lot of positive attributes. He was a kindly person who took events as they came, and he was always grateful for the therapy and the time that I gave him. He never appeared to regret his sexuality, although in that subculture one seldom hears opinions other than "Gay is beautiful." I prayed with him once, but he seldom showed interest in spiritual matters. It is difficult to think about spiritual realities when your stomach is empty and there is no one to share the burden of life.

Gary had a lonely death. The only people who came into his room were his nurses and doctors—there were no visitors, no family. He died estranged, lonely, unforgiven by his family, totally abandoned. He lived only three months from the time of his first illness, and I wondered if his isolation hastened his passing.

* * * * * *

Eric is a fourteen-year-old hemophiliac I met two years ago. Being a youth with hemophilia is tough. Seemingly innocuous bumps and bruises turn into life-threatening bleeding because of the absence of Factor VIII, a protein essential for clotting. Eric's activity has been necessarily curtailed all his life, excluding him from contact sports and other normal childhood activities.

Eric was a quiet child who was chronically discouraged because of his illness. No one could blame him for that. In addition to his hemophilia, Eric had other marks against him. His parents were divorced. Eric recently had been diagnosed with regional enteritis, a chronic, debilitating disease of diarrhea and abdominal pain. Periodic flares of asthma further complicated his life. Although a teenager, he had not yet entered puberty and appeared more like a ten-year-old. He was small for his age, and the bigger kids teased him about his size and sickliness; he compensated by becoming shy and introspective. One of the manifestations of this was his enjoyment of video games, which gave him a sense of control that he lacked in his life. I liked him and enjoyed the times he would open up to me.

Because Factor VIII is prepared from thousands of donated units of plasma, its recipients are exposed to several blood-borne viral infections. Eric had already contracted hepatitis B (serum hepatitis) and soon afterwards, HIV. For two years he had been infected with this second virus, and already one could see the effects on his diminutive body. He would lose weight and not be able to gain it back quickly. The medication for his chronic bowel inflammation was a steroid, which stopped his fever and diarrhea but further compromised his immune function, setting him up for bouts with opportunistic infections.

Because no one can predict when the immune system will become so damaged that the infections and cancers develop, Eric lives more day-to-day than most teenagers. He has no sense of the future. Teenagers think they're going to live forever and attempt to have as much fun as possible, but not Eric. His day is filled with the task of living and trying to feel healthy. The hopes that keep him going are small ones: to keep attending school, to grow a little bit in size, and to have his immune system remain strong. The invincibility of the teenager's approach to life is absent, for he doesn't know when he will next bleed into one of his joints or when a severe infection will strike. Eric is already a frail person, like other hemophiliacs. He spent about a month last year in the hospital, missing school, missing time with buddies, missing normal teenage activities.

Because of recent bouts with fever and diarrhea, he can go to school only part-time. He loses weight so easily, and I cannot discern why. Will he make the grades to continue to advance with his class? Will he live long enough to go to college?

In spite of his overwhelming problems, Eric is one of the fortunate young AIDS victims. He goes to school without fear of persecution, and his friends and small rural Texas community have rallied around him, hosting barbecue dinners to help with his medical bills.

Eric has not had many of the opportunities most kids enjoy. His has not been a normal childhood. Like the aged, he must wait with a type of "cancer" that could break out at any time. Twice in the last six months he nearly died of new infections. I only hope I can demonstrate the love of Christ as I minister to him in the coming months.*

* * * * * *

Many more stories could be told about the tragedies experienced by individuals with AIDS, but I hope these accounts have given you a new perspective on this disease, the perspective of the infected and dying. But how did this terrible new pestilence come about, leading to the situation we now face with the AIDS epidemic? To understand this, we will turn to history to see what led to these shattered dreams.

*Eric died March 5, 1990 from complications of HIV disease.

For since the creation of the world God's invisible qualities—his eternal power and divine nature— have been clearly seen, being understood from what has been made, so that men are without excuse (Romans 1:20).

Do not lust in your heart after [the immoral woman's] beauty[i]
* or let her captivate you with her eyes. . . .*
Can a man scoop fire into his lap
* without his clothes being burned?*
Can a man walk on hot coals without his feet being scorched?
So is he who sleeps with another man's wife;
* no one who touches her will go unpunished*
(Proverbs 6:25, 27-29).

Speak and act as those who are going to be judged by the law that gives freedom, because judgment without mercy will be shown to anyone who has not been merciful. Mercy triumphs over judgment! (James 2:12-13).

"You have heard that it was said, 'Do not commit adultery.' But I tell you that anyone who looks at a woman lustfully has already committed adultery with her in his heart" (Matthew 5:27-28).

Chapter Four

The Shattered Dreams of the Sexual Revolution

*T*here comes an hour in the afternoon when the child is tired of "pretending"; when he is weary of being a robber or a Red Indian. It is then that he torments the cat. There comes a time in the routine of an ordered civilization when the man is tired of playing at mythology and pretending that the tree is a maiden or that the moon made love to a man. The effect of this staleness is the same everywhere; it is seen in all drug-taking and dram-drinking and every form of tendency to increase the dose. Men seek stranger sins or more startling obscenities as stimulants to their jaded sense. They seek after mad oriental religions for the same reason. They try to stab their nerves to life, as it were with the knives of the priests of Baal. They are walking in their sleep and try to wake themselves up with nightmares.[1]

G. K. Chesterton, 1925

THE BEGINNING OF THE AIDS EPIDEMIC

The AIDS epidemic is a direct result of the sexual revolution. That is incontestable from an epidemiological standpoint. AIDS is a sexually transmitted disease first and foremost, and a difficult one to spread compared to other such illnesses. Though a smaller percentage of the cases of AIDS in the United States have been transmitted through shared needles, transfusions, and birth, the disease entered this country, spread throughout the rest of the world, and grew to frightening proportions due to sexual promiscuity. The cost of the epidemic in America, the one to two million people who will die from the disease by the end of the century, are living sacrifices to the "new morality."

According to many, the sexual revolution was caused by penicillin and the Pill. Penicillin, which became widely available after World War II, did predate the sexual revolution of the sixties and seventies. But predating does not necessarily mean causation, although many people make that assumption.

> In 1956, the Italian ship *Andrea Doria* collided with a Swedish ship in the Atlantic, sinking to the bottom of the ocean as a result. On the night of the collision, a woman who was retiring to her cabin flicked on the light switch. Immediately a great crashing noise and grinding of metal ensued. Passengers and crew members ran screaming through the ship as bedlam resulted. But this lady burst from her cabin with the simple explanation to calm the panicked passengers—she claimed to have engaged the ship's emergency brakes![2]

Penicillin as a cause of the sexual revolution has little more to recommend it, as we will show, than the confident explanation of the slightly confused lady on board the *Andrea Doria*.

The Pill as a cause of the sexual promiscuity of recent times has a better foundation—barely. Another story is in order. In an important Little League baseball game, the home team was behind 1-0 with one more time at bat. Fortunately for the team, their three best hitters were due up. But the first player grounded out to the shortstop, and the next batter fouled out to the catcher. The final batter struck out and forlornly returned to the dugout, amid the jubilation of the other team. He was surprised to hear his teammates complain that he had lost the game. Some of the loudest catcalls came from the two players who had made outs just before his. Perhaps the moral of the story should be: Do not make the last out of the game, for undue importance will be placed on it.

The Pill may not have been the last out of the game called Sexual Sanity, but it was the loudest heard. Consequently, it has been given undue credit as *the reason* for the discarding of traditional values by many in the sixties and seventies. However, it no more caused the sexual revolution than giving guns to everyone in a neighborhood would automatically cause a local war. Firearms might make it easier to fight, but war would break out only if individuals decided to use the guns for destructive purposes.

People had to choose to use the Pill; it was not an aphrodisiac placed in the West's water supply that overcame individual moral inhibitions. It was merely a method to carry out the value judgments people had already made. Its convenience is of minor importance. If I have made a lifetime vow of fidelity to my wife, I do not change the vow because of a more convenient method of breaking it. A whole ball game has been played in my mind before I make such a decision.

If neither penicillin nor the Pill was a direct cause, what did bring about the sexual revolution and the carnage of the AIDS epidemic? It is a complex history involving people, ideas, and many irreversible social changes. To understand this history is to grasp that the church has plenty to do to reverse the misery caused by immorality. It is also to acknowledge that the church's approach until now has been ill-conceived.

SEXUAL NEGATIVISM IN THE CHURCH AND SOCIETY

The church's negative view toward sex, even within marriage, was an energizing factor in the revolt. Most of the church fathers tolerated sex as an urge of the lower nature. Augustine, a licentious man prior to his conversion, wanted to limit the fervor within sex so as to reduce its dangers. But passionless sex is a contradiction in terms. The dominant Catholic church in the Middle Ages made monasticism the recommended ideal. Celibacy was a higher calling; sex was but a necessary evil. Aquinas, in the thirteenth century, allowed passionate sex within marriage, but only for procreation.[3] But passion cannot be turned on and off so easily.

The Reformers had a better attitude toward sexuality. Martin Luther, who was chaste for years while a Catholic priest, determined that absolute celibacy was almost impossible for most people. He married after he began the Reformation, as did most of the priests who joined him. However, ambivalence toward sexuality remained with Luther, since he concluded that sex was never devoid of sin. The Puritans, in contrast to the modern impression of them, had a healthy attitude toward sex within marriage while condemning it outside of wedlock.[4] Still, they had a wariness about sex as if passion within marriage invariably spilled over into immorality.

Victorian social norms, unfairly identified with Christian thought, were hypocritical toward sexuality. The Victorians valued chastity in women while allowing men an underground infidelity involving hordes of prostitutes.[5] As a result, sexually transmitted diseases rose to an all-time high in nineteenth century England. Victorian society was governed by social propriety, not Christian purity. But many thinkers could not see the difference, and Victorian hypocrisy supplied much of the impetus for the intellectual revolt.

The church could have blunted the rebellion by honoring sex for both men and women as God does. Scripture from start to finish, including the teaching of Christ and Paul, has a positive view of sex within marriage. Yet

Christians in the twentieth century continue to have difficulty treating sexuality positively. Isn't it possible to hold up the marriage ideal while showing the dangers and destruction of immorality? Ironically, as we will show later, the sexual revolution caused many Christians to swing too far, going beyond the simple goodness of marital sexuality to make it a form of salvation.

THE INTELLECTUAL REVOLT

Historically, many people in the West have rebelled against biblical sexual morality, but usually in small groups for short periods of time.[6] Earlier rebellions were unsuccessful because social and religious constraints until the twentieth century reinforced fidelity in marriage. Consider how little negative impact Bertrand Russell would have had on sexual morality had he lived early in Victoria's reign. Had Margaret Mead lived in Puritan New England, she would have been placed on trial rather than on the "Tonight Show" for her advocacy of sexual freedom. The current general rejection of biblical standards would not have occurred without changes in thought, for "As [a man] thinketh in his heart, so is he" (Proverbs 23:7, KJV).

The immorality advocated by the following intellectuals was not new; their ideas were old seeds sown in the fertile soil of a changing society, blossoming into anti-Christian thinking. These men and women were products as well as influencers of their culture. Their thoughts will be examined here. The more important and long-neglected social conditions which led to those thoughts will occupy us in the final part of this chapter.

The Thoughts

As modern science successfully explained many of the mysteries of the universe, most nineteenth century intellectuals had no need for God. One problem remained: the explanation for the existence of humans. This was deftly provided by the English naturalist *Charles Darwin* (1809-82) in the mid-1800s. Although lacking scientific support, he traced man's heritage to lower species. One secular scientist spoke for many when he said that evolution is a theology, not a science: "There's no evidence for any of the basic tenets of Darwinian evolution. I don't believe that there was any evidence for it. It was a social force that took over the world in 1860. . . ."[7]

Whatever the scientific merits of Darwin's work, the theory of natural selection, as applied to man, had some nasty side effects, including the tendency for intellectuals to apply survival of the fittest to society. Love for people was unimportant, and sexuality became a mere animal drive, in the same category as eating and drinking. Darwinism formed the foundation for subsequent secular thought on sexuality.

Karl Marx (1818-83) had many apt criticisms of capitalism but no reasonable solutions, as history has shown. His dialectical materialism paralleled evolution, with history and thought progressing to higher levels, as animals were in Darwinism.[8] Marx hated religion and marriage as institutions that maintained the prevailing social injustices. He was more successful than we realize, for "all modern politicians are Marxist in orientation, inasmuch as they believe that all problems are primarily economic."[9] Marxism, along with secular capitalism, has caused most people in the West, not just politicians, to think first of money and only secondarily of family, morality, spirituality, community, or esthetics, the other driving forces of society.

Psychiatrist *Sigmund Freud* (1856-1939) was also influenced by Darwin.[10] His emphasis on the unconscious was important and profound, but most of his other theories have since been questioned. As an atheist, he believed religion was the mass-delusion of all time. As a doctor he thought repressed sexual thoughts were the leading cause of neurosis, suggesting that restraining sexual urges until marriage was unhealthy. Freud was a philosopher, not a scientist, and his observations were deeply flawed. His theories were vague and constantly being reformulated as conflicting evidence arose.[11] But he never doubted the importance of his ideas, which had profound effects on the West by undermining traditional morality, paving the way for so-called scientific treatises on sex, and allowing sex to enter everyday conversation, even in mixed company.[12]

Atheist philosopher *Friedrich Nietzsche* (1844-1900) saw the coming age without God as a time of catastrophe, not progress. A new order of man, the superman, would assert himself out of this chaos. "God is dead," claimed Nietzsche, and in a sense he was right. God had become a casualty of history,[13] no longer necessary to explain the secrets of the universe. But as a secular prophet, Nietzsche understood that when God died, so did the support for the whole of Western culture. That insight cost him his sanity: "Alas, grant me madness. . . . By being above the law I am the most outcast of outcasts."[14] Nietzsche died in an asylum. Around the turn of the century the "earth was unchained from the sun" and everything (including sexual anarchy) became possible because the West was no longer rooted in the ethics of Christianity.

Without a divine being to provide order for the world, knowledge became fragmented and morality became mere personal preference. Rather than a golden age of freedom, the twentieth century became a series of genocides. More people died in the wars of this century than in all previous wars combined[15]—the inevitable results of the death of God and loss of morality. Only Nietzsche, among a few other prominent non-Christians, saw this coming. Out of this epistemological vacuum, further trends developed in sexuality.

Few minds in history can match the accomplishments of *Bertrand Russell* (1872-1970) in such diverse areas as philosophy, mathematics, ethics, politics, history, education, and religion. Russell spent most of his ninety-seven years attempting to bring down religion, and particularly Christianity, through essays, debates, and advocacy of changes in morality.[16] In the sexual arena, Russell advocated living together, nonbinding marriage until the first pregnancy, decriminalization of homosexuality, and tolerance of adultery. His life reflected his thinking, as his four wives and many mistresses attest.[17]

Planned Parenthood's founder, *Margaret Sanger* (1883-1966), was an untiring crusader for contraception. Largely through her efforts, birth control became acceptable in the twentieth century. Although portrayed as an advocate for the poor, she was an elitist who championed involuntary birth control to limit the numbers of "human weeds." She desired to legalize trial marriage, adultery, homosexuality, and abortion, some of which she herself tried.[18]

Ernest Hemingway (1899-1961), like Russell, won the Nobel prize for literature, but was of a completely different mind-set. Russell was a secular evangelist; Hemingway, a hedonist. Hemingway never campaigned for a change in morality, but his life was a thorough statement of a man defiant of God. He acted out Beethoven's dictum of taking life by the throat, and he did it in war, in hunting, in womanizing, and in drinking. Hemingway lived for himself, not for his four wives, many lovers, and the friends he discarded when they were no longer useful.[19] As age encroached on his virility, he ended his life with a shotgun blast to the head.

Hemingway is a dramatic example of the many twentieth-century men and women living out the results of the loss of absolute morality. For Hemingway, the void was filled with excitement and tests of manhood. For others literary expression, painting, political power, material gains, or sexual conquests filled the void. It is a mistake to separate the sexual hedonists from other rebels. It is all part of the same game—to fill the space of an absent divinity. Only the manifestations remain to be personalized. When these men and women are caught in times of honesty, their laughter becomes silence, the drugs wear off, and they are alone. The agnostic historian Will Durant said it best in a moment of despair, "You and I are living on a shadow . . . because we are operating on the Christian ethical code which was given us unfused from the Christian faith. . . . But what will happen with our children? . . . We are not giving them ethics warmed up with a religious faith. They are living on the shadow of a shadow."[20] Pity, not wrath, is the proper response for the child of God, for wrath is God's alone to give. How can we be angry at those living on a shadow?

Pseudoscience

Given this intellectual climate, it was not long before sexual mores were challenged by supposed men of science. Freud paved the way for the movement of sexuality from the moral and private realm to the "scientific" and public. But science cannot choose what is good; it can only describe and measure. Immorality in all its forms became acceptable because it was quantifiable. Chastity or abstinence, by purely linguistic manipulation, became unhealthy sexual repression.

After Freud, sex manuals became more erotic and concentrated on technique and position. Sex became the vital factor in making marriages supremely happy.[21] In correcting the repression of the Victorians, the pendulum had swung to the mistake of Casanova. Shared experiences, the joy of children, and accomplishments within family and community were subordinated to activity in the bedroom. Freud was the first of the pseudoscientists who took sexuality and love from their traditional arenas of morality and religion and tried to control them by giving their study an appearance of objectivity. Regrettably, he was not the last.

English physician Havelock Ellis (1859-1939) sought to overturn all sexual restrictions. For Ellis, sex was the central function of life to be gratified as one wished.[22] He recommended premarital sex, trial marriage, masturbation, a low age of consent, and homosexual acts, including the lesbian affairs of his wife. He also advocated eugenics, including sterilization of the "feeble-minded," a fact his admirers conveniently omit.[23] The ban of his seven-volume set, *Studies in the Psychology of Sex* (1897-1910), increased his notoriety. When the first volume landed him in court, the judge said Ellis's claims for scientific validity were "a pretense, adopted for the purpose of selling a filthy publication."[24] The judge was mistaken only in that Ellis was selling ideas more than books.

In 1925 *Margaret Mead* (1901-78) arrived for a nine-month stay on the island of Samoa. What she said she found was an island of peace, with loose family ties and free love among teens, without guilt or sexual violence. Mead parlayed that experience and others in the Pacific into a career of public denunciation of traditional family values. Russell and Ellis cited her findings frequently to support their positions. But criticism of her work has come out steadily since the 1940s, including some scientific publications from the second of her three husbands. The culmination of the criticism occurred in 1983 in a book by Samoan authority Derek Freeman, who accused her of "imposing her ideology on the evidence," a grievous charge against a scientist. Mead was deceitful, not merely mistaken. Samoan society was puritanical and anxiety-filled. Rape occurred twice as often as in America.[25] Unfortunately, despite its mistakes, Mead's 1927 book, *Coming of Age in Samoa*, captured the public's imagination and further desensitized Americans to radical views on sexuality.

What was begun by Freud and continued by the sex manuals and Mead's myth of sexual innocence in the Pacific islands was accomplished by *Alfred Kinsey* (1894-1956) in his *Sexual Behavior in the Human Male* (1948). Kinsey's report on the female came out in 1953. Both were publishing sensations and greatly influenced the accelerating decline of moral standards. They were supposedly scientific surveys demonstrating that Americans were far more liberal in sexual behavior than most thought. The reports claimed that most men had visited prostitutes, nearly half had been unfaithful to their wives, and over a third had experienced at least one homosexual affair.[26] Half the women had practiced premarital intercourse and a fourth had committed adultery. Written in the neutral language of science, the Kinsey reports removed sex from the personal, moral, and spiritual spheres it had occupied. Said an editorial in *Look* at about the same time: "What [Americans] have learned and will learn may have tremendous effect on the future social history of mankind. For they are presenting facts. They are revealing not what 'should' be, but what 'is'."[27]

Actually the surveys did nothing of the sort. Kinsey was trained as an observer of insects, not humans. He had no experience in conducting scientific surveys. The studies were badly skewed in their selection of people; most were college students and prisoners, who would tend to be far more liberal than the average American. Also, the intimate questions asked in the surveys would more likely be answered by those with sexual experience; in the forties, for most people, sex was a private matter.[28] Kinsey's interpretation was also biased by his personal views. He favored the male "sexual athlete"; the more sex, the better.[29] A more representative recent survey confirmed that Kinsey was wrong. In the highly sexualized eighties, people had less homosexual experience than what Kinsey said they had in the forties! Only half as many men had ever experienced a homosexual act as Kinsey had reported, and only about 3 percent of men were practicing homosexuals,[30] a figure far below the 10 percent claimed by homosexual activists or Kinsey. Regardless of what was true, people believed the Kinsey reports and thought themselves undersexed.

Physician *William Masters* (1915-) and self-proclaimed psychologist *Virginia Johnson* (1925-), who merely has a high school diploma, carried the drift to its ultimate conclusion by observing couples during sex play and intercourse. They recorded this voyeurism using photography and measurements of brain waves, body temperatures, and tumescence of sex organs.[31] Their research and books in the sixties and seventies brought sex full circle, from personal enjoyment within marriage to a depersonalized process studied on the exam table. Somehow this was supposed to make things better. A whole group of "sexologists" arose with their own journals and conventions. Psychiatrist Thomas Szanz demonstrated that the so-called research of Masters and Johnson was in reality promotion of prostitution, adultery, and fornication.[32]

The Consequences of These Anti-Christian Ideas

We are all thankful for the scientific advancements of the last two centuries. Unfortunately, one unintended consequence of these achievements was the arrival of attempted imitators, who were actually philosophers in laboratory white. Being shoddy scientists did not prevent these charlatans from pushing their agendas to alter society. In the process, millions have been harmed due to the overturning of heaven's sound guidelines on sexuality.

The moral slide in the past was held in check more by social constraints than by personal convictions. The ideas promoted by these intellectuals became important because concurrent changes in society made them acceptable. As we will soon discover, these technical and social changes were the most basic cause of the sexual revolution.

The Rise of Modern Medicine

Modern medicine began a century ago when Pasteur and Koch demonstrated that bacteria cause many diseases and Lister proved the effectiveness of sterile technique. Previously, surgeons failed to wash their hands before surgery or wear gloves while operating. Development of better care followed rapidly in many areas; the unintended moral consequences followed quietly.

Sexually Transmitted Diseases

With the indiscriminate use of prostitutes in Victorian society, syphilis and gonorrhea became more frequent.[33] Syphilis was the more feared illness because about 15 percent of the cases advanced to long-term neurologic problems, even death. No significant treatment was available until 1910 when Paul Ehrlich released an arsenic compound that was a relatively safe treatment of syphilis.[34] In so doing, a large curb to immoral sexuality was eliminated thirty-five years before the release of penicillin.

Gonorrhea, in contrast, was a relatively mild disease. Although painful, it was not life-threatening and eventually resolved without treatment. Sterility of women was its biggest complication. When penicillin became available in the forties, even these problems were treatable. Sexual intercourse was no longer dangerous—at least for a time.

With the arrival of the sexual revolution in full force in the sixties, new sexually transmitted diseases were discovered, while the old problems of syphilis and gonorrhea became increasingly common. Most of these new illnesses were mere nuisances, since existing antibiotics or therapies were available to treat them. As the sexual revolution moved from a small fringe in the sixties to the mainstream in the seventies, the types of venereal diseases continued to increase, now numbering about two dozen. Herpes gained the most notoriety because it was incurable. Suddenly young adults had to be concerned about who they slept with, since sex could again have lasting consequences.

Birth Control

A remarkable reversal in the twentieth century has been the public perception of birth control. One hundred years ago, it was a radical idea restricted in the U.S. by the Comstock laws.[35] Condoms, coitus interruptus, and douching were the main forms of contraception until the introduction of the Pill in 1960. Vulcanized rubber in the nineteenth century made condoms more acceptable, but they were not widely used until liquid latex and automation brought the price down.[36] The American Medical Association considered birth control sordid and opposed it until 1937, when it reversed its position after hard lobbying from Margaret Sanger.[37]

Some have suggested that the release of the birth control pill in 1960 was the downfall of traditional morality. Although not true, the Pill was a revolutionary development because it was the first form of contraception that separated the act of sex from the contraceptive method. Strongly supported by the medical community (which had come along way since 1937) and by the media, it had a "diplomatic immunity" that kept its safety from being questioned for several years, despite many health hazards.[38] The Pill became the favored form of birth control, with more and more women using it. The response by Catholic women was especially remarkable. In 1955, seven out of ten complied with their church's prohibition on the use of artificial contraception. By 1970, seven out of ten were using contraceptive methods (primarily the Pill) despite the 1968 papal encyclical continuing the ban.[39] As the Pill's side effects became more apparent, other forms of birth control, such as intrauterine devices, cervical caps, and sterilization, became more common.

Abortion

The Pill facilitated the sexual revolution by preventing pregnancy, but as the level of sexual activity increased, so did the pressure by some to allow abortions for the "mistakes." The historical opposition to abortion goes back to the earliest years of Christianity.[40] As recently as one hundred years ago abortion was considered murder by most of society, including women activists, who believed that abortion encourages men's sexual promiscuity and control of women.[41] Society's opposition was still high in the forties as shown by the World Health Organization's charter forbidding it and by the indictment of ten Nazi leaders at Nuremburg for encouraging it.[42] But the forties are an eternity from the sixties, where pragmatic considerations softened opposition, and both the American Medical and American Bar Associations campaigned for legal abortions.

SOCIAL CHANGES

Although modern medicine reduced certain complications of sexuality, the social changes between the 1880s and the present were far more important in promoting immorality. Many of these changes were not evil in themselves, but fallen people turned them to profane uses. This true story about the use of the car provides but one example:

> A teenage son came to his father to ask permission to take his girlfriend in his father's car to a party in the next town. The son explained that because of the distance, he would have to be back

after his usual curfew time. The father's answer was brief, but clear: "Absolutely not." To which the son gave the age-old protest, "Why not, Dad? Don't you trust me?" The father responded, "In a car, alone with a girl you care for, in another town, until 2 o'clock in the morning?—I wouldn't trust myself. Why should I trust you?"[43]

This wise father is not worried about his son pondering the thoughts of Darwin, Freud, or Mead when he is alone with his girlfriend in the car. He is worried that the morally neutral automobile will remove his son from the usual constraints on natural temptation. Although the rebel thinkers have had an effect, their influence would have been insignificant without this and the following changes through the decades.[44]

The 1890s

The United States was a far different place one hundred years ago. The country was largely rural and the towns were small, making it difficult to commit adultery privately. Moreover, men and women moved in separate spheres, with most married women working in the home. Their teen daughters were taught domestic chores at home, while their daughters' future husbands learned trades in small stores and businesses.[45] The first girls' high school in Great Britain opened in 1880, and later in the U.S. In 1890, only 7 percent of all children between fourteen and seventeen years old attended high school.[46] Girls matured later at the turn of the century, with the average onset of menses occurring at age sixteen. With greater nutrition, that average age has dropped to twelve and a half years. Marriage occurred at an earlier age, about eighteen for girls compared to around twenty-three now. Marriage occurred earlier because few people went to college and each sex accomplished their respective tasks of domestic or business training at an earlier age. The gap between sexual maturity in girls and time of marriage is especially impressive. Usually, a girl had only two years of physical maturity before she married in the 1890s; she now has over a decade.[47]

There were no automobiles, no telephones, no movies, and few phonographs. Mixing of the sexes was carefully monitored by adults, pregnancy during intercourse was still probable, condoms were expensive and frowned upon, syphilis was still a dreaded disease. In short, the possibility for sexual intimacy before marriage was much more difficult and risky than it is today.

1900-1920

This was a period of transition, as many of the changes of the 1890s were having increasing effect. More of the U.S. became industrialized, exerting pressure on traditional values. More people moved to the cities, increasing the opportunities for adultery and prostitution. Both were more likely to occur after 1910, when the first effective treatment for syphilis, salvarsan, became available. The year 1920 marked the first time more people lived in America's cities than in her rural areas.[48] Industrialization now also created a larger working class that was antagonistic toward the business class, especially prior to unionization. Workers began to develop new values, feeling squeezed out of many social situations.[49] Industrialization provided more disposable income and leisure for entertainment—and sin. Men and women were interacting more in and out of public schools.

Henry Ford's assembly line and Model T dramatically decreased the cost of cars, making them available to more families. The first nickelodeon, a precursor to the movie theater, opened in 1905. By 1912, five million people a day were going to "moving pictures." The inexpensive camera was available to more families and to more peddlers of pornography. Electric washing machines and air conditioners were invented around 1910, starting the revolution in housework that would make women seem less needed in the home. The first radio broadcast occurred in 1910, when Enrico Caruso performed live from New York City.[50]

Ideas of entertainment were going through a dramatic transformation. In the nineteenth century, dancing was done in family gatherings or formalized settings involving large segments of the community. Song lyrics were about daily life, not sentimentalized love. But by the 1910s, the cabaret, the precursor to today's singles bar, was in fashion. Men and women could meet informally in the cabaret, while they listened to the syncopated dance music of black musicians. Dancing acquired more erotic meaning for dating couples.[51]

The Roaring Twenties

What was at the periphery in the two decades before moved into the mainstream in the affluent 1920s. Manufacturers produced more cars, radios, telephones, home appliances, processed foods, and ready-made clothing, which had been scarce during the War. Wages were up, and hours worked were down, allowing more leisure time. Advertising came into its own; what was not available a decade before now became a need. Previously, ads explained the function of a product. Now they claimed a product would make you more attractive. Women were told that their "first duty . . . is to attract," and a number of products were made for that purpose. The cosmetics industry grew from sales of $17 million in 1914 to $141 million in 1925,[52] even while prices generally were trending downward.[53] Amidst this plenty, everything was becoming commercialized, even sexuality.[54] Part of this was driven by Freud's popularity as his thought filtered down to the general populace.[55] Americans were transformed from a society that never talked about sex to one obsessed with it, at least in liberal circles.[56] This new public sexuality lacked the pervasiveness it would later hold in the seventies, yet it was the same spirit.[57] The tendency toward self-gratification would later be inflamed by the self-actualizing psychologies.[58]

The mass media influenced society faster than expected, spreading the new ideas and encouraging conformity in the "global village" just as small communities in the past had squeezed their inhabitants into a common mold.[59] However, this new "village" encouraged immorality. Newspapers became centralized in the hands of "progressives."[60] The radio came in rapidly, much like VCRs today. In

1920, the public owned only five thousand radios. Four years later, the number had grown to two and a half million.[61] Radio displaced newspapers as the strongest media influence, only to be supplanted by the movies in the thirties. Movies in turn became subordinate to television by the late fifties. Although the accent in movies was on love and marriage, it was with a different bent. Women became enticing sex objects rather than the companions of the biblical model of marriage.[62] The schools strived for a homogeneous civil religion, following John Dewey's goals of making "good American citizens." Being a good Christian had been the goal before.[63] Dewey accomplished his goal of minimizing Christianity by making public school secular, controlled by the state rather than by religious groups.

All revolutions involve young people, otherwise the revolutions wither and die. The twenties were becoming more youth-oriented. Three-fourths of the teenagers now attended high schools, enabling boys and girls to mingle many hours each day. Easy access to cars made movies the common meeting place on dates. Weekend dances were strictly for youth, and afterwards lovers' lanes were convenient for "parking." Teenagers had the money and leisure to take advantage of these opportunities. Although only 12 percent of eighteen- to twenty-year-olds attended college in the 1920s, this was three times what it was a generation before. The college scene, with less parental supervision and more progressive elements, laid the foundation for a less traditional future. Although sexuality at all levels was more available, it was not consummated to the degree it is today. Kissing and petting were common, but intercourse was unusual unless a couple was planning marriage. One sexual partner was still the norm, so venereal diseases did not proliferate except with the use of prostitutes. The spirit of the twenties was like that of the sixties in pushing back the boundaries on sexuality.[64]

The Great Depression

Illicit sexuality does not require money and leisure, but having them makes it more available. The thirties was a time of survival, not experimentation. If anything, tradition forced the clock back a degree. Motion pictures had become more explicit over the years, but in 1934 the Catholic hierarchy in America established the Legion of Decency, which began a rating system for all movies. Although the Legion was concerned about violence, sexual content received 95 percent of its censure. Moreover, the ratings were not segregated according to age as today; censored movies were censored for all. Two-thirds of the dioceses posted the ratings prominently in the local parishes. The movie industry, controlled by a few moguls, could hardly ignore this attention, and the movies were cleaned up. The Catholic bishops attempted to do the same with written works, with less success. Prose of the time used street language for body parts, portrayed illicit sexuality sympathetically, and brought homosexuality into the open.[65]

Although the New Deal failed to solve the Depression (unemployment was still almost 20 percent in 1938)[66], it dramatically increased governmental power, resulting in some unintended consequences. If the power of the federal government is increased, then power must be decreased elsewhere. In this case it decreased in the family and in small communities, affecting traditional values. As media analyst Marshall McLuhan said, American society moved into "1984" in the 1930s without anyone noticing the Orwellian landscape.[67] Roosevelt began the government's social protection with good intentions, but as it became more far-reaching, it uncoupled the dependency of family members on one another.[68] Children depended less on their parents as young adults; parents no longer needed their children for support in their old age. The financial responsibility of Mom and Dad was acquired by Uncle Sam, devoid of the love, wisdom, and community that goes with family. Churches, though providing greater poverty assistance than any other group, allowed the welfare system to predominate.

During the Depression, American society appeared more traditional, but it was a superficial appearance that would change once society had an economic upturn.

World War II

War may be the most unsettling thing that can happen to a society. Families are split apart; anxiety creates a live-for-today mentality; young men are displaced from the stabilizing influence of their hometowns and families. For America, the First World War was brief, lasting about a year once America entered the war. The Second World War lasted four years, causing great changes at home as the country mobilized its war economy. Millions of men went overseas; young women went to the cities to find employment.[69] Prostitutes abounded, frequented by lonely, frightened soldiers not sure whether that day might be their last. Being farther away from home, compared to the European soldiers, made the GIs' loneliness that much more acute. The army attempted to discourage prostitution not for reasons of purity, but because of sexually transmitted illnesses.[70] One famous poster promoted by the government showed a skeleton in a dress high-stepping with Hitler and Tojo, and proclaimed: "VD, Worst of the Three."[71]

The war was particularly important to the homosexual movement that would blossom later. Bringing millions of men and thousands of women together fomented homosexual relationships and a homosexual identity they did not want to lose. Consequently, many of them settled in budding homosexual communities after the war. Gay bars proliferated in the forties, a trend that would lead to the bathhouses of later years.[72]

The sexual openness of the twenties made a comeback. Pin-up girls on barrack walls and the noses of airplanes gave pornography the opening to move from the margin to a more standard place in male life. Names of planes like "Grin and Bear It," in which the pin-up actually did (bare it) were commonplace.[73] Pornography was readily available in Europe; American soldiers often brought back armloads of it. The inexpensive paperback appeared in 1939 and led to the pulp novels with suggestive covers and stories.[74] Romance novels became progressively more graphic in their portrayal of premarital sex, teaching the more reserved gender that romance leads to sex rather than to marriage.[75]

As the war came to a close and Europe began rebuilding its devastated cities, the great military production of the U.S. turned to a feverish output of consumer goods, encouraged by people's desires to live a little after the Depression and war-rationing. Many soldiers, already worldly from fighting in foreign lands, returned to America with GI Bill funds, allowing them to go to college with its liberal emphasis and opportunities for immoral sex.

The Postwar Years

Prosperity increased more dramatically than ever. Conservatism appeared reborn as couples married early, fathers worked hard, and the baby boom started. But big problems loomed ahead, because the goals were motivated by self-desire. The humanistic psychologies of Rollo May, Carl Rogers, and others emphasized "self-actualization," which was merely selfishness in disguise.[76] More people went to church than ever before, but the religion was "so empty and contentless, so conformist, so utilitarian, so sentimental, so individualistic, and so self-righteous."[77] It was also mostly for women.[78] Fathers were working too hard to be concerned about spirituality. Mothers alone could not raise their children to be Christians, and the fifties' youth "graduated from their Sunday schools and their faith at the same time."[79] This was confirmed by the sixties' revolts against the emptiness of prosperity and the hypocrisy of religion and government. Much of this revolt was valid, but it eventually degenerated into promiscuous behavior, drug abuse, and political violence.

After the Kinsey reports, the Supreme Court softened its stance on obscene materials, saying they had to be "utterly without redeeming social value" before being banned,[80] a criterion impossible to prove. Smut became mainstream with the publication of *Playboy* and its imitators, which taught that women are bodies for gratification rather than people for companionship. French feminist Simone de Beavoir rejected this demeaning trend, advocating instead complete independence from men, economic advancement, and abortion, and so laid the groundwork for the feminism of the sixties. Kinsey also influenced books published in the fifties that depicted homosexuals as a persecuted minority. Alan Ginsberg published his graphically homosexual poem, "Howl,"[81] and with his counterculture friends laid the foundation for the "flower children" of the next decade. Affluence gave youth greater freedom than they had in the twenties, and the music of Elvis Presley continued the sexualized atmosphere. Despite the renewed sexual expression, it was still the boys who pushed for more intimate behavior and the girls who held back.[82] Perhaps the final change leading to the sexual casualness of the seventies was to destroy this female resistance. Consequently, marriage's protection for women and children was weakening. The nineteenth-century feminists were right: In a permissive society, the female is the loser.

The Sixties

Society's foundation had crumbled and the rockslide began in earnest with the revolt against the Vietnam War and the sterility of the middle class. The Pill was released in 1960, making pregnancy unlikely in illicit unions. Modern feminism began in 1963 with Betty Friedan's *The Feminine Mystique*. Rather than calling men to compassion, it suggested that women should demand their rights also. Rock music came into its own in the sixties, eventually advocating free love, drugs, violence, and Satanism.[83] The youth thought they were different from those over thirty, but were simply selfish in a different way. They graduated from their love-ins in the sixties to become the "me generation" of the next decade. Since the self-sacrifice necessary for family life was passé, divorces skyrocketed. Movies contained more graphic sex and violence; goodness seems boring on the silver screen.[84] Television invaded the home and soon would show the same sexuality and violence. A full 44 percent of men went to college in the sixties,[85] creating a milieu not only for alternate values but also alternate practices. Great Society programs led to disintegration of the black family by giving women welfare, and by making the man convenient but not necessary. Children could escape home by having babies.[86] Credit cards multiplied and taught Americans they did not have to wait to buy things. So why should they wait for sex?

Gay liberation began dramatically with the "Stonewall Inn Riot" in New York in 1969. Homosexuals at this gay haunt threw rocks and bottles at police who had come to arrest them under New York sodomy laws. The riot continued far into the night and through the weekend with "Gay power" scribbled on the walls in Greenwich Village. Within weeks, new homosexual organizations formed and called for homosexuals to come "out of the closet."[87] The political ascendancy of homosexuals was remarkable, unimpeded by a country that no longer believed in sin.

The Seventies and Eighties

The 1970 President's Commission on Pornography said pornography was harmless. Though events have shown otherwise, the impression was given that smut was no longer dirty, just adult. On cue, the industry produced more and raunchier magazines and movies which included homosexuality, sadomasochism, rape and violence, child sex, bestiality and, unbelievably, "snuff" movies, where the actual murder of a woman occurred on screen. Growing evidence showed that pornography was addictive and led to violence against women.[88] The VCR made pornography even more available; 40 percent of VCR owners rented X-rated movies in 1984.[89] The American Psychiatric Association (APA) took homosexuality off its disease list in 1973 despite protests by many psychiatrists. The homosexual political machinery had actively lobbied for acceptance throughout this time and had threatened to disrupt APA conventions and research if the association did not change its stance.[90] They succeeded not because of scientific evidence but because of these strong-arm tactics and the values bias of the antireligious psychiatrists.

No-fault divorce hurt women and children by dramatically lowering their income while elevating the living standard of the divorced men. Women were almost obligated to have sex on the first or second date to be considered normal. There was more and more sex, but people were less and less satisfied. Distinctions between adult and child were blurred as young teen girls appeared in ads looking like sophisticated women.[91] Some groups pushed for lowering the age of consent to below ten.[92] Children's television programs became less common, particularly for those eight and older, so they watched the same programs their parents did with their sexual innuendoes and overt sexual behavior. One scholar noted, "Traditional restraints against youthful sexual activity cannot have great force in a society that does not, in fact, make a binding distinction between childhood and adulthood."[93] Planned Parenthood took out an ad that said, "They did it 20,000 times on television last year. How come nobody got pregnant?"—then exacerbated the teen pregnancy problem with their permissive sex education programs.[94] The young were being brainwashed by the graphic sex, violence, and revolt against traditional values in movies and television. Half the mothers with preschool children were working by 1988[95] (compared to one out of ten in the sixties), with many more working as their children became older. Not only did this make the children less secure, it made it easier for teens to have sex after school while their parents were out of the house.[96] By 1976, 27 percent of the sexually active white teenage girls and 45 percent of the sexually active blacks had become pregnant by the time they were eighteen.[97]

THE CHURCH

The church failed to hold back the moral landslide. The conservative church was fighting the liberalizing tendencies in theology, unaware that society was changing dramatically. By the twenties and thirties, the liberal church had taken over most mainline denominations, which led to much of the irrelevance of the church in the fifties. Liberalizing tendencies in sexuality were slower in coming than in the secular world, but they came in a rush when they did. In 1955, Anglican theologian Derrick Bailey argued for acceptance of homosexuals. In 1963, eleven Quakers produced a document that accepted premarital sex, allowed adultery under certain circumstances, and said that homosexuality was all right. This was significant because it came from a traditionally conservative group.[98] Joseph Fletcher extended this with his controversial *Situation Ethics*, which said the only guidance for morality was what was done in love. Soon many were justifying abortion, adultery, infanticide, divorce, and the sexual abuse of children—all in the name of love. The Catholics changed more slowly, but with liberalization of the church under Vatican II, they soon joined the immoral free-for-all. In 1979, going against the conservative John Paul II, some American Catholic theologians proclaimed that adultery, homosexuality, and pornography were acceptable, at least under some circumstances. H. Richard Niebuhr, a liberal theologian himself, characterized liberalism in the church as teaching that "a God without wrath brought men without sin into a kingdom without judgment through the ministrations of a Christ without a cross,"[99] to which we might add "by the teaching of men without common sense."

CONCLUSIONS

Changes in sexual morality did not occur because of innovative ideas developed by radicals; none of their proposals were original. The sexual revolution did not arrive spontaneously in the sixties; a revolution had been evident at least since the twenties. Church leaders, wrongly assuming that ideas were the root cause of the sexual revolution, opposed it only at that level and thus failed. Morality declined steadily, despite the church's intervention. Moreover, Christians have sinned sexually almost as often as nonbelievers, even while accepting biblical morality. Immoral ideas are not the sole problem.

If I am locked in isolation, I can still commit sexual sin in my mind, but I cannot impregnate a woman or spread venereal disease. Compared to recent times, most people in 1890 were locked in figurative rooms, unable to act on the sexual sins of their imagination. Their imprisonment was caused by limited exposure to the opposite sex, insignificant leisure time or funds, lack of privacy, and the unified persuasion of family, church, and state to live by traditional values. That unity is essentially gone, and the walls have come tumbling down.

But this change occurred over generations. As the social restraints decreased, the persistence of the radicals increased, acting in conjunction with an emerging brave new world. A cry for "free love" in the regulated life of a small town a hundred years ago would have been offensive. The same appeal in a university city two generations later, where the sexes mingled and pregnancy was avoidable, was enticing. Our society embraces its own wisdom while castigating traditional morality. When we preach, "Thou shalt not . . . ," the secular world is merely amused at this voice out of the past. They have the same response as the modern man who visits an Amish town. He understands that some people dress in odd ways and ride horse-drawn carriages, but why on earth would anyone want to?

The church needs more than pat answers. Christians must show that purity is still desirable and possible in our sexualized world. Christians ought to spend time with their families, exhibiting the fulfillment of marriage. We need to provide creative alternatives for our teenagers to be together in a de-sexualized atmosphere, while giving them strong reasons to wait for sexual expression within marriage. We need to reach out compassionately to the tens of millions of victims ravaged by the sexual revolution.

But we will be inept in these tasks if we do not recognize the pervasive conditions encouraging us to fall. It is not just sinful ideas against which we war, but the very social structure itself. Reversing the sexual revolution will be like climbing a tall peak. We will scale it only with determined wills and the grace of God.

Chapter 4, Notes

1. G. K. Chesterton, *The Everlasting Man* (Garden City, N.Y.: Image Books, 1955), 164.

2. David Fisher, *Historians' Fallacies* (New York: Harper and Row, 1970), 166.

3. Tim Stafford, *The Sexual Christian* (Wheaton, Ill.: Victor Books, 1989), 45.

4. Ibid., 46-47.

5. Randy Alcorn, *Christians in the Wake of the Sexual Revolution* (Portland, Ore.: Multnomah Press, 1985), 34-35. Much of the framework of our chapter is taken from this excellent book. We depart from Alcorn, however, in that we see the problems as being much more difficult to eradicate and not simply in the realm of conscious choice. We also see the social changes outside of specific sexuality as being much more important than does Alcorn or virtually any other writer we have read.

6. Various anarchists and freethinkers throughout human history have lived in "free-love" communes or in open adultery. Denis De Rougement, "Love," in *Dictionary of the History of Ideas*, ed. Philip P. Wiener (New York: Charles Scribner's Sons, 1973), 3:103-8.

7. Professor Chandra Wickramasinghe quoted in *The Intellectuals Speak Out about God*, ed. Roy Abraham Varghese (Washington, D.C.: Regnery Gateway, 1984), 30-31; see also Michael Denton, *Evolution: A Theory in Crisis* (Bethesda, Md.: Adler and Adler, 1986).

8. *Encyclopedia Britannica*, 15th ed., s.v. "Marx, Karl."

9. C. Northcote Parkinson quoted in Herbert Schlossberg, *Idols for Destruction* (Nashville: Thomas Nelson Publishers, 1983), 61.

10. *Encyclopedia Britannica*, 15th ed., s.v. "Freud, Sigmund"; Alcorn, *Sexual Revolution*, 37.

11. Paul Johnson, *Modern Times* (New York: Harper and Row, 1983), 6.

12. Ibid., 7.

13. Ibid., 48.

14. Os Guiness, *The Dust of Death* (Downers Grove, Ill.: InterVarsity Press, 1973), 24.

15. It has been estimated that one hundred million men, women, and children have been killed by fellow men in the twentieth century. See Roger Rosenblatt, "What Really Mattered," *Time*, 5 October 1983, 24-27.

16. Paul Johnson, *The Intellectuals* (New York: Harper and Row, 1988), 197-224.

17. Alcorn, *Sexual Revolution*, 39.

18. Ibid., 39-40.

19. Charles Colson, *Kingdoms in Conflict* (Grand Rapids:

Zondervan Publishing House, 1987), 51-56; Johnson, *Intellectuals*, 138-72.

20. Will Durant quoted by Norman Geisler, "The Collapse of Modern Atheism," in *Intellectuals Speak Out*, 149.

21. John D'Emilio and Estelle B. Freedman, *Intimate Matters* (New York: Harper and Row, 1988), 265.

22. Ibid., 224.

23. Ibid., 224-26; Alcorn, *Sexual Revolution*, 37-38.

24. *Encyclopedia Britannica*, 15th ed., "Micropedia," vol. 3, 860.

25. John Leo, "Bursting the South Sea Bubble," *Time*, 14 February 1983, 68-70. For a detailed analysis of the many mistakes Mead made and why her personal convictions induced her to major fallacies, see Derek Freeman, *Margaret Mead and Samoa: The Making and Unmaking of an Anthropological Myth* (Cambridge, Mass.: Harvard University Press, 1983).

26. Reay Tannahill, *Sex in History* (New York: Stein and Day, 1982), 404.

27. D'Emilio and Freedman, *Intimate Matters*, 286.

28. Alcorn, *Sexual Revolution*, 44.

29. D'Emilio and Freedman, *Intimate Matters*, 270.

30. Robert Fay et al., "Prevalence and Patterns of Same-Gender Contact among Men," *Science* 243 (1989): 338-48. The biases of Kinsey included a large number of college students, prisoners, and members of homosexual groups. See Edward Sagarin, "Prison Homosexuality and Its Effect on Post-Prison Sexual Behavior," *Psychiatry* 39 (1976): 245-57. Over half of the black women interviewed had criminal records. See Gail Wyatt et al., "Kinsey Revisited, Part 2: Comparisons of the Sexual Socialization and Sexual Behavior of Black Women Over 33 Years," *Archives of Sexual Behavior* 17 (1988): 289-332. Also, Lois Downey, "Intergenerational Change in Sex Behavior: A Belated Look at Kinsey's Males," *Archives of Sexual Behavior* 9 (1980): 267-317. Several surveys of sexual activity, which were reported at the 1990 meeting in New Orleans of the American Association for the Advancement of Science, also concurred that Americans are more traditional than Kinsey reported. For example, only 1 percent of males are exclusively homosexual (Thomas Maugh II, Los Angeles Times News Service, "U.S. Sex Surveys Find More Smoke than Fire," *Austin American-Statesman*, 19 February 1990).

31. Alcorn, *Sexual Revolution*, 44-45.

32. Thomas Szanz, *Sex by Prescription* (Garden City, N.Y.: Anchor Press, 1980).

33. Alcorn, *Sexual Revolution*, 35.

34. Alexander Hellemans and Bryan Bunch, *The Timetables of Science* (New York: Simon and Schuster, 1988), 417.

35. D'Emilio and Freedman, *Intimate Matters*, 242.

36. Tannahill, *Sex in History*, 411.

37. D'Emilio and Freedman, *Intimate Matters*, 244.

38. Margaret White, *AIDS and the Positive Alternatives* (Basingstoke, U.K.: Marshall Pickering, 1987), 28-30.

39. D'Emilio and Freedman, *Intimate Matters*, 252.

40. John Whitehead, *The Second American Revolution* (Elgin, Ill.: David Cook Publishing Co., 1982), 138; Michael Gorman, *Abortion and the Early Church* (Downers Grove, Ill.: InterVarsity Press, 1982).

41. D'Emilio and Freedman, *Intimate Matters*, 64.

42. John W. Whitehead, *The Stealing of America* (Westchester, Ill.: Crossway Books, 1983), 46.

43. Adapted from a story told by Henry Brandt in Elisabeth Elliot, *Passion and Purity* (Old Tappan, N.J.: Fleming H. Revell Co., 1983), 147.

44. Os Guinness, *The Gravedigger File* (Downers Grove, Ill.: InterVarsity Press, 1983), 41.

45. D'Emilio and Freedman, *Intimate Matters*, 239.

46. Rosenblatt, "What Really Mattered," 24-27.

47. McDowell, *Why Wait?*, 56.

48. Bruce L. Shelley, *Church History in Plain Language* (Waco, Tex.: Word Books, 1982), 456.

49. D'Emilio and Freedman, *Intimate Matters*, 199.

50. Laurance Urdang, ed., *The Timetables of American History* (New York: Simon and Schuster, 1981), 272-84.

51. D'Emilio and Freedman, *Intimate Matters*, 231, illus. nos. 49 and 50.

52. Ibid., 278-79.

53. *Encyclopedia Britannica*, 15th ed., s.v. "inflation and deflation."

54. Ibid., 189.

55. Johnson, *Modern Times*, 5.

56. Alcorn, *Sexual Revolution*, 43.

57. D'Emilio and Freedman, *Intimate Matters*, 234.

58. Robert N. Bellah et al., *Habits of the Heart* (New York: Harper and Row, 1985), 141.

59. Schlossberg, *Idols for Destruction*, 310.

60. Marvin Olasky, *The Prodigal Press* (Westchester, Ill.: Crossway Books, 1988), 31ff.

61. Urdang, *Timetables of American History*, 307.

62. Tannahill, *Sex in History*, 403.

63. Whitehead, *Stealing of America*, 18.

64. D'Emilio and Freedman, *Intimate Matters*, 256-57.

65. Ibid., 281-82.

66. Johnson, *Modern Times*, 256-57.

67. Whitehead, *Stealing of America*, 2.

68. Allan Bloom, *The Closing of the American Mind* (New York: Simon and Schuster, 1987), 49.

69. D'Emilio and Freedman, *Intimate Matters*, 260.

70. Ibid., 212.

71. Allan Brandt, *No Magic Bullet* (New York: Oxford University Press, 1987), illus. facing p. 164.

72. Ibid., 290.

73. Ibid., illus. 60 following p. 274.

74. Ibid., 280.

75. Alcorn, *Sexual Revolution*, 88-89.

76. Kirk Kilpatrick, *Psychological Seduction* (Nashville: Thomas Nelson Publishers, 1983). The entire book's thesis concerns the mistaken emphasis of modern psychology.

77. Colson, *Kingdoms in Conflict*, 212.

78. Bellah, *Habits of the Heart*, 223.

79. Guinness, *Gravedigger File*, 148.

80. John Vertefeuille, *Sexual Chaos* (Westchester, Ill.: Crossway Books, 1988), 100.

81. D'Emilio and Freedman, *Intimate Matters*, 276.

82. Ibid., 262.

83. Vertefeuille, *Sexual Chaos*, 132-33.

84. K.L. Billingsley, *The Seductive Image* (Westchester, Ill.: Crossway Books, 1989), 64.

85. Johnson, *Modern Times*, 643.

86. George Gilder, *Wealth and Poverty* (New York: Basic Books, 1981), 109-11. Also see the interview with Robert Bellah, author of *Habits of the Heart*, by Rodney Clapp, "Habits of the Hearth," *Christianity Today*, 3 February 1989, 213.

87. D'Emilio and Freedman, *Intimate Matters*, 318-19.

88. Vertefeuille, *Sexual Chaos*, 106-7.

89. Ibid., 102.

90. Stanton Jones, "Homosexuality According to Science," *Christianity Today*, 18 August 1989, 26.

91. D'Emilio and Freedman, *Intimate Matters*, 329.

92. See statements of North American Man-Boy Love Association and the 1980 Gay Rights Platform at the Democratic National Convention in San Francisco. Also Joseph Sobran, "Why Don't Journalists Expose the Pederasty Lobby?" *The Dallas Times Herald*, 24 January 1983.

93. Neil Postman quoted in Whitehead, *Stealing of America*, 70-71. Also see Postman interview in *U.S. News & World Report*, 19 January 1981, 43-45.

94. D'Emilio and Freedman, *Intimate Matters*, 274. See also Jeff Nesbit, "Teen Pregnancy Found to Rise Despite Sex Education, Prevention Efforts," *Austin American-Statesman*, 10 February 1986.

95. D'Emilio and Freedman, *Intimate Matters*, 332.

96. The first act of sex most often happens at the home of one of the teens between 3 and 5 P.M. when the parents are away. See Josh

McDowell and Dick Day, *Why Wait?* (San Bernardino, Calif. : Here's Life Publishers, 1987), 366.

97. D'Emilio and Freedman, *Intimate Matters*, 342.

98. Alcorn, *Sexual Revolution*, 54.

99. Niehbuhr quoted in Bruce Shelley, *Church History in Plain Language* (Waco, Tex.: Word Books, 1982), 416.

When the Lamb opened the fourth seal, I heard the voice of the fourth living creature say, "Come!" I looked, and there before me was a pale horse! Its rider was named Death, and Hades was following close behind him. They were given power over a fourth of the earth to kill by sword, famine and plague, and by the wild beasts of the earth (Revelation 6:7-8).

"I will send famine and wild beasts against you, and they will leave you childless. Plague and bloodshed will sweep through you, and I will bring the sword against you. I the LORD have spoken" (Ezekiel 5:17).

"I sent plagues among you as I did to Egypt.
I killed your young men with the sword,
    along with your captured horses.
I filled your nostrils with the stench of your camps,
    yet you have not returned to me," declares the
    LORD (Amos 4:10).

What has been will be again,
    what has been done will be done again;
    there is nothing new under the sun
(Ecclesiastes 1:9).

Chapter Five

In the Beginning: The History of the AIDS Epidemic

April 4, 1981
Centers for Disease Control
Atlanta

In her tiny office in the cluster of red brick buildings that served as nerve center for the federal government's monitoring of the public health, technician Sandra Ford did a second take on the pentamidine request form. Pentamidine was one of the dozen drugs that were used so rarely that the federal government stockpiled the nation's supply through special arrangement with the Food and Drug Administration. Not only were the drugs not yet officially licensed for widespread use, but not enough profit existed in their production to interest commercial firms. When doctors needed them, they called Sandy Ford. . . .

This guy should go back to medical school if he can't find some simple [cancer], Sandra Ford thought. Maintaining her professional air, however, Ford asked the doctor again, in a different way:

How did he come to have not one but two patients with *Pneumocystis carinii* pneumonia [PCP] who needed pentamidine? This was a simple question, Ford thought. What was the underlying cause of the immune suppression that had brought on the pneumonia?

The Manhattan physician, again, answered he didn't know why the two young men had PCP. In fact, there didn't seem to be any reason for the immune system to be so out of whack. Still, they needed pentamidine because they weren't reacting well to the sulfa drugs more commonly used for *Pneumocystis*.

Ford figured the doctor was either incompetent or lazy. He probably didn't have the patients' charts in front of him and didn't want to move ... into another room to get them. But in the last eight weeks, she had filled five orders for adult male patients with unexplained *Pneumocystis*. All but one of them lived in New York.[1]

* * * * * *

E arly in 1981, one of the keys to the new epidemic was about to be discovered by an unknown technician doing a mundane job in a city hundreds of miles from the centers of the epidemic. Such is one of the many paradoxes that have occurred throughout the fascinating, though tragic, history of the AIDS epidemic. At that very moment, many medical investigators across the U.S., and a few in Europe, were closing in on a new disease that would eventually be called Acquired Immunodeficiency Syndrome.

The history of this epidemic is notable in discerning the intricate involvement of medicine, politics, and social and sexual changes in society. Few diseases have been so heavily affected by nonmedical decisions that displayed poor judgment. To grasp some of these poor decisions is to know how to avoid future mistakes.

The Concealed Train: 1980 and Before

No one knows when or where AIDS began, but accumulating evidence suggests the disease has existed for several decades at least. Although the first report on AIDS occurred in 1981, subsequent research indicates that AIDS existed in sporadic cases prior to the mid-seventies throughout Europe, North America, and Africa.[2] This evidence includes HIV-positive blood samples from the fifties and dozens of cases of people who died of illnesses suspiciously like AIDS. The growing scientific consensus is that changes in sexual habits as well as new social conditions in Africa unleased this scourge.

Several obstacles intrinsic to AIDS made discovery unlikely before the 1980s. First, the long incubation period made it difficult to trace people and their symptoms. If a person dies of a rare illness and then a friend dies within days with similar symptoms, it is easy to make the connection. But if the second death occurs five to ten years later, after moves, change of doctors, and the forgetfulness of time, follow-up is much more difficult, if not impossible.

Second, the chance of a second person infected with AIDS having the same symptoms as the first person is small, since the secondary infections and cancers are several dozen and each can be revealed in different ways. So the first man might die suddenly of a rare pneumonia, his female sexual contact might die slowly of a fungal infection five years later, and a blood donation from her might kill another man with cancer ten years afterwards.

Third, research capabilities for viral and immune disorders are far advanced over what they were in the fifties. If the AIDS epidemic had begun in the seventies, some scientists believe the state of viral research at that time could not have made the rapid discoveries that occurred in the eighties.[3]

Finally, an increase in cases with consistent symptoms was needed for AIDS to be identified. Newly identified diseases have a number of similar cases that notify physicians of the novelty of the ailment. With Legionnaire's disease, many men at one convention became ill with pneumonia. Toxic shock syndrome was identified when a number of menstruating women became ill with fever and a characteristic rash. Conforming to this pattern, the first report of AIDS had multiple cases of *Pneumocystis* pneumonia. A subsequent article described multiple patients with Kaposi's sarcoma.

Since HIV has a low rate of contagiousness compared to other sexually transmitted illnesses, and the incubation of the virus is five to ten years, the sexual changes of the late sixties led to the AIDS cases of the late seventies. By 1978, physicians were seeing patients with rare pneumonias, unusual cancers, and enlarged lymph nodes. In retrospect, fifty-five men in the U.S. and ten in Europe had symptoms of AIDS by 1980, although the disease was unknown in the medical community.[4] After a time, enough HIV existed in certain isolated groups that it took fewer sexual contacts to make infection possible. AIDS then exploded onto the scene in the eighties when this critical mass was reached. Escalating cases and the higher research sophistication on retroviruses increased the amount of information accordingly.

By 1980 homosexuals were a significant political power, especially in California. San Francisco had become the great mecca for male homosexuals in the seventies, with thousands migrating there every year. The annual Gay Freedom Day parade drew hundreds of thousands of spectators each July. Homosexuals in San Francisco became the largest single voting block in the city, and they were not lax in using their new-found political power. In 1980, Governor Brown of California declared Gay Freedom Week and presidential candidate Ted Kennedy gave a ringing endorsement for gay rights at the Democratic National Convention.[5]

The meteoric rise in homosexual promiscuity was documented by huge increases in other sexually transmitted diseases, such as herpes, syphilis, and gonorrhea. Homosexual bathhouses became popular gathering places for the newly liberated homosexual men in cities like San Francisco and

New York. Promiscuous, anonymous sex was occurring in these bathhouses at an enormous rate, which became part of a $100-million-a-year industry. The bathhouses concentrated the people at risk for sexually transmitted diseases so that one-third of the time that a patron went there, he left with syphilis or gonorrhea. New York City, scene of the Stonewall Inn riot of 1969, was further along in this moral degeneration than San Francisco—only more quietly so. Physicians were treating increasing numbers of venereal diseases in male homosexuals and were very concerned. On purely medical grounds, they counseled their patients to have fewer partners, but the homosexual community ignored the doctors' advice.[6]

Concentrate too much plutonium in a small place, and a nuclear explosion occurs. Concentrate too many infected people in a closed community, and a biological explosion occurs. The chain reaction had just begun.

A Runaway Train Suspected: 1981

A Los Angeles physician first described AIDS in June 1981 in the weekly report of the Centers for Disease Control (CDC). About the same time, other doctors were also concluding that an undescribed disease existed. Michael Gottlieb, the UCLA physician who wrote the first report, was merely the quickest to get the information out in a respected medical publication.[7]

Two illnesses were the major signposts that something new was on the horizon. *Pneumocystis carinii* infects virtually everyone in the world, but is easily suppressed, causing no greater problem than the numerous bacteria that reside in the mouth and large intestines. However, when one loses the vitality of the immune system, as in the treatment of certain cancers and organ transplant patients, this microorganism can produce a severe, often lethal, pneumonia. Since *Pneumocystis* pneumonia (PCP) was rare in the pre-AIDS era, Sandra Ford mistakenly attributed the requests for pentamidine to misdiagnosis. To see PCP in supposedly healthy males was unprecedented.

Less than two months after the original report of PCP in homosexual men, two articles appeared in the CDC weekly about a rare form of cancer seen with increasing frequency in young male homosexuals.[8] Normally this cancer, called Kaposi's sarcoma, is mild as cancers go, since it seldom shortens the life expectancy of the older men who normally contract it. However, it was a much more serious cancer in these young males, frequently threatening the life of its victims within a year or two.[9]

These reports of two unusual illnesses in homosexual men were the opening for the scientific community to investigate this new immune disorder. Various theories were advanced as to its cause, including persistent viral infections, "recreational drug" usage such as amyl nitrates (used to enhance sexual intensity), or overexposure to sperm.[10] However, by December 1981, investigators from the CDC, by studying sexual partners of homosexual men with AIDS, deduced that the new disease must be caused by an infectious agent.[11] The men who originally developed AIDS were among the most sexually active of an already promiscuous group of people and were also the men most likely to come down with other venereal diseases.[12] Apparently a new one had appeared. In similar fashion, hepatitis B and chlamydia in the seventies had became prominent sexually transmitted diseases due to the marked increase in immoral sex.

The probability of an infectious agent as the cause was also substantiated by two factors. First, cases of AIDS were now being seen in other parts of the world, mostly in Europe, with some of these cases originating in Africa.[13] These patients were not in the same environment as the American homosexuals nor had they been using a postulated bad batch of amyl nitrates from America. But an infectious agent transported across the world by modern air travel could cause disease worldwide. Second, new cases of AIDS were being discovered in a whole new group of people: IV drug users and possibly their infants. The vast majority of drug users with AIDS were heterosexual, used no amyl nitrates, and had no association with the homosexual community.

But IV drug users do exchange blood, which suggested that blood was a contagious fluid. This fact was reminiscent of the past and suggestive of something terrifying for the future. As for the past, the pattern for AIDS was like the hepatitis B epidemic among homosexual men and IV drug users in the seventies. This implied that AIDS was caused by an agent transmitted by sex and by blood exchange. For the future, it suggested a new group of victims was to come: those who had received blood transfusions and infants of infected mothers. The victims would not take long to make their appearance.

Many in the homosexual community originally denied the existence of this new threat and claimed the media was exaggerating the danger.[14] They made no significant change in their sexual behavior, and many more young men were infected. The homosexual physicians who had attempted to modify the rampant sexual activity of the homosexual community were seeing their worst fears come true: a new virulent illness with lethal results that was unresponsive to treatment.

By the end of 1981, experts had come to a substantial understanding of the transmission of AIDS and were recommending that male homosexuals limit their sexual contacts. By December, the first articles appeared in the prestigious *New England Journal of Medicine*. At the same time, *Newsweek* and *Time* carried their first stories on AIDS. The new disease had gone national.[15]

THE TRAIN INCREASES SPEED: 1982

Information about AIDS accumulated rapidly in 1982. In addition to *Pneumocystis* pneumonia and Kaposi's sarcoma, new secondary illnesses were coming to light, including parasitic, viral, and bacterial infections. Some patients exhibited neurologic and gastrointestinal symptoms that seemed unrelated to secondary infections. It was later demonstrated that these symptoms are direct effects of the virus.

Homosexuals continued to resist change in their lifestyles. Many thought the hoopla about the new disease was all a media creation; others thought the government had conspired against them by infecting them with a new illness. The few homosexual physicians who gave appropriate advice were roundly chastised by homosexual publications for causing an "epidemic of fear."[16] This denial increased the number of victims at a time when prevention could have kept AIDS to the level of a minor tragedy, rather than the national calamity it is today. Through May 1982 the CDC reported 355 cases;[17] by the end of the year there were almost twice that number. Tragic as those victims were, the numbers pale beside the 100,000 in the U.S. by mid-1989.

The CDC confirmed the increased risk of acquiring AIDS through sexual contact by studying a cluster of AIDS cases, linking 40 of the first 248 AIDS patients to sexual contact with one man.[18] Gaetan Dugas, a Canadian flight attendant with AIDS, was very promiscuous, having 250 different male sexual partners per year from 1979 through 1981. Labeled "Patient Zero," he refused to stop having sex even when the experts warned him that he was infecting other men. Dugas was probably not the first case in America, but he became the most prominent.

A common place to contract AIDS was one of the large bathhouses where homosexual men would have sex with multiple partners. Most of the early cases of AIDS were in men who frequented those places. Many doctors unsuccessfully recommended that homosexual men reduce their visits to the bathhouses. Even the tepid suggestion to put up posters about the dangers of multiple partners brought anger from the homosexual community and the bathhouse owners. These owners gave millions of dollars to homosexual magazines and political causes which served to insulate them from criticism. Cries of civil rights violations were often used by the owners to cover up their own self-interests. Moreover, the bathhouses were a symbol for many of the civil rights homosexuals had won over the last decade.[19] So it was difficult to close them down, even though it made medical sense.

Three new groups predicted at risk to acquire AIDS were confirmed in 1982. Hemophiliacs, transfusion recipients, and babies born to infected mothers were risk groups the medical community expected to emerge because of the previous experience with hepatitis B. Hemophiliacs, after having their lives transformed by Factor VIII, saw this boon of medicine become a nightmare. Factor VIII is prepared from pooled blood involving upwards of several thousand donors. The method of preparation used cold filtering methods that excluded bacteria and certain toxins but allowed small particles such as viruses to come through. The transfusion victims came to light more slowly but were expected, since, like hemophiliacs, they are recipients of blood products. The newborns, in a sense, are also transfusion recipients since mixing of maternal and infant blood often occurs before or during delivery. The first babies with HIV were primarily the infants of IV drug-using mothers.[20] The diagnosis of AIDS in these infants initially was doubted, since the signs of AIDS in children are different from adults. The new groups at risk confirmed that AIDS was an infectious illness. That it passed through the filter plates used for Factor VIII suggested it was viral.

An unexpected high risk group was Haitians, since they fit no pattern with other illnesses. Over time, Haitians with AIDS were reconciled to one or more of the established risk categories.[21]

One of the most disgraceful parts of the AIDS epidemic was the lack of appropriate screening by the blood banks to exclude high-risk blood after AIDS was suspected to be caused by a virus. This failure will cost thousands of lives. Members of the scientific community argued vehemently that the blood of donors who are homosexual, who show evidence of past hepatitis B infection, or have low T-helper cells should be discarded. Homosexual leaders vigorously opposed these suggestions, saying that they stigmatized them as a group. Blood banks also opposed any screening techniques, citing the high costs and the lack of indisputable evidence for a viral cause.[22] The lawsuits have already begun and will be numerous.

Large, blood-red letters spelling a sexually spread disease appeared on the cover of the August 2, 1982, issue of *Time*. The word was *herpes*, not *AIDS*. The painful genital sores were more of a concern to the general reader than the "gay plague." The media gave scant coverage to the AIDS epidemic early on and usually cited unwarranted concerns that AIDS was rapidly entering the heterosexual population. Other news reports about new breakthroughs gave false hopes to the homosexual community, weakening the impetus to change.[23] Although reports on promising drugs and on vaccines for AIDS made good press, they were not realistic. A strong call for abstinence then would have saved tens of thousands of lives—if it had been heeded.

The Train Out of Control: 1983

By June 1983, 1,641 AIDS cases had been reported to the CDC; two years before, AIDS was not even recognized in the medical community.[24] The CDC admitted that the number of cases was doubling every six months. On schedule, a total of three thousand cases had been diagnosed by December of the same year.[25] No longer were only the most promiscuous homosexual men getting the illness.

Early in 1983 the term AIDS Related Complex or ARC was coined to describe the syndrome of enlarged lymph nodes, fever, diarrhea, and thrush.[26] It was hoped that this was a healthier reaction to the causative agent with little mortality compared to AIDS. That dream, like many in this epidemic, was not to be fulfilled.

Most homosexual leaders opposed any restrictions on the homosexual life-style. One radical declared that society was responsible to find a cure; he was not obligated to alter his promiscuity.[27] In spite of such harsh rhetoric, some homosexuals dramatically reduced their sexual contacts; others denied that the illness was at all important. Most opposed the screening of blood, thinking it would make scapegoats of the homosexual community. Bathhouse owners opposed any regulation of their businesses, even though the CDC called the bathhouses "an amplification system" for the spread of the illness. In San Francisco, the baths were required to post warnings that sex with strangers could be dangerous. These posters were usually placed in out-of-the-way places, deceptively downplaying the dangers.[28] It is eerie how closely this response parallels a passage in *The Plague*:

> [The doctor] observed that small official notices had just been put up about the town, though in places where they would not attract much attention. It was hard to find in these notices any indication that the authorities were facing the issue squarely. The measures enjoined were far from Draconian and one had the feeling that many concessions had been made to a desire not to alarm the public.[29]

Some homosexuals valiantly tried to oppose the disease, only to be vilified as "homophobic," a swear word among homosexuals. Larry Kramer, a well-known homosexual writer, wrote an article called "1,112 . . . and Counting," which chastised homosexuals for being more concerned about sex than about their lives. Although his article tried to shake up the denial within the homosexual community, it mostly brought a wave of criticism from homosexual leaders.[30]

In 1983, northern New Jersey and the ghettos of New York City became the first place in the world where more people were acquiring AIDS from needles than through homosexual activity. Nine out of ten intravenous drug users with AIDS were from this location,[31] though the problem existed in other areas too. The CDC also reported that a number of women with immunodeficiency had been habitual sexual partners of men with AIDS, suggesting a new form of transmission.[32] The disease could be spread from man to woman through sex rather than just through blood.

The race for the discovery of the viral culprit was on, and it was rumored to be full of fouls. Investigators at the Pasteur Institute in France, led by Luc Montagnier, isolated a retrovirus from a lymph node of a patient with ARC in January 1983. Their report appeared in the May 20, 1983, issue of *Science*. In that same issue were three articles from American investigators, led by Robert Gallo of the National Cancer Institute, which suggested that the family of retroviruses called human T-cell leukemia viruses were closely related to the AIDS virus. Almost a year later Gallo, then Jay Levy in San Francisco, reported isolating the virus in the United States.[33] Gallo was a better-known virologist than his foreign competitors, and the French had trouble getting recognition for their achievement. The conflict over who first isolated the agent causing AIDS apparently was resolved prior to their first collaborative article in the fall of 1988.[34]

Scientists openly complained that not enough funds were available for AIDS research. One said he had to "beg, borrow, and steal people away from other projects."[35] The CDC continued to be at the center of breakthroughs, despite their limited funds. Experts there complained that not enough money was available because most people did not see the delayed effect of this infection. Their statisticians now estimated that the incubation period was at least five and a half years.[36] This meant that AIDS cases appearing in 1983 were contracted in 1978 or earlier. The number of casualties would skyrocket, because from 1981 to 1983 most male homosexuals denied AIDS was a major problem and continued high-risk behavior.

A brief letter in the British journal *Lancet*[37] described the earliest known case of AIDS (at the time). It occurred in a woman doctor who died in 1977. She had worked four years in central Africa and was exposed repeatedly to the blood of Africans during surgery. Because of this and reports of previously healthy Africans succumbing to AIDS in Europe, teams of epidemiologists were dispatched to that area. Their reports were not encouraging.[38] An epidemic of large proportions was occurring there, and no one knew about it in the West. Although the number of AIDS victims in Africa was vastly overestimated at that time, Africa clearly was an additional center of the new epidemic.[39]

The controversy surrounding the nation's blood supply continued. The public suppliers of blood seemed unconcerned about the growing evidence for AIDS transmission through blood. Private drug companies, who supplied commercial blood products such as Factor VIII, heeded the warnings of the hemophiliac lobby and began excluding the blood of high-risk groups. One San Francisco hospital also began screening blood by checking the number of T-helper cells, a marker for good immune function. It was the only public supplier of blood to do so.[40] Some people called for designated donors, where a person having elective surgery could have blood given for him by a relative or friend. Those few calls of 1983 became a roar later on. The blood banks remained some what cavalier—a Congressional act protected them from product liability, since transfusions are vital though inherently risky even prior to AIDS. Negligence was another matter. The blood bank community was also concerned about what new guidelines might do to supplies of blood.

Media coverage went up dramatically when a national expert wrote an editorial describing how severe AIDS would be if it were casually transmitted.[41] The author of that editorial later repudiated any chance of casual spread, but the damage was done. The public became convinced that scientists did not know how the disease was spread, and AIDS hysteria, always a near possibility, became reality. Police in San Francisco were seen wearing yellow gloves and masks. Emergency teams refused to assist people suspected of AIDS, and even physicians became selective about whom they treated.[42]

THE TRAIN CRASHES: 1984

The cumulative cases of AIDS continued to rise rapidly. By summer there were five thousand; almost half were dead. AIDS had become the leading cause of death among hemophiliacs—only three years after the initial report of AIDS. The CDC director shocked many by announcing that he expected twenty-five thousand cases of AIDS within five years. But he was wrong; that depressing body count was reached in two years. Equally sobering was the realization that a high percentage of those infected with the virus eventually would develop full-blown AIDS.[43] At one time, it had been hoped that only a small portion would be progressive.[44] Because 1984 was an election year, AIDS became more political. President Reagan was criticized for not uttering a single public statement about AIDS. He probably saw it as a no-win situation. Anything he said would be considered too little by the liberals and too much by the conservatives. Many Christians were now saying that AIDS was God's judgment on homosexuals, even though homosexuals were not the only ones infected.

The largest issue in the homosexual political community was the possible closure of bathhouses. The CDC had decided the baths should be closed, but had no enforcement power.[45] Despite the accumulating evidence about the danger of the baths, all but one homosexual organization in San Francisco opposed closure. Thus homosexual men were betrayed by their own leaders. Eventually the baths did close, first in San Francisco and then in New York and Los Angeles, because the reality of the epidemic overcame political stonewalling. But the forced closures were probably unnecessary; the baths were already failing economically as more homosexual men were staying away. However, homosexual politicians persuaded a judge to reopen the baths if they used patrolling monitors to curtail privacy and eliminate sexual activity. The changes were the death blow to the reopened baths; homosexual men would not go if they could not have sex.[46] Ironically, some community health officials did not close baths in their area, considering it too late to stem the tide of the epidemic.[47]

Scientists continued their rapid assault on the illness. Dr. Robert Gallo and Margaret Heckler, head of the U.S. Department of Health, announced the isolation of the virus, which incensed the French scientists who had isolated the virus earlier. A lawsuit resulted over the valuable patent rights for the HIV blood test. The test to detect AIDS antibodies was used in 1984 for research purposes. One of its more vital functions was to show that many of the children of IV drug addicts with immune disorders also had the AIDS virus, although only 15 percent satisfied the clinical definition of AIDS.[48] In certain areas of Africa, the test showed a positive rate about fifteen times higher than that of the U.S. This data proved to be off substantially, due to false positive readings, but at the time it pointed to Africa as the origin of the disease.[49]

The controversy over blood donor screening and testing continued. In May 1984, blood banks in the San Francisco area finally agreed to test for indirect evidence of infected blood by looking for antibodies to hepatitis B. Since these antibodies were present in over 80 percent of the patients with HIV infection, to discard blood containing hepatitis B antibodies would eliminate four-fifths of the HIV-contaminated blood. This was a full twenty months after the CDC's recommendation that such action be taken.[50] Slowly other blood banks began testing as the evidence mounted for transfusion-acquired AIDS. Ironically, some people claimed that testing blood was a politically motivated decision. In reality, testing donated blood was one of the few nonpolitically motivated decisions during the early AIDS epidemic.

THE RESULTS OF THE CRASH: 1985

Only four years after the first cases of AIDS were described, the CDC reported that over ten thousand people had been diagnosed in the U.S. alone. About one-half were dead or near death. In Europe over a thousand cases had been diagnosed. The homosexual community there initially denied the importance of the disease. Sweden and Britain were more realistic about the danger of spread, passing a law which could quarantine an infected person for having sex with an unknowing partner.[51]

Early in March, the first deliveries of the HIV-antibody test arrived at blood banks. No longer was there any question about the need to test blood; many cases of transfusion-related HIV disease had been proven. Once the blood supply was protected, the test became available to doctors. Now the debate dramatically shifted focus: Who should be tested and what should be done with the gathered information? Recommendations ran the whole spectrum, from testing everyone in the nation (with complete quarantine for those who tested positive) to anonymous testing (with no contact tracing and no penalties for spreading the disease). What has actually occurred is somewhere in between and varies from state to state.

The federal government continued to be criticized for its limited expenditures on AIDS, particularly since the new budget recommended a decrease.[52] Although spectacular progress had been made in the description, diagnosis, and causes of AIDS, it was not a time to cut back on funding when a lethal illness was more than doubling each year.

An underground industry peddled miracle cures to HIV patients. Some of these remedies included vitamins to increase immune function, psychic surgery, meditation techniques, visits to Lourdes, and black market experimental drugs that might have legitimate uses in the illness. Desperation therapies will likely increase as the number of victims increases and as traditional medicine's lack of success becomes more apparent.

Two major events of the year came from the entertainment industry. Both helped to catapult AIDS into the mainstream of society. Homosexual activist Larry Kramer, who wrote the article "1,112 . . . and Counting," wrote a critically acclaimed play about mistakes made in the AIDS epidemic. When *The Normal Heart* played on Broadway, it was called "deeply affecting, tense and touching"[53] and generated both sympathy for the homosexual community and new funds from New York City to assist in the epidemic.[54] More notable because of its international impact was the announcement that Rock Hudson had AIDS. Hudson portrayed a rugged man in film and was the opposite of the stereotypical homosexual male. Suspicions began when he appeared on television with Doris Day, looking so haggard that viewers were concerned he was dying. His spokesman denied he had

AIDS until Hudson collapsed while in Paris to receive exper-imental chemotherapy. People now realized that almost any-one could be keeping homosexual activity secret regardless of how masculine he seemed. One writer said this announce-ment was the turning point of the epidemic; AIDS had come out of the closet and was now acceptable for middle-class America.[55] Rock Hudson's disclosure under duress and sub-sequent death gave the epidemic much needed publicity.

A great irony became apparent about this time. A dis-ease that was devastating an infamous group was not mak-ing them less popular, although there was some antihomosexual backlash. America's traditional support for the underdog was converting AIDS into political capital for the homosexual community. "AIDS is our strength," they shouted even as the funerals mounted.[56] AIDS, which ini-tially caused splits in the homosexual community, now started to bring them together.

THE NORMALCY OF AIDS: 1986 TO THE PRESENT

One of the great abilities of American society is to adapt to new problems. AIDS has now become integrated into everyday life. News reports on AIDS, rare early in the epidemic, are more common than any other medical subject. Blood banking includes autologous transfusions of one's blood for elective surgery. The frenetic activity of the sexual revolution has slowed, giving way to deliberate planning by sexually active men and women. Subjects that were unspeakable only a few years ago are being heard by our children in everyday conversation. Knowledge of AIDS will be widespread; common sense concerning what to do about it may still be uncommon.

"The nightmare accelerates" is the best description for the period between 1986 and the present. The CDC pre-dicted in 1986 that 270,000 Americans would have AIDS by 1991 and 179,000 would be dead. We are on track for those totals. In the middle of 1989 100,000 people in the U.S. alone had been diagnosed with AIDS. In expected years of life lost, AIDS will be the biggest killer of men in the U.S. by 1991, surpassing cancer, heart disease, and accidents.[57] Since 1986, many celebrities have died of AIDS, usually while claiming they had something else. These included choreographer Michael Bennett, clothing designer Perry Ellis, lawyer Roy Cohn, French philosopher Michel Foucault, Republican fundraiser Terry Dolan, national newscaster Max Robinson, and Liberace.

Since 1985, the virus has been described biochemically, demonstrating its methods of destruction of the immune system. Treatment of the secondary infections is improving and at least one antiviral drug (AZT) has been effective in slowing the course of the illness. Several attempts at vaccines have begun, although most scientists are pessimistic about their long-term effectiveness. The lawsuit between the French and American investigators over the recognition (and royalties) for the discovery of the virus was resolved through a compromise signed by the presidents of France and the U.S. in 1987.[58] That signing underscored how much politics has been involved in this sexually transmitted disease.

One of the biggest stories was the role played by former Surgeon General C. Everett Koop. His controversial AIDS report in 1987 included suggestions for sex education, condom use, and confidential testing. His proposals were strongly opposed in some circles and hailed in others. In mid-1988, Koop authorized the unprecedented mailing of the "Understanding AIDS" letter to every American household. He felt obligated to give out as much information as possible so that Americans could protect themselves. The merits of these ideas will be examined later in this book.

We have said little about the rest of the world, yet the World Health Organization (WHO) estimates that by 1991, three million cases of AIDS will have been acquired worldwide. It is to the rest of the world that we now briefly turn.

CENTRAL AFRICA

Many people have tried to place the origin of AIDS in Africa. Their evidence includes the high number of HIV-positive blood samples in African cities going back to the

1950s plus the existence of another retrovirus, which can cause an AIDS-like illness in monkeys. However, blood testing in Africa has been mistake-filled, and the retrovirus is not that similar to AIDS genetically.[59] The suggestion that the HIV spread from animals to humans via tribal rites, exposure during butchering, or bestiality is without evidence. The attempt to blame Africa for AIDS is another example of the West's refusal to accept responsibility for its sexual immorality. Africans believe AIDS began in the First World countries and then spread to them.[60] Experts admit that the origin of AIDS is unknown.[61]

Some news reports have stated that seventy-five million Africans are infected with HIV. These numbers are enormously inflated for several reasons. First, early testing was done among sexually active groups in cities. The urban areas, which contain only 25 percent of the African population, have much higher rates of infection than the countryside, which in many areas is virtually AIDS-free. A similar mistake would be to assert that eighty million Americans are infected with syphilis because one-third of the prostitutes in New York have syphilis. Second, the HIV test often reads positive in uninfected people in developing countries because of interference from tropical infections, such as malaria. Third, many Africans have been diagnosed with AIDS without the use of valid tests. This overestimates the number of AIDS cases several-fold since many illnesses mimic the weight loss and diarrhea seen in African AIDS.[62]

Many changes in Africa in the last thirty years have encouraged the spread of AIDS regardless of its origin. The continent has modernized, allowing easy access to most areas. Urban numbers have doubled, contributing to immorality due to anonymity and availability of prostitutes.[63] Frequent famines and wars have increased migration of people, breakdown of the family, and prostitution. The sexual revolution has been imported from the West concurrently with technology.[64] Economic necessity often forces husbands to work away from their families for months at a time, increasing the risk of contracting sexually transmitted diseases (STD) from prostitutes.[65] Untreated STDs that produce genital ulcers increase the ease of spread.[66] Limited medical funds cause improper diagnoses, poor education of the infected, inadequately screened blood, and poorly sterilized needles. In central Africa annual medical expenditures per person are only about fifteen dollars, less than one-hundredth of what is spent in the U.S.[67]

AIDS in central Africa is spread primarily by heterosexual activity, since homosexuality and IV drug use are rare. The disease is distributed equally among males and females. In the U.S. and Europe, where homosexuals make up the primary risk group, the ratio is ten or fifteen males to each female, although this ratio will likely even out somewhat in the future. Due to the large percentage of infected females of child-bearing age in Africa, many more infants have HIV disease than in the countries that have primarily homosexual spread. A second virus, HIV-2, has been found in Africa, although it still constitutes a minority of the cases.[68] Due to secondary intestinal parasites and severe tuberculosis, African AIDS usually takes the form of a wasting disease called "slim disease" because the person loses dramatic amounts of weight. With so many other lethal illnesses endemic to Africa, an occasional death from an unknown, debilitating disease caused little alarm initially. Much less treatment is available for AIDS in African countries than in industrialized nations. Most patients die at home essentially untreated.[69]

Central Africa is the worst place in the world for AIDS to occur because of the multitude of other problems. Malaria, sleeping sickness, and respiratory and diarrheal diseases kill millions in Africa each year. About a hundred thousand children die *every week* in Africa from starvation, diarrhea, parasites, and other tropical diseases.[70] This weekly devastation is more than all the tabulated deaths from AIDS over the first ten years of the HIV epidemic. AIDS will never kill as many a year as these other problems. Yet not only will there be over one million deaths from AIDS in the next decade, the deflection of scarce resources, the loss of key personnel, and the reduction in tourism will make chronic problems on the continent into multiple disasters.

The narcissistic West cares about Africa only when it can obtain some material or political advantage or shift blame for its own problems. The sudden interest in AIDS in Africa is seen aptly by native Africans as a self-serving attempt by Western nations to protect their own domain.

Fortunately Christians have done better. Although some missionary health professionals were infected with the virus prior to the understanding of AIDS, no decrease in volunteers has been seen. Some missionaries are "scared out of their wits" about AIDS but continue to put compassion for people ahead of themselves. Moreover, missionaries, who form the backbone of medical care in Africa, have been at the forefront in education showing how biblical morals will preserve life.[71]

WESTERN AND NORTHERN EUROPE

Europe has AIDS patterns virtually identical to the U.S. except that their epidemic began about two years later. Homosexuality and IV drug abuse are the primary forms of spread. The Mediterranean countries such as Spain and Italy have a greater portion of IV drug related cases. Scandinavia, with its sexual "freedom," has a higher incidence of homosexually spread HIV. France has the greatest number of AIDS cases on the continent in large part due to its central African connections, which allowed the European epidemic to start first in France. [72]

ASIA AND AUSTRALIA

Few cases have been reported so far on these continents. Most cases were imported from foreign blood bought for transfusions or by travelers to HIV-infected areas. As in the West, the disease is spread in Australia and New Zealand primarily through homosexual activity and IV drug abuse.[73]

THE CARIBBEAN AND SOUTH AMERICA

Although some people suggested that AIDS began in Haiti before coming to the U.S., some Haitians believe American homosexuals brought it to the island in the 1970s when Haiti was a well-known homosexual resort.[74] Haiti may be the first country in the world where AIDS contributed to a revolution. Tourism, a main source of income for this poor nation, dropped in 1983 to one-seventh its previous level due to the news reports about AIDS. The resulting loss of income and food shortages caused riots, which led to the overthrow of the government.[75] This country and most of the Caribbean are now places of heterosexual spread predominantly, thus affecting more women and infants.[76]

Brazil has the largest number of infected people in Central and South America, having almost as many cases as France. Originally, most of these cases involved homosexuals and IV drug users, but now include more and more heterosexuals.[77] Virtually all the nations in the Western hemisphere have reported some cases.

The World Health Organization reports that over 80 percent of the countries in the world have cases of AIDS. It will eventually spread to all countries on earth. However, the spread could be arrested if the world followed some simple public health measures given two to three thousand years ago:

"You shall not commit adultery" (Exodus 20:14).

"Do not lie with a man as one lies with a woman; that is detestable" (Leviticus 18:22).

"Flee from sexual immorality" (1 Corinthians 6:18).

The world has not listened to the words of the Most High. Let's hope and pray it listens now.

Chapter 5, Notes

1. Randy Shilts, *And the Band Played On* (New York: St. Martin's Press, 1987), 54, 61.

2. H. P. Katner and G. A. Pankey, "Evidence for a Euro-American Origin of Human Immunodeficiency Virus (HIV)," *The Journal of the National Medical Association* 79 (1987):1068-72; D. Huminer, J. B. Rosenfeld, and S. D. Pitlik, "AIDS in the Pre-AIDS Era," *Reviews of Infectious Diseases* 9 (1987):1102-8. Subsequent evidence submitted by the same authors strengthened their "assumption that unrecognized cases of AIDS have occurred sporadically before the start of the current epidemic" (*Reviews of Infectious Diseases* 10 [1988]:1061); A. J. Nahmias et al., "Evidence for Human Infection with an HTLV-III/LAV-like Virus in Central Africa, 1959," *Lancet* 1 (1986):1279-80; and R. F. Garry et al., "Documentation of an AIDS Virus Infection in the United States in 1968," *The Journal of the American Medical Association* 260 (1988):2085-87.

3. W. A. Blattner, "A Novelistic History of the AIDS Epidemic Demeans Both Investigators and Patients," *Scientific American* 259 (1988):149.

4. Shilts, *Band Played On*, 49.

5. Ibid., 15, 30.

6. Ibid., 13-20.

7. Centers for Disease Control, "*Pneumocystis* Pneumonia—Los Angeles," *Morbidity and Mortality Weekly Report* 30 (1981):250-52; M.S Gottlieb et al., "*Pneumocystis carinii* Pneumonia and Mucosal Candidiasis in Previously Healthy Homosexual Men: Evidence of a New Acquired Cellular Immunodeficiency," *The New England Journal of Medicine* 305 (1981): 1425-31.

8. Centers for Disease Control, "Kaposi's Sarcoma and *Pneumocystis* Pneumonia among Homosexual Men—New York City and California," *Morbidity and Mortality Weekly Report* 30 (1981):305-8; and Centers for Disease Control, "Follow-up on Kaposi's Sarcoma and *Pneumocystis* Pneumonia," *Morbidity and Mortality Weekly Report* 30 (1981):409-10.

9. D. T. Durack, "Opportunistic Infections and Kaposi's Sarcoma in Homosexual Men," *New England Journal of Medicine* 305 (1981):1465-67.

10. U. Hurtenbach and Wm. Shearer, "Germ Cell-induced Immune Suppression in Mice: Effect of Innoculation of Syngeneic Spermatozoa on Cell-mediated Immune Responses," *Journal of Experimental Medicine* 155 (1982):1719-29; and J. Sonnabend, S. S. Witkin, and D. T. Purtilo, "Acquired Immunodeficiency Syndrome, Opportunistic Infections and Malignancies in Male Homosexuals— A Hypothesis of Etiologic Factors in Pathogenesis," *The Journal of the American Medical Association* 249 (1983):2370-74.

11. W. Heyward and J. W. Curran, "The Epidemiology of AIDS in the U.S." *Scientific American* 259 (1988):72-81. This was formally published in 1984: D. M. Auerbach et al., "Cluster of Cases of the Acquired Immune Deficiency Syndrome—Patients Linked by Sexual Contact," *The American Journal of Medicine* 76 (1984):487-92.

12. H. W. Jaffe et al., "National Case-control Study of Kaposi's Sarcoma and *Pneumocystis Carinii* Pneumonia in Homosexual Men: Part 1, Epidemiology Results," *Annals of Internal Medicine* 99 (1983):145-51.

13. Shilts, *Band Played On*, 111.

14. Ibid., 78.

15. See "Opportunistic Diseases," *Time*, 21 December 1981, 68, and Matt Clark with Mariana Gosnell, "Diseases that Plague Gays," *Newsweek*, 21 December 1981, 51-52.

16. Shilts, *Band Played On*, 149, 182.

17. Centers for Disease Control, "Update on Karposi's Sarcoma and Opportunistic Infections in Previously Healthy Persons: United Ststes," *Morbidity and Mortality Weekly Report* 31 (1982): 294, 300-301.

18. Shilts, *Band Played On*, 147; and D. M. Auerbach et al., "Cluster of Cases of the Acquired Immune Deficiency Syndrome—Patients Linked by Sexual Contact," *The American Journal of Medicine* 76 (1984):487-92.

19. Shilts, *Band Played On*, 180.

20. Centers for Disease Control, "Unexplained Immunodeficiency and Opportunistic Infections in Infants—New York, New Jersey, California," *Morbidity and Mortality Weekly Report* 31 (1982):665-67.

21. "The Collaborative Study Group of AIDS in Haitian-Americans. Risk Factors for AIDS among Haitians Residing in the United States—Evidence of Heterosexual Transmission," *The Journal of the American Medical Association* 257 (1987):635-39; and Mann et al., "International Epidemiology of AIDS," 82-89.

22. Shilts, *Band Played On*, 207.

23. Ibid., 184.

24. Centers for Disease Control, "Acquired Immunodeficiency Syndrome (AIDS) Update—United States," *Morbidity and Mortality Weekly Report* 32 (1983):309-11.

25. Ibid., 688-91.

26. See "AIDS-Related Complex" in R. Yarchoan and J.M. Pluda, "Clinical Aspects of Infection with AIDS Retrovirus: Acute HIV Infection, Persistent Generalized Lymphadenopathy, and AIDS-Related Complex," in *AIDS: Etiology, Diagnosis, Treatment, and Prevention*, 2d ed., ed. V.T. Devita, S. Hellman, and S.A. Rosenberg (New York: J.B. Lippincott, 1988), 111-13.

27. Shilts, *Band Played On*, 378.

28. Ibid., 306, 318.

29. Albert Camus, *The Plague* (New York: Random House, The Modern Library, 1948), 48.

30. Shilts, *Band Played On*, 244-45.

31. H. W. Jaffe, D. J. Bregman, and R. M. Selik, "Acquired Immune Deficiency Syndrome in the United States: The First 1000 Cases," *The Journal of Infectious Diseases* 148 (1983):339-45.

32. Centers for Disease Control, "Immunodeficiency in Female Sexual Partners of Males with Acquired Immune Deficiency Syndrome (AIDS)—New York," *Morbidity and Mortality Weekly Report* 31 (1983):697-98; and C. Harris et al., "Immunodeficiency in Female Sexual Partners of Men with the Acquired Immunodeficiency Syndrome," *The New England Journal of Medicine* 308 (1983):1182-84.

33. R.C. Gallo et al., "Frequent Detection and Isolation of Cytopathic Retroviruses (HTLV-III) from Patients with AIDS and at Risk for AIDS," *Science* 224 (1984):500-503; J.A. Levy et al., "Isolation of Lymphocytopathic Retroviruses from San Francisco Patients with AIDS," *Science* 225 (1984):840-42.

34. R. C. Gallo and L. Montagnier, "AIDS in 1988," *Scientific American* 259 (1988):41-48.

35. Jean Seligmann, Vincent Coppola, and Mary Hager, "The AIDS Epidemic: The Search for a Cure," *Newsweek*, 18 April 1983, 78.

36. Shilts, *Band Played On*, 402.

37. I.C. Bygbjerg, "AIDS in a Danish Surgeon (Zaire, 1976)," *Lancet* 1 (1983):925.

38. J. B. Brunet et al., "Acquired Immunodeficiency Syndrome in France," *Lancet* 1 (1983):700; N. Cluymeck et al., "Acquired Immunodeficiency Syndrome in Black Africans," *Lancet* 1 (1983):642; N. Clumeck et al., "Acquired Immunodeficiency Syndrome in African Patients," *The New England Journal of Medicine* 310 (1984):492-97; P. Van de Perre et al., "Acquired Immunodeficiency Syndrome in Rwanda," *Lancet* 2 (1984):62-65; and P. Piot et al., "Acquired Immunodeficiency Syndrome in a Heterosexual Population in Zaire, *Lancet* 2 (1984):65-69.

39. Cynthia Haq, "Data on AIDS in Africa: An Assesment," in *AIDS in Africa*, ed. Norman Miller and Richard Rockwell (Lewiston, N.Y.: Edwin Mellen Press, 1988), 9-29.

40. Shilts, *Band Played On*, 249, 308.

41. A. S. Fauci, "The Acquired Immunodeficiency Syndrome: The Ever-broadening Clinical Spectrum," *The Journal of the American Medical Association* 249 (1983):2375-76.

42. Shilts, *Band Played On*, 301-2.

43. M. Melbye et al., "Long-term HTLV-III Seropositive Homosexual Men without AIDS Developing Measurable Immunologic and Clinical Abnormalities: A Longitudinal Study,"

Annals of Internal Medicine 104 (1986):496-500; J. J. Goedert et al., "Effect of T4 Count and Cofactors on the Incidence of AIDS in Homosexual Men Infected with Immunodeficiency Virus," *The Journal of the American Medical Association* 257 (1987):331-34; J. E. Kaplan et al., "Lymphadenopathy Syndrome in Homosexual Men: Evidence for Continuing Risk of Developing the Acquired Immunodeficiency Syndrome," *The Journal of the American Medical Association* 257 (1987):335-37; and H. W. Murray et al., "Progression to AIDS in Patients with Lymphadenopathy or AIDS-related Complex: Reappraisal of Risk and Predictive Factors," *The American Journal of Medicine* 86 (1989):533-38.

44. U. Mathur-Wagh et al., "Longitudinal Study of Persistent Generalized Lymphadenopathy in Homosexual Men: Relation of Acquired Immunodeficiency Syndrome," *Lancet* 1 (1984):1033-38; D. I. Abrams et al., "Persistent Diffuse Lymphadenopathy in Homosexual Men: Endpoint or Prodrome?" *Annals of Internal Medicine* 100 (1984):801-8; H. W. Jaffe et al., "The Acquired Immunodeficiency Syndrome in a Cohort of Homosexual Men: A Six-year Follow-up Study," *Annals of Internal Medicine* 103 (1985):210-14; and Centers for Disease Control, "Update: Acquired Immunodeficiency Syndrome in the San Francisco Cohort Study, 1978-1985," *Morbidity and Mortality Weekly Report* 34 (1985):573-75.

45. Shilts, *Band Played On*, 306.

46. Ibid., 464, 499.

47. Ibid., 454.

48. The Centers for Disease Control later changed the criteria for AIDS to incorporate children who are probably infected.

49. M. Essex and P. J. Kanki, "The Origins of the AIDS Virus," *Scientific American* 259 (1988):64-71.

50. Shilts, *Band Played On*, 433.

51. Ibid., 564-65.

52. Matt Clark, Deborah Witherspoon, and Mary Hager, "AIDS," *Newsweek*, 12 August 1985, 20-27.

53. William A. Henry III, "A Common Bond of Suffering," *Time*, 13 May 1985, 85.

54. Shilts, *Band Played On*, 556.

55. Ibid., xxi-xxiii.

56. Enrique Rueda and Michael Schwartz, *Gays, AIDS, and You* (Old Greenwich, Conn.: Devin Adair Company, 1987), 8.

57. San Francisco AIDS Conference, December 1988.

58. Shilts, *Band Played On*, 593.

59. Essex and Kanki, "AIDS Virus," 69.

60. Gloria Waite, "The Politics of Disease," in *AIDS in Africa*, 154.

61. Mann et al., "International Epidemiology of AIDS," 82.

62. Tom Barton, "Sexually Related Illness in Eastern and Central Africa," in *AIDS in Africa*, 270.

63. Waite, "Politics of Disease," in ibid., 153.

64. Barton, "Sexually Related Illness," in ibid., 289.

65. Marc H. Dawson, "AIDS in Africa: Historical Roots," in ibid., 59.

66. Mann et al., "International Epidemiology of AIDS," 86.

67. Gregg Easterbrook, "The Revolution in Medicine," *Newsweek*, 26 January 1987, 40. This article revealed that about $1700 per person is spent for medical care in America whereas most African nations spend less than $15 per person (cited in "Introduction," *AIDS in Africa*, xxvii).

68. Mann et al., "International Epidemiology of AIDS," 82.

69. Gary Merritt, William Lyerly, and Jack Thomas, "The HIV/AIDS Pandemic in Africa, " in *AIDS in Africa*, 127.

70. Frank Jansen, *Target Earth: The Necessity of Diversity in a Holistic Perspective on World Mission* (Kailua-Kona, Hawaii: University of the Nations, 1989), 20.

71. Sharon E. Mumper, "AIDS in Africa: Death Is the Only Certainty," *Christianity Today*, 8 April 1988, 38.

72. Mann et al., "International Epidemiology of AIDS," 87-89.

73. Ibid., 86.

74. Margaret White, *AIDS and the Positive Alternatives* (Basingstoke, U.K.: Marshall Pickering, 1987), 63.

75. Ibid., 52.

76. Mann et al., "International Epidemiology of AIDS," 88.

77. Ibid., 89; and T.C. Quinn, F.R.K. Zacarias, and R.K. St. John, "AIDS in the Americas: An Emerging Public Health Crisis," *The New England Journal of Medicine* 320 (1989):1005-7.

PART 2

THE MEDICAL DESCRIPTION OF AIDS

"They sow the wind
and reap the whirlwind"
(Hosea 8:7).

"For God did not send his Son into the world to condemn the world, but to save the world through him. Whoever believes in him is not condemned . . ." (John 3:17).

Praise be to the God and Father of our Lord Jesus Christ, the Father of compassion and the God of all comfort, who comforts us in all our troubles, so that we can comfort those in any trouble with the comfort we ourselves have received from God. For just as the sufferings of Christ flow over into our lives, so also through Christ our comfort overflows (2 Corinthians 1:3-5).

Jesus straightened up and asked [the adulteress], "Woman, where are they? Has no one condemned you?"

"No one, sir," she said.

"Then neither do I condemn you," Jesus declared. "Go now and leave your life of sin" (John 8:10-11).

Chapter Six

The Spread of AIDS

I met a man in the fall of 1988 who affected me deeply. Richard Sanders is a university professor in his mid-forties who greatly enjoys teaching. He is a good lecturer and well respected by his colleagues. Students are not intimidated by him because he does not consider himself more important than they are. Dr. Sanders is a man of passion in all the positive senses of the word. He is also a homosexual.

I had no idea that he was the first several times I was with him. We had talked pleasantly a few times, and I had heard him give an impressive lecture. It hardly prepared me for what was to follow, for during the conversation in which he admitted his homosexuality to me, I had one of the most moving experiences of my life.

Dr. Sanders had discovered that I was writing a book on AIDS and he began asking me many questions. He had strong opinions on everything we discussed, as would be expected of a tenured college professor. Knowing that I was an evangelical, he had many probing questions on the AIDS epidemic and its effect on the Christian community. I presented some of my ideas and awaited his response.

What I had said touched him, and he chose to increase

the depth of our relationship. He began, "Let's end this subterfuge. I am gay and know I have been gay all my life despite having been married for thirteen years." He then criticized some of my ideas, though without much emotion. He suddenly seemed weary. He said, "You know, Glenn, we gays have suffered more than anyone else." He recounted the gay-bashing he had seen and experienced; he thought it was cruel for people like me to try to convert the homosexual from what he truly was. He conveyed no animosity, although his voice faltered at points.

Then he lowered his voice and said, with tears in his eyes, "Glenn, two weeks ago I went to a funeral for a friend. It was my thirty-second." He paused to gather himself. "No one I know outside of the gay community has gone to anywhere near that many funerals." He considered this for a moment and said, "Oh, perhaps my grandmother—but she is in her late eighties, and for her it is a social occasion." He smiled, then quickly became serious again, and I could see his body quivering with emotion. "Glenn, what does it do to a man in his forties to see so much suffering and death? It has to change such a man. It has to have scarred me deeply."

I was hardly breathing. To my lasting shame I forced back the tears, though I was weeping inside. I marveled at this man's openness with me and his willingness to share his grief. I knew he was right. He had been changed in ways I could only imagine.

We sat quietly for a few more minutes. The strength in his voice returned as we talked about more mundane issues. As I rose to leave, I thanked him for his willingness to relate such personal details to me. I knew he was a vanquished man, beaten by a disease that had never touched his body. But I also knew I had been transformed in that thirty-minute conversation. I had vicariously experienced the pain of another human being, who like me bears the image of his Maker. A small part of me died that day, but by the grace of God and the openness of a fellow mortal, I gained new insight into the anguish of this world.

* * * * * *

I wish Richard Sanders's story was an unusual one, but it is not unique. In the geographic centers of homosexual life, such as San Francisco, Los Angeles, and New York, the misery is accumulating. In some places the AIDS virus has spread to over 50 percent of the male homosexual population.[1] Even homosexuals outside the fast track have close connections to these areas and are seeing many friends die. Since the vast majority of these infected men will likely develop AIDS[2], given enough time, the situation will only worsen. Before my conversation with Dr. Sanders I knew the death rate in the homosexual community was going to be devastating. I now understand that life and survival are devastating for many homosexuals as well.

We have already seen how HIV spread into the homosexual and IV-drug subcultures through sexual transmission and the sharing of needles. We will now discuss the biological aspects of the virus that have caused it to spread so thoroughly into specific groups.

What Is a Virus?

Viruses are the smallest of all microorganisms, hundreds of times smaller than bacteria. Their existence was suspected for decades before proof was established in 1915.[3]

It is difficult to think of viruses as living organisms, at least in the conventional sense. Although all are composed of genetic material and proteins like ordinary plant and animal cells, no virus can function apart from a living cell. They do not produce energy, use oxygen, or have mobility. Viruses are difficult to destroy, since they reside inside cells and use the host cell's energy and molecules to reproduce. Therefore, any drug that interferes with the virus usually disrupts the host cell and is quite toxic. Viruses are simple organic chemicals, except that, like all genetic material, they have a message that can "tell" the parasitized cell what to do. Although viruses contain one hundred thousand times less information than that in the genes of an average human cell, it is enough in the case of HIV to cause the eventual destruction of the person who has it.

THE HUMAN IMMUNODEFICIENCY VIRUS

Beginning in 1983, HIV was first isolated in three separate laboratories around the world.[4] It has been classified among the retroviruses because of its tendency to reverse the flow of genetic information, causing viral genetic material to be incorporated into the nucleus of the host cell. Normally information flows from the DNA of the host's nucleus to outside the nucleus. Although retroviruses have been studied in animals for decades, it was not until 1980 that the first one was described in humans. It was called Human T-Cell Leukemia Virus (HTLV-I) because it causes an unusual leukemia in the T white blood cells. A second type of human retrovirus was isolated prior to the discovery of the AIDS virus.

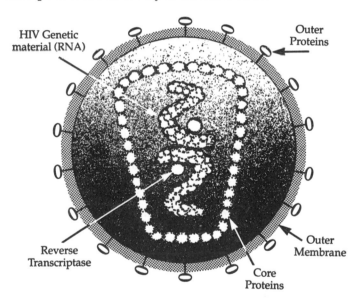

THE HUMAN IMMUNODEFICIENCY VIRUS

Illustration by Rosanne Avilar

When the HIV enters a new host's bloodstream, say after a transfusion, millions of viruses float in the bloodstream. Since they have no motility of their own, the viruses follow the natural course of the host's circulation. They would continue this journey endlessly, except that the viruses are attracted by chemical forces to receptors on certain cells of the immune system. If they get close enough to one of these cells, they dock like a spacecraft on a space station. The match has to be chemically exact. Different viruses are attracted to different types of cells: the hepatitis viruses attach to liver cells, the influenza virus attaches to cells in the respiratory system, and viruses that cause diarrhea attach to cells in the intestines.

One of the unique characteristics of the AIDS virus is that it attaches to two cells within the body's immune system: the macrophage and the T-helper cell.[5] Both of these are types of white blood cells. The macrophage would usually be a poor place for the virus to attach because these cells normally engulf (phagocytose) and destroy foreign invaders such as viruses and bacteria. But the HIV is not destroyed by this defense cell; instead it is able to survive and reproduce slowly, converting the macrophage into a reservoir of infectious viral particles.

The T-helper cell is a more critical place for HIV to attack, because this cell is the main controlling cell in the immune system. Once these cells are destroyed by the virus, the immune system is crippled and unable to fight off certain usually mild infections. HIV attaches to other cell receptors in the body. It has a strong affinity for certain brain cells, suggesting that the dementia or premature senility in AIDS patients is primarily caused by the presence of the virus itself.[6] It also attaches to cells in the intestines and may directly cause chronic diarrhea, rather than requiring a parasite as in most AIDS patients.

THE INVASION OF THE CELL

The life cycle of HIV begins when the virus is floating free in the blood (#1 in the drawing below). It becomes chemically attracted to the T-helper cell, attaches, and empties its proteins and genetic material into the cell (#2). The HIV has two strands of ribonucleic acid (RNA), one of which is used as a template or model on which mirror images of deoxyribonucleic acid (DNA) are formed (#3). The new

DNA strands, carrying viral genetic information, penetrate the T-helper cell nucleus (#4). All of these steps are activated by viral proteins which also entered the cell.

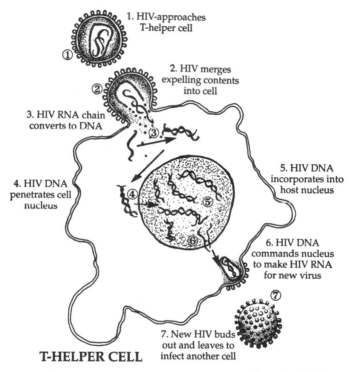

1. HIV-approaches T-helper cell

2. HIV merges expelling contents into cell

3. HIV RNA chain converts to DNA

4. HIV DNA penetrates cell nucleus

5. HIV DNA incorporates into host nucleus

6. HIV DNA commands nucleus to make HIV RNA for new virus

7. New HIV buds out and leaves to infect another cell

T-HELPER CELL

Illustration by Nancy Wood

Once inside the nucleus, the control center of the cell, the viral DNA strands, which have become double stranded, incorporate into the host's normal DNA (#5). This ability of the virus to become a permanent part of the instructions of the cell gives it two advantages over other viruses: first, it is doubly protected from the body's normal defenses (and man-made antiviral agents) by being within the cell and within the nucleus. Second, it in effect becomes part of the cell, so that every time the host cell reproduces, the daughter cells contain the genetic material of HIV.

The final steps occur when the viral DNA gives instructions to produce more viral particles. Genetic material exits the nucleus with instructions to produce all the components of the virus (#6) which then assemble and exit the cell ready to infect another T-helper cell (#7)(see photo below). The viral genes may remain latent within a cell, they may produce viral particles slowly, or they may produce thousands

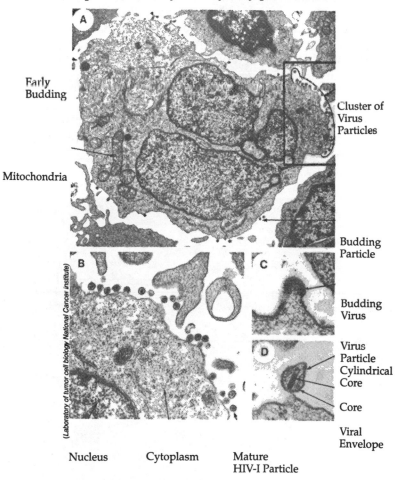

A. An electron micrograph showing viral particles exiting from a white blood cell.
B. An enlargement of section from photograph A.
C. A single budding virus.
D. A complete virus ready to infect another cell.

of particles in a burst of activity. The rate of viral particle production probably depends on the type and activity of the cell infected and the instructions of viral regulatory genes.

THE DESTRUCTION OF THE CELLS

HIV tends to reproduce slowly within the macrophages and so typically does not destroy them. On the other hand, the important controllers of the immune system, the T-helper cells, are more likely to be destroyed due to more rapid viral production. When enough of the T-helper cells are eliminated, the immune system no longer functions well, and opportunistic infections occur, eventually killing the infected individual.[7]

The manner in which the virus kills the cell can vary. If new viruses are being produced rapidly, holes will be produced in the cell membrane, causing it to rupture (note the hundreds of small spherical viruses budding off the T-helper cell in the photo below). Sometimes the virus will instruct

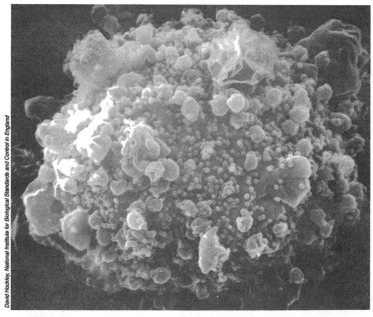

INFECTED T-HELPER CELL WITH VIRUS PARTICLES (SMALL SPHERES) COMING FROM THE SURFACE

the cell to fuse with other cells forming giant, abnormal masses of fifty to five hundred cells called syncytia. These giant cells cannot function normally in part because they have too many instructions (a committee of five hundred), so they eventually die. Another way of destruction is that the cell may be altered enough to be labeled as foreign by the body, bringing the body's immune system upon it. In this way the immune system targets its own demise.

THE EXPLOSION OF KNOWLEDGE ON HIV

In the short number of years of the AIDS epidemic, scientists have learned much about the virus and its operation. We have seen it under the electron microscope. We have described the viral genes and their function. We have identified at least eight proteins contained within the virus and their various functions (structural support, regulation of reproduction, and incorporation of viral genes into the host's DNA). We know how the viral membrane appears biochemically and where it attaches to the host cell. In short, scientists know an enormous amount about HIV's structure and operation. Yet we do not fully know why the virus is at times quiet, only to become active in viral production later. We do not understand why the body's immune system is so ineffective at destroying the virus. We do not understand the complex interactions between the cell and the virus. However, these intricate details are understood incompletely in virtually all viruses and many bacteria.

THE SPREAD TO OTHERS

Early in the epidemic, physicians realized that AIDS was not spread by casual contact in the manner of colds or sore throats. Since these illnesses are easily spread by sneezing, coughing, or touch, everyone gets them, regardless of age, sexual activity, or the use of drugs. But AIDS in the U.S. has been largely confined to homosexual men, IV drug users and their sexual contacts, and children born to infected women.[8]

An explanation for this must exist at the microscopic level, the virus's habitat so to speak. In addition to the cells in the blood (T-helper cells and macrophages), HIV can attack certain cells in the brain, lymph nodes, bone marrow, and thymus gland. These are not cells that other people come in contact with. The spread of any infection requires not only an infectious agent, but also a method of getting that agent to a second person. That is why the spread of any infection is almost always caused by fluid, whether saliva, nasal mucous, blood, diarrhea, semen, or vaginal fluids. We do not worry about a virus that is only in body tissues, since that is where it will stay.

HIV is free-floating in the blood for a short time before antibodies are made against it, but most often spread occurs through infected T-helper cells and macrophages in the fluid exchanged with another person.[9] These cells are found in three places in sufficient concentration to spread the virus: the blood, semen, and vaginal fluids. The AIDS virus and its infected cells are found in saliva, phlegm, urine, or diarrheal fluid only when they are contaminated by blood, which is seldom. Thus, the spread of the HIV is limited to sex, transfusions, sharing needles, and pregnancy, since these are the times people come in contact with blood, semen, and vaginal fluids.

SPREAD THROUGH SEXUAL ACTIVITY

About 70 percent of the spread of HIV in the U.S. occurs through sexual contact involving semen or vaginal fluids.[10] All but 4 percent of this spread occurs in male homosexuals, at least within the United States. Although this is a high percentage of sexual spread, it was even higher earlier in the epidemic before the virus had spread among IV drug abusers. The virus has been documented to be spread from male to male, male to female, and female to male.[11] Female to female spread is rare, but can occur during traumatic sexual practices between lesbians.

Male homosexuals spread HIV efficiently for three reasons. First, they are more promiscuous than other segments of the population. It was common for homosexual men to have sex with fifty to a hundred different men a year, especially in certain areas of New York and California. The first men diagnosed with AIDS were among the most promiscuous.[12] The more sexual partners, particularly within an isolated subculture, the greater the likelihood of contracting the AIDS virus. Although homosexual men have reduced their sexual contacts,[13] HIV infection is so widespread among male homosexuals in geographic pockets that anything other than monogamy with an uninfected partner is risky.

Second, homosexual practices, especially receptive anal intercourse, maximize spread of the virus.[14] The semen, containing infected white blood cells, must enter the blood stream to cause infection. Anal intercourse is traumatic to the rectal lining, which is not made to stretch like the vagina. Consequently, tears and fissures occur and act as entry points for the HIV-infected cells. Although the receptive partner in genital-anal sex is at highest risk for infection, the one who penetrates can acquire HIV by exposure of his penis to blood from the tears in the partner's rectum. It is not clear how much oral-genital contact or other homosexual practices influence the infection rate, since most homosexual men practice more than one type of sexual activity.

Third, homosexual men contract many other sexually transmitted diseases such as herpes, chancroid, and syphilis, which provide openings into the body for the virus.[15] Also these large numbers of infections may impair the immune system, making the transmission of the virus easier.

Although heterosexual spread of HIV is less likely than spread in homosexual men,[16] transmission has occurred in the U.S.[17] Tears and abrasions of the vagina and penis can sometimes happen during normal heterosexual intercourse. But vaginal sex is safer than anal intercourse. The transfusion victim described in chapter 3 failed to transmit the virus to his wife during two years of normal sexual activity. Also, assuming one is not intimate with an IV drug user, a heterosexual partner is less likely to be infected than a homosexual. Despite these factors, the number of heterosexuals with HIV in the U.S. is slowly rising, and heterosexual couples who practice anal intercourse increase the risk of spread.[18]

Spread of HIV by Contaminated Needles and Transfusions

Within the first year of the identification of AIDS among homosexuals, other risk groups became apparent, including heterosexual partners of AIDS patients, IV drug users, hemophiliacs, and blood transfusion recipients.[19] These observations suggested early in the epidemic that the causative agent of AIDS was spread similarly to hepatitis B and was probably a virus.[20]

As we've already seen, hemophiliacs were particularly hard hit by HIV. By the time screening of blood and heat treatment of Factor VIII to inactivate the virus became routine in 1985, nine out of ten hemophiliacs were infected.[21] AIDS is now their most frequent cause of death.

Approximately twelve to fifteen thousand individuals in the U.S. acquired HIV infection from transfusions between 1978 and 1985, before the blood was screened.[22] About 90 percent of these were infected by a single transfusion, because a single unit of whole blood contains several billion white blood cells, which are capable of being infected by the AIDS virus.[23] Now that we can test for HIV-infection and good screening exists for high risk groups, the chance of receiving a contaminated unit of blood is about 1 in 40,000 to 1 in 250,000.[24] Since physicians are giving blood more sparingly, and banking of one's own blood or that of family members for elective surgery is common, infection rates should drop even lower.[25] Better ways of detecting viral contamination are also being developed.

While transfusions are becoming much safer, blood exchange through sharing of needles and syringes is becoming more dangerous.[26] Intravenous drug users are the second largest AIDS group in the U.S.[27] One-third of all AIDS cases can be traced to IV drug users, their sexual partners, or children born to either. AIDS cases are increasing the fastest in these groups, and they serve as a bridge for HIV spread to other heterosexuals and unborn children, accounting for most of the heterosexual and pediatric AIDS cases.[28] Once introduced into IV drug users, HIV spreads rapidly because of the high concentration of drug users in close-knit urban communities.[29] The amount of risk is directly related to the frequency of drug usage and sharing of needles and syringes.[30] When drug users share a common needle, a small transfusion of blood cells occurs with each injection. The number of blood cells involved is a hundred times greater than the number of cells medical personnel sometimes receive through accidental needle sticks.[31] AIDS may become a bigger problem for IV drug users and their sexual partners than for homosexual males, because the latter are more reachable by education and more likely to change high-risk behavior.[32] HIV infection becomes another contributor to the high death toll among IV drug users.[33]

Doctors, nurses, and laboratory workers can be exposed to HIV in the course of their jobs.[34] An accidental needle stick involving HIV-infected blood is the predominant mechanism of HIV transmission for medical personnel.[35] The risk of HIV infection from an accidental needle stick with contaminated blood is approximately 1 in 250 or 0.4 percent.[36] Blood spillage on open wounds or mucous membranes leading to HIV infection is rare.[37] Numerous studies fail to support transmission of HIV from routine or close physical contact with HIV-infected patients.[38] Practicing medicine is now much safer than prior to the discovery of antibiotics and vaccines. However, the small potential for acquiring AIDS accidentally is a reminder that some occupational risk always accompanies the privilege of being in medical practice.

PERINATAL SPREAD OF HIV INFECTION

Although accounting for only 1.7 percent of all cases,[39] children represent the fastest increasing age group of AIDS patients. Only 20 percent of these children were infected through transfusions of HIV-infected blood products.[40] The rest were born to HIV-infected women, most of whom are either IV drug abusers or have had sexual contact with an addict.[41] About three-fourths of the children with AIDS are black or Hispanic,[42] reflecting the predominance of IV drug usage among minorities in the ghettos and barrios.

HIV can be transmitted from mother to baby in three ways: through the placenta to the unborn child, at the time of labor and delivery, or through breast-feeding.[43] The circulatory systems of the infant and mother are designed to be completely separate. Tiny capillaries of the maternal and fetal circulation come exceedingly close at millions of points to allow oxygen and nutrients to be passed to the infant and the fetal waste products and carbon dioxide to be given to the mother for disposal. It is common for some tiny mixing of blood to occur, which might allow infected maternal white blood cells or the AIDS virus in the maternal serum to be transmitted to the developing baby. HIV has been found in fetal tissues confirming such a spread.

During labor a great deal of trauma occurs to the baby and mother that often leads to bruising, abrasions, and local swelling. These areas of trauma produce visible and microscopic openings that might allow the virus to enter the infant's bloodstream. If the mother's perineum tears or if she receives an episiotomy, large amounts of blood may be ingested or get into the baby's eyes, mouth, rectum, or vagina, which might lead to infection.

Breast-feeding is another means of potential exposure. Breast-feeding is a known method of spreading hepatitis B from mother to infant. In both hepatitis and AIDS this is thought to occur when the infant ingests its mother's blood through cracked and bleeding nipples. This method of spread has been suspected in the few cases of mothers who received transfusions of contaminated blood right after delivery and whose infants later came down with AIDS.

Diagnosing HIV infection in infants is complicated because the test for AIDS detects antibodies against the virus.[44] If the mother has the antibody, she will pass it to the infant (just as she passes antibodies against other illnesses she has had) and the baby will be HIV-positive for a few months. The only sure way to diagnose AIDS in infants is to culture HIV from the baby's blood or to have the child develop symptoms of immune deficiency suggestive of full-blown AIDS. Since culturing the virus from the blood is difficult, all one can do in most circumstances is to retest for the AIDS antibody when the baby is a year old. New tests are being developed for detecting the virus itself rather than the antibody against the virus. Studies suggest that about one-third of the infants of mothers infected with HIV will develop AIDS, which is much lower than originally feared.[45]

WHAT ABOUT THE UNIDENTIFIED CAUSES OF AIDS?

Between 3 and 5 percent of all AIDS patients have acquired HIV from undetermined causes.[46] Are these the casually spread cases that some authors have warned us about? They are nothing of the sort.[47] Through September 1989, 6,048 AIDS patients (or 5 percent of the total 107,308 cases in the U.S.) were unclassifiable at some point in time. Ten percent of these 6,048 cases were patients who could not be investigated because they died quickly, refused to talk, or ceased contact with researchers. Of the patients in which adequate follow-up was attainable, almost all were reclassified into the usual high risk groups.[48]

Of all 107,308 cases of AIDS, only 383 (0.35 percent) patients could not be identified with the usual risk groups after a thorough investigation. Although a much smaller group than the original 6,048, it would still be reassuring if they could be classified. In fact, most of them can be by indirect means. A large number of these 383 patients had past histories of sexually transmitted diseases other than AIDS or admitted sexual contact with prostitutes.[49] Therefore, these patients are most likely at increased risk for HIV disease because of sexual activity. Some of the other unclassified patients are probably past or present intravenous drug users.

In other words, many of the "undetermined" group are

people who became infected by sexual activity or IV drug use but lied about their risky behavior. A dramatic example of this was the bishop in Houston who came to the hospital with AIDS but heatedly denied any homosexual activity. When homosexual leaders threatened to expose him, the clergyman was forced to admit that he frequently cruised the gay bars. The homosexual leaders placed pressure on him to avoid panic among heterosexuals concerned about the "mysterious" spread of AIDS.[50] (See chapter 9 for further evidence against casual contagiousness.)

CHRIST AND THE SPREAD OF AIDS

At the time Jesus walked the land of Palestine, a disease existed that was as much a stigma as AIDS. Leprosy was much more contagious than AIDS (although not easily spread) and carried with it the stain of uncleanness. Some were lepers through no fault of their own. Some may have contracted it because of sin in their life, as did Moses' sister Miriam (Numbers 12:10). Yet whether or not sin was the cause of the leprosy (or of other forms of pain and suffering) made no difference in Christ's response to the sufferers. He did not, like some celestial Santa Claus, ask whether they had been bad or good, and then have compassion depending on the answer. He had compassion on all who came to him with open hearts, regardless of their lack of perfection.

Even more significantly, he touched them. In that simple act Jesus did three things. First, he demonstrated tangibly to the lepers that they were significant as human beings despite their condition and the way others treated them. Second, Jesus identified with the lepers by becoming ritually unclean in the process of touching them. He desired more to love these ostracized individuals than to have high standing in the Jewish community. Third, he threw down a gauntlet to which we must respond. Choose the way of the world and yell "Leper! Unclean!" at another person created in God's image, or choose the way of Christ and the cross and identify with those who suffer and with their loss of dignity.

May we cast our lot with the Carpenter and become stigmatized and unclean in the world's eyes that we might minister to the lost sheep of the world.

Chapter 6, Notes

1. Please see Table 3-5 in J. J. Goedert and W. A. Blattner, "The Epidemiology and Natural History of Human Immunodeficiency Virus," in *AIDS: Etiology, Diagnosis, Treatment, and Prevention*, 2d ed., ed. V. T. Devita, S. Hellman, and S. A. Rosenberg (New York: J.B. Lippincott, 1988), 43; H. W. Jaffe et al., "The Acquired Immunodeficiency Syndrome in a Cohort of Homosexual Men: A Six Year Follow-up Study," *Annals of Internal Medicine* 103 (1985):210-14; W. Winkelstein, Jr. et al., "Sexual Practices and Risk of Infection by the Human Immunodeficiency Virus: The San Francisco Men's Health Study," *The Journal of the American Medical Association* 257 (1987):321-25; and R. L. Berkelman et al., "Epidemiology of Human Immunodeficiency Virus Infection and Acquired Immunodeficiency Syndrome," *The American Journal of Medicine* 86 (1989):761-70.

2. K-J Lui, W. W. Darrow, and G. W. Rutherford, "A Model-based Estimate of the Mean Incubation Period for AIDS in Homosexual Men," *Science* 240 (1988):1333-35.

3. For a more technical and complete discussion on the complexities of viruses, see K. L. Tyler and B. N. Fields, "Introduction to Viruses and Viral Diseases," in *Principles and Practice of Infectious Disease*, 3d ed., ed. G. L. Mandell, R. G. Douglas, and J. E. Bennett (New York: Churchill Livingstone, 1989), 1124-34.

4. R. Barre-Sinoussi et al., "Isolation of a T-lymphotropic Retrovirus from a Patient at Risk for Acquired Immune Deficiency Syndrome," *Science* 220 (1983):868-70; R. C. Gallo et al., "Frequent Detection and Isolation of Cytopathic Retroviruses (HTLV-III) from Patients with AIDS and at Risk for AIDS," *Science* 224 (1984):500-502; and J. A. Levy et al., "Isolation of Lymphocytopathic Retroviruses from San Francisco Patients with AIDS," *Science* 225 (1984):840-42.

5. D. D. Ho, R. J. Pomerantz, and J. C. Kaplan, "Pathogenesis of Infection with Human Immunodeficiency Virus," *The New England Journal of Medicine* 317 (1987):278-86; A. S. Fauci, "The Human Immunodeficiency Virus: Infectivity and Mechanisms of Pathogenesis," *Science* 239 (1988):617-22; J. N. Weber and R. A. Weiss, "HIV Infection: The Cellular Picture," *Scientific American* 259 (1988):101-9; J. A. Levy, "Human Immunodeficiency Viruses and the Pathogenesis of AIDS," *The Journal of the American Medical*

Association 261 (1989):2997-3006; and H. Z. Streicher and R. J. Joynt, "HTLV-III/LAV and the Monocyte/Macrophage," *The Journal of the American Medical Association* 256 (1986):2390-91.

6. D. D. Ho, moderator, "The Acquired Immunodeficiency Syndrome (AIDS) Dementia Complex," *Annals of Internal Medicine* 111 (1989):400-410.

7. A. S. Fauci, "The Human Immunodeficiency Virus: Infectivity and Mechanisms of Pathogenesis," *Science* 239 (1988):617-22.

8. R. Detels, "Epidemiologic Perspectives," in "The Acquired Immunodeficiency Syndrome," M. S. Gottlieb, moderator, *Annals of Internal Medicine* 99 (1983):214-16; H. W. Jaffe, D. J. Bergman, and R. M. Selik, "Acquired Immune Deficiency Syndrome in the United States: The First 1000 Cases," *The Journal of Infectious Diseases* 148 (1983):339-45; R. M. Selik, H. W. Haverkos, and J. W. Curran, "Acquired Immune Deficiency Syndrome (AIDS) Trends in the United States, 1978-1982," *The American Journal of Medicine* 76 (1984):493-500; A. M. Hardy et al., "The Incidence Rate of Acquired Immunodeficiency Syndrome in Selected Populations," *The Journal of the American Medical Association* 253 (1985):215-20; W. A. Blattner et al., "Epidemiology of Human T-lymphotropic Virus Type III and the Risk of Acquired Immunodeficiency Syndrome," *Annals of Internal Medicine* 103 (1985):665-70; G. H. Friedland and R. S. Klein, "Transmission of the Human Immunodeficiency Virus," *The New England Journal of Medicine* 317 (1987):1125-35; W. L. Heyward and J. W. Curran, "The Epidemiology of AIDS in the U.S.," *Scientific American* 259 (1988):72-81; Centers for Disease Control, "Update: Acquired Immunodeficiency Syndrome: United States, 1981-1988," *Morbidity and Mortality Weekly Report* 38 (1989):229-35; and Centers for Disease Control, "First 100,000 Cases of Acquired Immunodeficiency Syndrome: United States," *Morbidity and Mortality Weekly Report* 38 (1989):561-63.

9. J. A. Levy, "The Transmission of AIDS: The Case of the Infected Cell," *The Journal of the American Medical Association* 259 (1988):3037-38.

10. Berkelman et al., "Epidemiology of Human Immunodeficiency Virus," 761-70; and Heyward and Curran, "Epidemiology of AIDS," 72-81.

11. H. W. Jaffe and A. R. Lifson, "Acquisition and Transmission of HIV," in *The Medical Management of AIDS*, ed. M. A. Sande and P. A. Volberding (Philadelphia: W.B. Saunders Company, 1988), 20; and N. Clumeck et al., "A Cluster of HIV Infection among Heterosexual People without Apparent Risk Factors," *The New England Journal of Medicine* 321 (1989):1460-62.

12. H. W. Jaffe et al., "National Case-control Study of Kaposi's sarcoma and *Pneumocystis carinii* Pneumonia in Homosexual Men:

Part 1, Epidemiologic Results," *Annals of Internal Medicine* 99 (1983):145-51; and J. J. Goedert et al., "Determinants of Retrovirus (HTLV-III) Antibody and Immunodeficiency Conditions in Homosexual Men," *Lancet* 2 (1984):711-15.

13. W. Winkelstein et al., "The San Francisco Men's Health Study: Continued Decline in HIV Seroconversion Rates among Homosexual/Bisexual Men," *American Journal of Public Health* 78 (1988):1472-74.

14. J. E. Groopman et al., "Seroepidemiology of Human T-lymphocyte Virus Type III among Homosexual Men with the Acquired Immunodeficiency Syndrome or Generalized Lymphadenopathy and among Asymptomatic Controls in Boston," *Annals of Internal Medicine* 102 (1985):334-37; L. A. Kingsley et al., "Risk Factors for Seroconversion to Human Immunodeficiency Virus among Male Homosexuals: Results from the Multicenter AIDS Cohort Study," *Lancet* 1 (1987):345-48; Winkelstein et al., "Sexual Practices and Risk of Infection," 321-25; J. S. Chmiel et al., "Factors Associated with Prevalent Human Immunodeficiency Virus (HIV) Infection: the Multicenter AIDS Cohort Study," *American Journal of Epidemiology* 126 (1987):568-75; J. McCusker et al., "Behavioral Risk Factors for HIV Infection among Homosexual Men at a Boston Community Health Center," *American Journal of Public Health* 78 (1988):68-71; and R. A. Coates et al., "Risk Factors for HIV Infection in Male Sexual Contacts of Men with AIDS or an AIDS-related Condition," *American Journal of Epidemiology* 128 (1988):729-39.

15. S. D. Holmberg et al., "Prior Herpes Simplex Virus Type 2 Infection as a Risk Factor for HIV Infection," *The Journal of the American Medical Association* 259 (1988):1048-50; and W. E. Stamm et al., "The Association between Genital Ulcer Disease and Acquisition of HIV Infection in Homosexual Men," *The Journal of the American Medical Association* 260 (1988):1429-33.

16. N. S. Padian, "Heterosexual Transmission of Acquired Immunodeficiency Syndrome: International Perspectives and National Projections," *Reviews of Infectious Diseases* 9 (1987):947-60.

17. R. R. Redfield et al., "Frequent Transmission of HTLV-III among Spouses of Patients with AIDS-related Complex and AIDS," *The Journal of the American Medical Association* 253 (1985):1571-73; T. A. Peterman and J. W. Curran, "Sexual Transmission of Human Immunodeficiency Virus," *The Journal of the American Medical Association* 256 (1986):2222-26; M. E. Guinan and A. Hardy, "Epidemiology of AIDS in Women in the United States: 1981-1986," *The Journal of the American Medical Association* 257 (1987):2039-42; N. S. Padian et al., "Male-to-female Transmission of Human Immunodeficiency Virus," *The Journal of the American Medical Association* 258 (1987):788-90; M. E. Chamberland and T. J. Dondero, "Heterosexually Acquired Infection with Human Immuno-

deficiency Virus (HIV): A View from the Third International Conference on AIDS," *Annals of Internal Medicine* 107 (1987):763-66; H. W. Haverkos and R. Edelman, "The Epidemiology of Acquired Immunodeficiency Syndrome among Heterosexuals," *The Journal of the American Medical Association* 260 (1988):1922-29; and Friedland and Klein, "Transmission of the Human Immunodeficiency Virus," 1125-35.

18. Padian et al., "Male-to-female Transmission," 788-90. Heterosexually spread cases of AIDS were up 27 percent in 1989 according to a report from the Centers for Disease Control (Associated Press, *Austin American-Statesman*, 9 February 1990).

19. Centers for Disease Control, "*Pneumocystis carinii* Pneumonia among Persons with Hemophilia A," *Morbidity and Mortality Weekly Report* 31 (1982):365-67; Centers for Disease Control, "Possible Transfusion-associated Acquired Immune Deficiency Syndrome (AIDS): California," *Morbidity and Mortality Weekly Report* 31 (1982):652-54; Selik, "Trends in the United States, 1978-1982," 493-500; B. L. Evatt et al., "The Acquired Immunodeficiency Syndrome in Patients with Hemophilia," *Annals of Internal Medicine* 100 (1984):499-504; J. W. Curran and L. F. Barker, "The Acquired Immunodeficiency Syndrome Associated with Transfusions: The Evolving Perspective," *Annals of Internal Medicine* 100 (1984):298-300; T. A. Peterman et al., "Transfusion-associated Acquired Immunodeficiency Syndrome in the United States," *The Journal of the American Medical Association* 254 (1985):2913-17; Friedland and Klein, "Transmission of the Human Immunodeficiency Virus," 1125-35; J. K. Stehr-Green et al., "Hemophilia-associated AIDS in the United States, 1981-1987," *American Journal of Public Health* 78 (1988):439-42; D. C. Des Jarlais et al., "HIV-1 Infection among Intravenous Drug Users in Manhattan, New York City, from 1977 through 1987," *The Journal of the American Medical Association* 261 (1989):1008-12; and T. F. Zuck, "Transfusion-transmitted AIDS Reassessed," *The New England Journal of Medicine* 318 (1988):511-12.

20. D. P. Francis, J. W. Curran, and M. Essex, "Epidemic Acquired Immune Deficiency Syndrome: Epidemiologic Evidence for a Transmissible Agent," *Journal of the National Cancer Institute* 71 (1983):1-4.

21. See Table 3 in Centers for Disease Control, "Human Immunodefiency Virus Infection in the United States: A Review of Current Knowledge," *Morbidity and Mortality Weekly Report* 36 (1987, suppl. no. S-6):27; and M. W. Hilgartner, "AIDS and Hemophilia," *The New England Journal of Medicine* 317 (1987):1153-54.

22. Centers for Disease Control, "Human Immunodeficiency Virus Infection in Transfusion Recipients and Their Family Members," *Morbidity and Mortality Weekly Report* 36 (1987):137-40; J.

D. Kalbfleisch and J. F. Lawless, "Estimating the Incubation Time Distribution and Expected Number of Cases of Transfusion-associated Acquired Immune Deficiency Syndrome," *Transfusion* 29 (1989):672-76; and T. A. Peterman and J. W. Ward, "What's Happening to the Epidemic of Transfusion-associated AIDS?" *Transfusion* 29 (1989):659-60.

23. J. W. Mosley and the Transfusion Safety Study Group, "The Transfusion Safety Study," Third International Conference on AIDS, Washington, D.C., 1987, 160; and J. W. Ward et al., "Risk of Human Immunodeficiency Virus Infection from Blood Donors Who Later Developed the Acquired Immunodeficiency Syndrome," *Annals of Internal Medicine* 106 (1987):61-62.

24. J. W. Ward et al., "Transmission of Human Immunodefiency Virus (HIV) by Blood Transfusions Screened as Negative for HIV Antibody," *The New England Journal of Medicine* 318 (1988):473-78; Zuck, "Transfusion-transmitted AIDS Reassessed," 511-12; P. D. Cumming et al., "Exposure of Patients to Human Immunodeficiency Virus through the Transfusion of Blood Components that Test Antibody-negative," *The New England Journal of Medicine* 321 (1989):941-46; and J. E. Menitove, "The Decreasing Risk of Transfusion-associated AIDS," *The New England Journal of Medicine* 321 (1989):966-68.

25. Council on Scientific Affairs, "Autologous Blood Transfusion," *The Journal of the American Medical Association* 256 (1986):2378-80; and D. M. Surgenor, "The Patient's Blood Is the Safest Blood," *The New England Journal of Medicine* 316 (1987):542-44.

26. R. A. Hahn et al., "Prevalence of HIV Infection among Intravenous Drug Users in the United States," *The Journal of the American Medical Association* 261 (1989):2677-84.

27. Centers for Disease Control, "Update: Acquired Immunodeficiency Syndrome: United States, 1981-1988," *Morbidity and Mortality Weekly Report* 38 (1989):229-35; and Centers for Disease Control, "HIV/AIDS Surveillance," December 1989.

28. D. C. Des Jarlais, S. R. Friedman, and R. L. Stoneburner, "HIV Infection and Intravenous Drug Use: Critical Issues in Transmission Dynamics, Infection Outcomes, and Prevention," *Reviews of Infectious Diseases* 10 (1988):151-58; and Haverkos and Edelman, "Acquired Immunodeficiency Syndrome among Heterosexuals," 1922-29.

29. Des Jarlais et al., "HIV-1 Infection," 1008-12.

30. G. H. Friedland et al., "Intravenous Drug Abusers and the Acquired Immunodeficiency Syndrome (AIDS): Demographic, Drug Use, and Needle-sharing Patterns," *Archives of Internal Medicine* 145 (1985):1413-17; and Friedland and Klein, "Transmission of the Human Immunodeficiency Virus," 1125-35.

31. P. N. Hoffman, D. P. Larkin, and D. Samuel, "Needlestick and Needleshare: The Difference," *The Journal of Infectious Diseases* 160 (1989):545-46.

32. Berkelman et al., "Epidemiology of Human Immunodeficiency Virus," 761-70.

33. Des Jarlais, Friedman, and Stoneburner, "HIV Infection and Intravenous Drug Use," 151-58.

34. D. K. Henderson et al., "Risk of Nosocomial Infection with Human T-cell Lymphotropic Virus Type III/Lymphadenopathy-associated Virus in a Large Cohort of Intensively Exposed Health Care Workers," *Annals of Internal Medicine* 104 (1986):644-47; Centers for Disease Control, "Update: Acquired Immunodeficiency Syndrome and Human Immunodeficiency Virus Infections among Health-care Workers," *Morbidity and Mortality Weekly Report* 37 (1988):229-39; and G. B. Kelen et al., "Human Immunodeficiency Virus Infection in Emergency Department Patients: Epidemiology, Clinical Presentations, and Risk to Health Care Workers: The Johns Hopkins Experience," *The Journal of the American Medical Association* 262 (1989):516-22.

35. R. Marcus and the CDC Cooperative Needlestick Surveillance Group, "Surveillance of Health Care Workers Exposed to Blood from Patients Infected with the Human Immunodeficiency Virus," *The New England Journal of Medicine* 319 (1988):1118-23.

36. C. E. Becker, J. E. Cone, and J. Gerberding, "Occupation Infection with Human Immunodeficiency Virus (HIV)," *Annals of Internal Medicine* 110 (1989):653-56.

37. Centers for Disease Control, "Update: Human Immunodeficiency Virus Infections in Health-care Workers Exposed to Blood of Infected Patients," *Morbidity and Mortality Weekly Report* 36 (1987):285-89.

38. J. L. Gerberding et al., "Risk of Transmitting the Human Immune Deficiency Virus, Cytomegalovirus, and Hepatitis B Virus to Health Care Workers Exposed to Patients with AIDS and AIDS-related Conditions," *The Journal of Infectious Diseases* 156 (1987):1-8; T. L. Kuhls et al., "Occupational Risk of HIV, HBV and HSV-2 Infections in Health Care Personnel Caring for AIDS Patients," *American Journal of Public Health* 77 (1987):1306-9; Friedland and Klein, "Transmission of the Human Immunodeficiency Virus," 1125-35; and Heyward and Curran, "AIDS in the U.S.," 72-81.

39. Centers for Disease Control, "HIV/AIDS Surveillance."

40. S. L. Katz and C. M. Wilfert, "Human Immunodeficiency Virus Infection of Newborns," *The New England Journal of Medicine* 320 (1989):1687-89.

41. L. F. Novick et al., "HIV Seroprevalence in Newborns in New York State," *The Journal of the American Medical Association* 261 (1989):1745-50.

42. M. E. Guinan and A. Hardy, "Epidemiology of AIDS in Women in the United States," *The Journal of the American Medical Association* 257 (1987):2039-42; and Centers for Disease Control, "Distribution of AIDS Cases, by Racial/Ethnic Group and Exposure Category, United States, June 1, 1981-July 4, 1988," *Morbidity and Mortality Weekly Report* 37 (1988, SS-3):1-10.

43. Friedland and Klein, "Transmission of the Human Immunodeficiency Virus," 1125-35; and Berkelman et al., "Epidemiology of Human Immunodeficiency Virus," 761-70.

44. Katz and Wilfert, "Infection of Newborns," 1687-89.

45. Task Force on Pediatric AIDS, "Perinatal Human Immunodeficiency Virus Infection," *Pediatrics* 82 (1988):941-44; and S. Blanche et al., "A Prospective Study of Infants Born to Women Seropositive for Human Immunodeficiency Virus Type I," *The New England Journal of Medicine* 320 (1989):1643-48.

46. Centers for Disease Control, "Update: Acquired Immunodeficiency Syndrome: United States, 1981-1988," 229-36; and Centers for Disease Control, "HIV/AIDS Surveillance," October 1989.

47. A. R. Lifson et al., "Unrecognized Modes of Transmission of HIV: Acquired Immunodeficiency Syndrome in Children Reported with Risk Factors," *Pediatric Infectious Disease* 6 (1987):292; and K. G. Castro et al., "Investigations of AIDS Patients with No Previously Identified Risk Factors," *The Journal of the American Medical Association* 259 (1988):1338-42.

48. Centers for Disease Control, "Update: Acquired Immunodeficiency Syndrome: United States, 1981-1988," 229-36.

49. Centers for Disease Control, "Update: Heterosexual Transmission of AIDS and HIV Infection: U.S.," *Morbidity and Mortality Weekly Report* 38 (1989):423-24, 429-34.

50. This case was discussed in the Houston AIDS conference in 1988.

While Jesus was having dinner at Matthew's house, many tax collectors and "sinners" came and ate with him and his disciples. When the Pharisees saw this, they asked his disciples, "Why does your teacher eat with tax collectors and 'sinners'?"

On hearing this, Jesus said, "It is not the healthy who need a doctor, but the sick. But go and learn what this means: `I desire mercy, not sacrifice.' For I have not come to call the righteous, but sinners" (Matthew 9:10-12).

Let the wicked forsake his way
    and the evil man his thoughts.
Let him turn to the LORD, and he will have mercy on him,
    and to our God, for he will freely pardon
(Isaiah 55:7).

"I am the First and the Last. I am the Living One; I was dead, and behold I am alive for ever and ever! And I hold the keys of death and Hades" (Revelation 1:17-18).

All of us have become like one who is unclean,
    and all our righteous acts are like filthy rags;
we all shrivel up like a leaf,
    and like the wind our sins sweep us away
(Isaiah 64:6).

Chapter Seven

The Course, Diagnosis, and Treatment of AIDS

M y name is Stephen. I am thirty-four years old and a professional man in a conservative part of the country. I accepted the Lord Jesus as my Savior about thirteen years ago. It was not a dramatic event compared to the conversion of some of my friends. It was a simple process whereby I came to realize that I was a sinner in need of God's grace.

I found out I was infected with the AIDS virus about two-and-a-half years ago. A friend was going to be tested and he convinced me to go as well. I was shocked when the results came back positive and now, at times, wish I had never gone for the test. I live under a cloud. My doctor has watched the slow decrease in the number of T-helper cells in my blood over the last two years. As the number progressively decreases, it is as if I am watching the curtain come down on my life. Sometimes I don't believe it because I am so young and healthy. Few people know I have the virus, including my many friends in the large Baptist church I attend. I also frequently visit a charismatic church and have many friends there, but none know about my illness. I am frightened about dying, but I accept it better than most people I know with AIDS because of my relationship with the Lord.

I have noticed a change in my attitude toward life. I no

longer plan long-term goals. If I have a chance to visit some place, I go, since I will never have another chance. A friend of mine says that if he ever becomes sick, he will go through a lot of money in a hurry. That is totally understandable, but I couldn't do that because I don't have much money. Besides, I want to leave as much money as I can to my parents; they have given me so much.

My big fear is the shame my death will bring to my family. They do not know that I have been involved in the gay life-style off and on over the years. My brother has suspected, but I don't think he wants to know. All my family are strong Christians, and it would make it doubly hard for them if they found out. I am afraid it would literally kill my parents, since they are such worriers anyway. Because of the shame this disease will bring to my family, I have considered having a friend put me to sleep. It might be easier on everyone that way.

I have known several people who have died of AIDS. It is not an easy way to die. I look at the people who were younger than I am when they died, and I am sad because they have not had as much of a chance to live as I have. Then again, I am sure others will think the same thing about me. My friends in the Sunday school class are always talking about what a great future and career I have ahead of me. Little do they know that I may not live to see my fortieth birthday. But I don't dwell on the shortness of my remaining life.

When I do think about death, I think about an older church friend who has terminal cancer. We have talked about death on a number of occasions. He has received a lot of emotional and spiritual support from our mutual friends. People go out of their way to help him because of the nearness of his death. I help too and am glad to do it, but I wonder what kind of support he would have if he were dying of AIDS instead of cancer. I am not expecting the same kind of support from our friends when my time comes. I have seen enough men die of AIDS to know that AIDS victims die alone. AIDS patients are lepers even within the gay community. The only support I might get is from other AIDS patients. Just the diagnosis of the infection with the virus is enough to chase most people away. That is why I have told virtually no one, and why other men who are HIV-infected do the same. I know of many respectable men, some of whom are married, who are gay and infected with the virus. A large number of them are in the churches but are afraid to ask for help. Many want help but are afraid they will get kicked out immediately if their churches find out they have the AIDS virus.

I don't understand why I have been attracted to men while my identical twin brother is straight. I am sure it is not something you are born with or something sociological, as a lot of other gays say. Doctor friends tell me that my genes are identical to my brother's; how can it be that I am gay and my brother straight? We both shared the same birthday, the same parents, and the same house. Somehow it had to be a choice that I made. I did not have anything traumatic happen to me that might have forced me into the gay life-style. I did not have an older man seduce me. I was not jilted by a woman. It was just something I drifted into. Getting out has been much harder. I am celibate now because I know that homosexual sex is a sin, and I do not want to give this terrible disease to someone else. Although I go through the motions of life, a lot of what I do is waiting.

I do share the love of Christ with other gays that I have known, but it is hard because the church has done nothing for gays. Christians sit in judgment, point their fingers and say "I told you so." If only they knew how many Catholic priests were gay. I know two Baptist preachers who are practicing gays. Many young men who look like the boy next door or husbands in happy marriages are gay. Many men who are active in their churches are gay and want help to escape, but fear they will be told to leave if they tell anyone. There is a huge spiritual vacuum now in the church when it comes to gays and AIDS. If there ever is a chance to bring someone into the kingdom, it is when the person is dying and knows it. But most Christians appear to be self-righteous and are reluctant to share the gospel with a homosexual dying of AIDS.

But I know the love of Jesus, and I know he would be different, so why not his followers?

* * * * * *

Most people infected with HIV are like Stephen and have no symptoms at all. This asymptomatic stage, which may last up to ten years and longer, is one of the main reasons this epidemic spread so extensively before AIDS was recognized as a new disease. Perhaps more chilling is that, unlike Stephen, most of the estimated one to two million HIV-positive Americans do not know they are infected. The effects of any social or medical change to reduce the spread of AIDS will not be seen for many years to come. This places tremendous importance on suggested actions now, such as "safe sex," because if the suggestions are mistaken, the consequences will be felt for many years.

Despite the current lack of symptoms, Stephen fears the future because the debilitating disease not only kills, but tends to reduce the person to helplessness in the process. It is common for sufferers of AIDS to die at only two-thirds of their normal weight due to the severe diarrhea, extensive mouth ulcers, poor nutritional intake, and recurrent infections. AIDS patients seldom die while still vigorous and healthy; death is usually a slow process and a welcomed comfort. The following descriptions of progressive HIV infection will show why.

THE HIV ANTIBODY TESTS

It was a great boon to the study and treatment of AIDS when an antibody test to identify HIV-infected people became available in 1985. Antibodies are proteins produced by the immune system in response to a specific foreign invader. Two different antibody tests are used to diagnosis infection with HIV.[1] The first test is called the *ELISA test* and is purposely designed to be overly sensitive to avoid missing anyone who is infected. It will say some people are infected who are not (false-positives).

To determine if a positive ELISA test is accurate, the *Western Blot* is performed. If it is also positive a person is confirmed to be infected with HIV. The reason the Western Blot is not done initially is that it is more expensive than the ELISA and more technically difficult to perform. Antibodies against HIV can usually be detected within three to six months after infection, but may take longer (up to one year or longer). Newer tests being developed will identify lower levels of antibody or part of the virus itself.

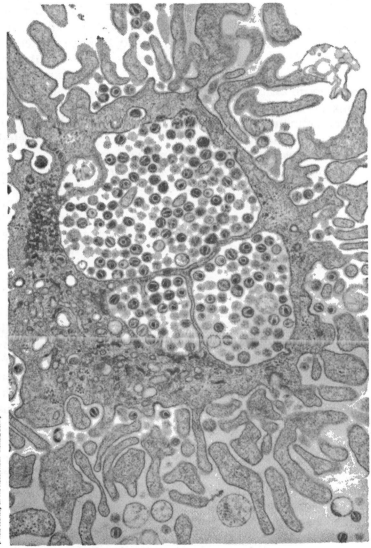

(Photo courtesy of: The Robert Koch - Institut, Berlin)

DOZENS OF HIV PARTICLES WITHIN A WHITE BLOOD CELL

THE STAGES OF INFECTION

When HIV enters someone's blood stream, the person may or may not become infected. If the number of viral particles introduced is small, if the susceptibility of the host is low, and if the immune defenses respond quickly, then the infection will not occur. The more frequent the exposure or the larger the amount of blood involved, then the greater the chances of infection. So an accidental needle stick with contaminated blood has only a 1 in 250 chance of transmitting the infection. Sharing a needle and syringe with an infected junkie is more likely to transmit HIV. Being transfused with a contaminated unit of blood almost guarantees infection because of the huge numbers of viral particles injected which overwhelm almost any person's defenses.

Since the virus becomes incorporated in the host's DNA, the infection and contagiousness are permanent. A slow decline in immune function ensues over months and years due to destruction of T-helper cells.[2] Eventually the immune system is so weak that mild infections become life-threatening. A series of stages is used to describe declining T-helper cells and clinical symptoms.

The First Stage (The Acute Retroviral Syndrome)

A few days to several weeks after exposure and infection with HIV, about half of newly infected persons will develop a sudden mononucleosis-type illness.[3] Symptoms vary but may include muscle aches, fever, headache, sore throat, fatigue, rash, and lymph node swelling. The patient is sick for a few days to three weeks, but will recover without treatment.[4] Because these symptoms may be mild, this first stage of infection may go unrecognized by patient or doctor. If HIV infection is suspected because of the illness and high risk, a physician will draw blood immediately and then several months later to determine if HIV antibodies have developed.

The Second Stage (The Asymptomatic Period)

The mono-like symptoms resolve as the immune system reduces viral reproduction, leading to a long period when the infected person feels well.[5] The virus slowly destroys T-helper cells (which direct much of the immune system), but survives inside macrophages without destroying them. These white blood cells are the "Trojan horse" that can carry the virus to other parts of the body, including the brain. Up to 80 percent of the one to two million people infected with HIV in the U.S. are unaware of their infection at this stage.

The Third Stage (Persistent Lymph Node Enlargement)

After a variable length of time, from months to years, more than 50 percent of those infected will progress from the asymptomatic stage to develop enlarged lymph nodes.[6] These swollen lymph nodes are usually not tender, but their presence signals progression of the disease. Opportunistic infections are unusual since T-helper cells are not completely depleted and the immune system is still working. However, a diagnosis of HIV infection is important at this stage since antiviral treatment to suppress HIV can prolong life.

The Symptomatic Stage of HIV Infection before AIDS

The length of time it takes an individual to go from initial infection to complete immune suppression varies.[7] HIV slowly reduces the number of T-helper cells by making holes in the membranes, by merging abnormal cells, and by causing the immune system to attack the T helper cells which appear foreign. When the number of these cells drops to about two hundred per cubic millimeter, more ominous problems occur.[8] Profound fatigue, prolonged fevers, night sweats, weight loss, and diarrhea all suggest advancing immune deficiency. At one time this stage was called AIDS Related Complex (ARC). Seemingly mild infections of the skin and mouth appear at this stage.[9] Although treatable, these abnormalities (discussed below) may herald the onset of serious attacks of opportunistic infections and cancers.

Oral thrush.[10] This fungal infection of the mouth is commonly seen in healthy babies, diabetics, and patients on steroids or antibiotics. Oral thrush is easily recognized by small white patches on the tongue, roof, and sides of the mouth. While treatable, thrush can be painful and even spread into the esophagus, causing severe eating difficulties.

Hairy leukoplakia.[11] This is a unique infection associated with the end-stages of HIV infection and is thought to be due to the same virus that causes mononucleosis. It is diagnosed by seeing characteristic raised, white plaques, usually on the sides of the tongue. This is not painful and is not treatable.

Gum disease. Inflammation of the gums from normal bacteria in the mouth can become painful, and teeth may be lost.

Oral and anal-genital herpes simplex infections.[12] About half of adults suffer with recurrent cold sores caused by the nonsexually transmitted form of the herpes virus. Millions suffer from recurrent genital herpes that is sexually transmitted. Most have mild symptoms that occur less and less often. However, the HIV-infected patient has increasing chances of severe attacks as his immune system deteriorates. Extensive, agonizing ulcers around the lips and mouth make eating unbearable. Large ulcers around the anus and genitals cause severe rectal pain, fever, and constipation. Painful recurrences are common. Treatment with an antiviral drug is helpful, but resistance can occur.

Shingles.[13] The virus causing chickenpox may relapse later in life, causing painful blisters on the skin called shingles. It is common in HIV-infected patients, and lesions may persist for months despite treatment. Pain interferes with sleep and productivity and often leads to addiction to pain medication.

HIV wasting syndrome.[14] This illness is defined as loss of greater than 10 percent of weight associated with prolonged diarrhea or fever. This wasting can develop despite the absence of any of the usual causes of weight loss in HIV-infected people (tuberculosis, cancers, or parasites). A patient may undergo exhaustive testing to determine the cause, yet no cause is found.

Although few of these ailments are life-threatening, they all contribute to the large amount of suffering inherent in the latter stages of HIV infection.

The Final Stage (End-Stage HIV Infection or AIDS)

When the number of T-helper cells drops below two hundred, the immune system can no longer function adequately. The person becomes almost defenseless, unable to effectively combat invaders it had previously held in check. Greater numbers of HIV circulating in the blood may increase the person's contagiousness. Susceptibility to opportunistic infections and cancers now appears. The patient has full-blown AIDS.

Many of the following opportunistic infections are relapses. The patient had been mildly infected with these illnesses before, but the normal immune system suppressed the infection, which became inactive. It is as if the body placed these parasites, funguses, and viral infections in life imprisonment surrounded by immune walls. Once the immune system is destroyed, several infections may break out at once. The person with AIDS has not caught *Pneumocystis* pneumonia, histoplasmosis, and herpes simultaneously. They have simply started growing since they are no longer opposed.

The following is not a complete picture of problems that can occur in the final stages of AIDS. The variety of infections and cancers that one can get is extensive. However, these are the most significant secondary problems.

Parasitic Infections in AIDS

Pneumocystis carinii pneumonia (PCP). This is the most common life-threatening opportunistic infection in AIDS patients in the U.S. PCP is present in two-thirds of all cases of AIDS at the time of diagnosis, ultimately developing in eight out of ten patients.[15] Its ability to cause lung disease is nonexistent in normal people, and it used to be seen only in immune deficiencies caused by certain cancers, chemotherapeutic drugs, or steroids. *Pneumocystis* infection of the lung likely represents reactivation of a previous infection.

The symptoms of PCP may be subtle or severe.[16] Fever lasting days to weeks, night sweats, and weight loss may herald shortness of breath and a dry, hacking cough. A chest

X-ray will be abnormal in 90 to 95 percent of cases. Confirmation occurs when sputum or lung tissue is examined microscopically to see the parasite.

Treatment of active PCP is difficult because of severe side effects from the two therapeutic medications.[17] The more advanced PCP is when diagnosed, the poorer the response to medication. PCP is the most common lethal opportunistic infection in AIDS patients. Although mentally alert, patients die slowly as their lungs are destroyed by the infection. PCP can be prevented to a degree in AIDS patients.[18] Therapy with sulfa tablets or inhaled pentamidine may be effective in preserving health and improving quality of life.

Toxoplasma gondii infection (toxoplasmosis). This protozoan is everywhere in nature and can infect most mammals. While cats perpetuate infection worldwide, the two major routes of spread to humans are ingestion of contaminated meat and transmission from an infected mother to her unborn child.[19] Most acquired infections of toxoplasmosis are asymptomatic and will resolve without problems. However, a form of the protozoan may persist in tissues such as the brain and heart for years, only to reactivate and grow once again when a patient's immunity becomes impaired.

In AIDS patients, reactivation of infection from cysts in the brain causes an inflammation called encephalitis.[20] Between 5 and 10 percent of patients in the U.S. will develop this brain infection prior to death. Diagnosis is suspected when patients develop severe headaches, seizures, altered mental state, coma, or paralysis. Computerized tomography (CT) usually reveals typical findings, but a brain biopsy may be required for diagnosis. Drugs are available but toxic, and the recurrence rate is high when the drugs are stopped. Death usually is a relief because the constant headache worsens with growth of the parasites in the brain.

Intestinal parasites. Cryptosporidium is a bowel parasite which was recently discovered to cause a mild diarrhea in people with normal immune function. About 4 percent of AIDS patients are infected with this parasite, having severe, prolonged diarrhea with up to twenty-five stools per day, abdominal pain, and dehydration.[21] One-half the AIDS patients in Haiti are infected. Sometimes it infects the gall bladder, requiring its removal. The cysts that spread the infection are often found in soil and are spread by anal sex. Drugs are not effective. The parasite *Isospora* causes similar symptoms, but is much less common in the U.S. It responds well to a common antibiotic although relapses can occur. Other bowel parasites such as amoeba and *giardia*, a common parasite in normal children, cause severe diarrhea. These are treatable, but recur.

Fungal Infections in AIDS

Fungal infections rarely cause serious problems in healthy individuals. Yeast infections in the diaper area or mouth of a baby and in the vagina of an adult woman are common but mild. Many people have mild flu-like symptoms when infected with other fungi. But if one develops AIDS, the infection may reactivate, often with lethal results.

Cryptococcus is the most common fungal infection in AIDS. Most of these patients have meningitis with headaches, low-grade fever, and clouded thinking for days to weeks prior to diagnosis.[22] Meningitis is diagnosed by seeing the fungus under the microscope or by doing lab studies on the spinal fluid. Pneumonia is frequent. The fungus can be found in the blood in more than 80 percent of patients with meningitis.

Histoplasma is a fungal infection that usually occurs near the great river basins of the central U.S. The fungus is found in the excrement of birds and bats, and is inhaled by people when the feces dry. Although lung disease is the main infection in normal people, AIDS patients likely have widespread disease with fever, weight loss, and cough.[23]

Coccidioides is located in dry areas of the Southwest. Symptoms are similar to histoplasmosis with fever, weight loss, weakness, and cough.[24] The illness is often diagnosed from sputum samples, but usually it has spread throughout the body and is lethal for those with AIDS.

Treatment of these fungal infections is difficult.[25] The current IV drugs used are toxic, although newer oral drugs are being studied. Symptoms may improve with treatment, but there is no cure since relapses are inevitable once therapy is withdrawn.

Tuberculosis (TB) and Related Infections in AIDS
     The TB and related bacteria grow slowly. The body controls the initial infection, but the bacteria may be alive though inactive. As the immune system weakens, reactivation occurs.
     Tuberculosis in 1900 was the biggest cause of death in the U.S. Since then, better living conditions and effective drugs made it an uncommon and rarely fatal illness. Yet TB is making a comeback through AIDS.[26] Most patients have reactivated TB, which often spreads from the lungs to the blood, bone marrow, kidneys, joints, lymph nodes, skin, and brain. Fortunately, even if widespread, it responds well to the common TB drugs. Usually two or more drugs need to be used at one time. Although TB in AIDS patients is mildly contagious, especially to family members and health care workers, it is easily treated in the healthy person.
     Other bacteria related to TB, such as *Mycobacterium avium-intracellulare,*[27] cause fever, night sweats, weight loss, and diarrhea. This bacteria can be isolated from water, soil, and birds. It grows unimpeded in AIDS patients and is found in the blood, bone marrow, lungs, intestines, and many organs. It does not respond to TB drugs nor does it cause problems in healthy people.

Other Bacterial Infections in AIDS
     Bacterial infections are more common in patients with AIDS.[28] Organisms that cause sinusitis, ear infections, and pneumonias are harder to treat. Skin infections may be recurrent. Gastroenteritis from salmonella, shigella, and *Campylobacter* is incurable, requiring daily antibiotics just to control the symptoms. Syphilis may help spread HIV through genital ulcers and is more difficult to eradicate than in healthy individuals.[29]

Opportunistic Viral Infections in AIDS
     Several related viruses (herpes, chickenpox, and cytomegalovirus) cause severe problems in AIDS patients.

Cytomegalovirus (CMV) infection causes a mono-like illness in normal adults. It can cause severe problems in AIDS patients and in unborn babies, who acquire CMV from their mothers.[30] Many homosexual men are infected with CMV, and up to 40 percent shed CMV in semen and urine,[31] but it seldom causes problems unless they develop AIDS.[32] It often causes blindness in AIDS patients through retinal infection. Although CMV spreads throughout the body in AIDS patients, it seldom causes other symptoms.[33] A new drug (gancyclovir) is available to treat the CMV eye infection, but it must be used perpetually. Some concern has been expressed that AIDS patients may spread CMV to mothers, leading to increased infections among newborns. But studies have shown that the most dangerous place for a woman to acquire CMV (and the danger is small) is not in a casual setting or even in a hospital setting, but in a day-care.[34]

Cancers Associated with AIDS

Since normal immune systems destroy malignant cells,[35] it should be expected that AIDS patients develop particular cancers more frequently than normal adults.[36]

Kaposi's sarcoma (KS) is the unusual cancer that increased dramatically in number in homosexual men in the early eighties, heralding this new epidemic.[37] Kaposi's sarcoma unassociated with AIDS was a rare mild cancer of older men which seldom shortened life. The new KS is much more aggressive, less responsive to chemotherapy and radiation, and more likely to be life-threatening.[38] This malignancy causes nodular skin lesions that are initially painless, blue to violet in color, and from one-fourth to one inch in diameter. The nodules can appear almost anywhere on the body, but are especially prone to affect the face and chest, clearly marking the patient as a person with AIDS.

The new KS also causes nodular growths internally on the bowels, the lungs, and other organs. Even if the cancer attacks internally, the patient is more likely to die from opportunistic infections than from KS. However, treatment may be ineffective, and uncontrolled growth of the nodules is painful. Three aspects of KS and AIDS are surprising. First, nonhomosexuals with AIDS rarely have KS. Second, the cancer develops while a good level of immune function remains. Third, the number of new cases is decreasing each year even as the epidemic advances. An unknown factor is probably necessary to develop KS in HIV patients.[39]

Lymphomas are a group of cancers composed of abnormal white blood cells called lymphocytes. Prior to the AIDS epidemic, it was proven that a person is thirty-five times more likely to develop this cancer if his immune system is working poorly due to drugs, radiation therapy, or an inborn deficiency. The lymphomas can begin at virtually any place in the body since lymphocytes occur in all lymph nodes and many organs.[40] Symptoms depend on the location of the tumor and arise from pressure and displacement of normal tissue. Treatment of the AIDS-associated lymphomas is similar to the treatment of tumors in normal individuals, but the response is much poorer.[41] Chemotherapy may predispose the patient to further immune deficiency.

HIV Infection in the Brain[42]

The brain, spinal cord, and nerves are directly affected by HIV. The virus can be detected in the spinal fluid in the earliest stages, although usually no neurological problems develop until later. The more advanced the HIV disease, the greater chance that the nervous system will be affected, reaching close to 90 percent of the patients in end-stage disease. Evidence of nerve or brain infection includes burning sensations in the arms and legs, memory loss, inappropriate emotions and behavior, unsteady gait, weakness, lack of coordination, inability to talk or walk, incontinence, decreased intellectual capacity, and psychosis.

CHILDREN WITH AIDS

Almost 2 percent of AIDS cases occur in children, and racial minorities constitute the majority of these (blacks, 53 percent; Hispanics, 24 percent; whites, 22 percent).[43] More children will be infected as more adult women of child-bearing age acquire HIV through IV drug use and heterosexual spread. Initially, many physicians were unsure if children were sick with AIDS because the symptoms were so different from adult patients. But these children were proven to have HIV when the antibody test became available in 1985.

Children are not merely little adults, and children with AIDS often manifest symptoms and illnesses different from those seen in adults.[44] Children can have almost all of the reactivated infections of adult patients. However, children also have many first-time infections with chickenpox, herpes fever blisters, and common bacterial infections which cause ear infections and pneumonias. These tend to be more severe in children with AIDS than in normal children.

About a 30 percent chance exists that an HIV-infected mother will transmit the virus to her infant.[45] Once the child develops symptoms from HIV infection, growth slows or stops; fever and diarrhea often begin. Once the antibodies transferred from mother to baby in the uterus disappear at around six months of life, the infant becomes vulnerable to most bacteria. Meningitis, blood infections, and pneumonias often occur and must be treated promptly to prevent the death of the child.

Opportunistic infections can occur, including the viral, parasitic, and fungal infections described above. Most children with AIDS suffer neurologic evidence of HIV infection, including developmental delays and regression.[46] Infants with AIDS usually die in less than a year once symptoms develop.

Children who acquire AIDS from transfusions usually have a longer asymptomatic period. Older children have developed antibodies to many infections, and these antibodies protect them from many of the illnesses infants with AIDS have. However, once they develop symptoms, their life expectancy is no longer than that of adults with AIDS.

Children with HIV infection are more difficult to care for than adults. The bacterial and opportunistic infections should be treated vigorously,[47] and prevention by using high-dose IV gamma globulin is under study and may be useful in the long-term health management of these children. Also, preventative antibiotics can reduce the chances of developing *Pneumocystis* pneumonia. All HIV-infected children should be immunized with the inactivated vaccines of diphtheria, tetanus, pertussis, and polio, and the attenuated (live but weakened) vaccines of measles, mumps, and rubella.[48] Giving the live polio vaccine to an HIV-infected patient is avoided since the vaccine could cause polio.

TREATMENT OF HUMAN IMMUNODEFICIENCY VIRUS

Viruses are more difficult to treat than bacteria, fungi, or parasites because they use the body's own molecules to reproduce. Drugs effective against a virus usually attack the host cells also. Only in the last decade have antiviral agents of proven effectiveness become available. Some mild to moderately effective drugs exist for herpes, chickenpox, a severe respiratory virus, and influenza. With the discovery of HIV in 1983, research for drugs that would delay or reverse the steady march toward death began at once.

As we saw in chapter 6, the human immunodeficiency virus is complicated. Drugs potentially could be effective if they attacked the virus directly, blocked the virus's entrance into the cell, or hindered reproduction of HIV inside the cell.[49] Research initially concentrated on finding drugs that could inhibit the unique viral enzyme, reverse transcriptase. Because HIV's genetic material cannot incorporate itself into the host cell nucleus without the proper functioning of this enzyme, a "reverse transcriptase inhibitor" would prevent reproduction of HIV and destruction of the T-helper cell. AZT works in this manner.

AZT has been proven to prolong survival even in patients with end-stage HIV disease. The problems with this treatment include high cost (hundreds of dollars a month), need for continuous dosing (every four hours for life), bone marrow toxicity, anemia, nausea, and headaches. AZT only inhibits viral replication and does not destroy HIV.

Therefore, it is not curative. The drug is being used earlier in the course of HIV infection. Newer drugs also are being studied individually and in combination with AZT. Although a cure is unlikely in our lifetime, HIV infection will probably be controllable like other chronic illnesses (diabetes, high blood pressure, heart disease, and Parkinson's disease).

SUMMARY

Take away a person's immune system, and he is at the mercy of many illnesses. The variety of secondary infections in AIDS patients is enormous—any one patient may have two or more infections or cancers at the same time. A patient might have a parasitic diarrhea and then develop a bacterial diarrhea. Another patient might have toxoplasmosis in the brain, dementia from HIV, and herpes in the mouth. A third patient might have a fungal meningitis, Kaposi's sarcoma, and then die from *Pneumocystis* pneumonia. This variety of problems increases the misery of the patient while making medical management very difficult.

CHRIST AND THE TREATMENT OF ILLNESS

In the past some people suggested that sexually transmitted illnesses such as syphilis are penalties for sexual sin and should not be treated. That same attitude is evident in some of the moral indignation directed against homosexual men with AIDS. However, those who say we should not treat homosexual men or spend millions of dollars on AIDS research are inconsistent. If sin stops therapy, doctors should stop treating people with cirrhosis of the liver caused by alcoholism, lung cancer and emphysema caused by smoking, and heart disease and high blood pressure caused by an unwise choice of foods. These are just a few of the illnesses provoked by sins against one's own flesh. Fully one-half of all deaths in the U.S. are due to the use of drugs, cigarettes, alcohol, and food in ways that are destructive.

Moreover, since all have sinned and fall short of God's glory, why should anyone be treated? But attempts at healing should occur for one simple reason: All people bear the image of God. Many people came to Jesus to be healed of sickness. No one was turned down. He didn't interview them beforehand to determine how worthy they were, for none were worthy. Even though they had strayed, the Good Shepherd would pursue them to reunite them with the flock. Jesus did not come into the world to condemn the world, but to save it (John 3:17).

A dying man will not understand our spiritual concerns for him if we are unwilling to attend to his needs. Jesus did this fully and had compassion on all who were ill regardless of their spiritual state. And so should we.

Chapter 7, Notes

1. Centers for Disease Control, "Update: Serologic Testing for Antibody to Human Immunodeficiency Virus," *Morbidity and Mortality Weekly Report* 36 (1988):833-45; J. P. Phair and S. Wolinsky, "Diagnosis of Infection with the Human Immunodeficiency Virus," *The Journal of Infectious Diseases* 159 (1989):320-23; Centers for Disease Control, "Interpretation and Use of the Western Blot Assay for Serodiagnosis of Human Immunodeficiency Virus Type 1 Infections," *Morbidity and Mortality Weekly Report (Suppl. 7)* 38 (1989):1-7; C. J. Schleupner, "Detection of HIV-1 Infection," in *Principles and Practice of Infectious Disease*, 3d ed., ed. G. L. Mandell, R. G. Douglas, and J. E. Bennett (New York: Churchill Livingstone, 1989), 1092-1102.

2. A.R. Lifson, G.W. Rutherford, and H.W. Jaffe, "The Natural History of Human Immunodeficiency Virus Infection," *The Journal of Infectious Diseases* 158 (1988):1360-67; H.W. Murray et al., "Progression to AIDS in Patients with Lymphadenopathy or AIDS-related Complex: Reappraisal of Risk and Predictive Factors," *The American Journal of Medicine* 86 (1989):533-38; D.P. Bolognesi, "Prospects for Prevention of and Early Intervention against HIV," *The Journal of the American Medical Association* 261 (1989):3007-13; and D. Baltimore and M.B. Feinberg, "HIV Revisited: Toward a Natural History of the Infection," *The New England Journal of Medicine* 321 (1989):1673-75.

3. B. Tindall et al., "Characterization of the Acute Clinical Illness Associated with Human Immunodeficiency Virus

Infection," *Archives of Internal Medicine* 148 (1988):945-49; B. Tindall et al., "Primary Immunodeficiency Virus Infection: Clinical and Serologic Aspects," in *The Medical Management of AIDS*, ed. M. S. Sande and P. A. Volberding (Philadelphia: W. B. Saunders Co., 1988), 75-89.

4. R. E. Chaisson and P. A. Volberding, "Clinical Manifestations of HIV Infection," in *Principles and Practice of Infectious Disease*, 1064.

5. R. R. Redfield and D. S. Burke, "HIV Infection: The Clinical Picture," *Scientific American* 259 (1988):90-98; and Centers for Disease Control, "Classification System for Human T-Lymphotropic Virus Type III/Lympadenopathy-associated Virus Infections," *Morbidity and Mortality Weekly Report* 35 (1986):334-39.

6. D. I. Abrams et al., "Persistent Diffuse Lymphadenopathy in Homosexual Men: Endpoint of Prodrome?" *Annals of Internal Medicine* 100 (1984):801-8; C. E. Metroka et al., "Generalized Lymphadenopathy in Homosexual Men," *Annals of Internal Medicine* 99 (1983):585-91; and Chaisson and Volberding, "Clinical Manifestations of HIV Infection," 1064-65.

7. A. R. Lifson, G. W. Rutherford, and H. W. Jaffe, "The Natural History of Human Immunodeficiency Virus Infection," *The Journal of Infectious Diseases* 158 (1988):1360-67.

8. J. J. Goedert et al., "Effect of T4 Counts and Cofactors on the Incidence of AIDS in Homosexual Men Infected with Human Immunodeficiency Virus," *The Journal of the American Medical Association* 257 (1987):331-34; B. F. Polk et al., "Predictors of the Acquired Immunodeficiency Syndrome Developing in a Cohort of Seropositive Homosexual Men," *The New England Journal of Medicine* 316 (1987):61-66; see Table 6 in Chaisson and Volberding, "Clinical Manifestations of HIV Infection," 1063; and Centers for Disease Control, "Guidelines for Prophylaxis against Pneumocystis Carinii Pneumonia for Persons Infected with Human Immunodeficiency Virus," *Morbidity and Mortality Weekly Report (Supp. 5)* 38 (1989):1-9.

9. J. S. Greenspan, D. Greenspan, and J. R. Winkler, "Diagnosis and Management of the Oral Manifestations of HIV Infection and AIDS," in *Medical Management of AIDS*, 127-40.

10. Ibid.; see also R. S. Klein et al., "Oral Candidiasis in High-risk Patients as the Initial Manifestation of the Acquired Immuno-deficiency Syndrome," *The New England Journal of Medicine* 311 (1984):354-58.

11. J. S. Greenspan et al., "Replication of Epstein-Barr Virus within the Epithelial Cells of Oral 'Hairy' Leukokplakia, an AIDS-associated Lesion," *The New England Journal of Medicine* 313 (1985):1564-71; and D. Greenspan et al., "Relation of Oral Hairy Leukoplakia to Infection with the Human Immunodeficiency Virus and the Risk of Developing AIDS," *The Journal of Infectious Diseases* 155 (1987):475-81.

12. G. V. Quinnan et al., "Herpesvirus Infections in the Acquired Immune Deficiency Syndrome," *The Journal of the American Medical Association* 252 (1984):72-77; and W. L. Drew, W. Buhles, and K. S. Erlich, "Herpesvirus Infections (Caused by Cytomegalovirus, Herpes Simplex Virus, Varicella-zoster Virus): How to Use Ganciclovir (DHPG) and Acyclovir," in *The Medical Management of AIDS* (Philadelphia: W.B. Saunders Co., 1988), 278-86.

13. Drew, Buhles, and Erlich, "Herpesvirus Infections," 278-86; and P. R. Cohen, V. P. Beltrani, and M. E. Grossman, "Disseminated Herpes Zoster in Patients with Human Immunodeficiency Virus Infection," *The American Journal of Medicine* 84 (1988):1076-80.

14. Centers for Disease Control, "Revision of the CDC Surveillance Case Definition for Acquired Immunodeficiency Syndrome," *Morbidity and Mortality Weekly Report (Suppl. 1)* 36 (1987):1-15.

15. J. A. Kovacs and H. Masur, "Opportunistic Infections," in *AIDS: Etiology, Diagnosis, Treatment, and Prevention*, 2d ed., ed. V. T. Devita, S. Hellman, and S. A. Rosenberg (New York: J. B. Lippincott, 1988), 203-5.

16. C. P. Kales et al., "Early Predictors of In-hospital Mortality for *Pneumocystis carinii* Pneumonia in the Acquired Immunodeficiency Syndrome," *Archives of Internal Medicine* 147 (1987):1413-17; P. D. Walzer, "*Pneumoscystis carinii*," in *Principles and Practice of Infectious Disease*, 2103-10; and P. C. Hopewell, "*Pneumocystis carinii* Pneumonia: Diagnosis," *The Journal of Infectious Diseases* 157 (1988):1115-19.

17. J. M. Wharton et al., "Trimethoprim-sulfamethoxazole or Pentamidine for *Pneumocystis carinii* Pneumonia in the Acquired Immunodeficiency Syndrome: A Prospective Randomized Trial," *Annals of Internal Medicine* 105 (1986):37-44; F. R. Sattler et al., "Trimethoprim-sulfamethoxazole Compared with Pentamidine for Treatment of *Pneumocystis carinii* Pneumonia in the Acquired Immunodeficiency Syndrome: A Prospective, Noncrossover Study," *Annals of Internal Medicine* 109 (1988):280-87; and J. A. Kovacs and H. Masur, "*Pneumocystis carinii* Pneumonia: Therapy and Prophylaxis," *The Journal of Infectious Diseases* 158 (1988):254-59.

18. Centers for Disease Control, "Guidelines for Prophylaxis against *Pneumocystis carinii* Pneumonia for Persons Infected with Human Immunodeficiency Virus," *Morbidity and Mortality Weekly Report (Suppl. 5)* 38 (1989):1-9.

19. R. E. McCabe and J. S. Remington, "Toxoplasma Gondii," in *Principles and Practice of Infectious Disease*, 2090-2103.

20. B. J. Luft and J. S. Remington, "Toxoplasmic Encephalitis," *The Journal of Infectious Diseases* 157 (1988):1-6.

21. R. Soave and W. D. Johnson, Jr., "Cryptosporidium and Isospora Belli Infections," *The Journal of Infectious Diseases* 157 (1988):225-29.

22. W. E. Dismukes, "Cryptococcal Meningitis in Patients with AIDS," *The Journal of Infectious Diseases* 157 (1988):624-28; and S. L. Chuck and M. A. Sande, "Infections with Cryptococcus Neoformans in the Acquired Immunodeficiency Syndrome," *The New England Journal of Medicine* 321 (1989):794-99.

23. P. C. Johnson et al., "Progressive Disseminated Histoplasmosis in Patients with Acquired Immunodeficiency Syndrome," *The American Journal of Medicine* 85 (1988):152-58; and J. R. Graybill, "Histoplasmosis and AIDS," *The Journal of Infectious Diseases* 158 (1988):623-26.

24. D. A. Bronnimann et al., "Coccidioidomycosis in the Acquired Immunodeficiency Syndrome," *Annals of Internal Medicine* 106 (1987):372-79.

25. A. E. Glatt, K. Chirgwin, and S. H. Landesman, "Treatment of Infections Associated with Human Immunodeficiency Virus," *The New England Journal of Medicine* (1988):1439-48.

26. R. E. Chaisson and G. Slutkin, "Tuberculosis and Human Immunodeficiency Virus Infection," *The Journal of Infectious Diseases* 159 (1989):96-100; and Centers for Disease Control, "Tuberculosis and Human Immunodeficiency Virus Infection: Recommendations of the Advisory Committee for the Elimination of Tuberculosis (ACET)," *Morbidity and Mortality Weekly Report* 38 (1989):236-50.

27. C. C. Hawkins et al., "Mycobacterium Avium Complex Infections in Patients with the Acquired Immunodeficiency Syndrome," *Annals of Internal Medicine* 195 (1986):184-88; and L. S. Young, "Mycobacterium Avium Complex Infection," *The Journal of Infectious Diseases* 157 (1988):863-67.

28. D. J. Witt, D. E. Craven, W. R. McCabe, "Bacterial Infections in Adult Patients with the Acquired Immune Deficiency Syndrome (AIDS) and AIDS-related Complex," *The American Journal of Medicine* 82 (1987):900-906; S. J. Sperber and C. J. Schleupner, "Salmonellosis during Infection with Human Immunodeficiency Virus," *Reviews of Infectious Diseases* 9 (1987):925-34; K. Krasinski et al., "Bacterial Infections in Human Immunodeficiency Virus-infected Children," *Pediatric Infectious Disease Journal* 7 (1988):323-28; M. A. Jacobson, H. Gellermann, and H. Chambers, "Staphylococcus Aureus Bacteremia and Recurrent Staphylococcal Infection in Patients with Acquired Immunodeficiency Syndrome and AIDS-related Complex," *The American Journal of Medicine* 85 (1988):172-76; "Haemophilus Influenzae Pneumonia in Young Adults with AIDS, ARC, or Risk of AIDS," *The American Journal of Medicine* 86 (1989):11-14; and H. M. Krumholz, M. A. Sande, and B. Lo, "Community-acquired Bacteremia in Patients with Acquired Immunodeficiency Syndrome: Clinical Presentation, Bacteriology, and Outcome," *American Journal of Medicine* 86 (1989):776-79.

29. D. R. Johns, M. Tierney, and D. Felsenstein, "Alteration in the

Natural History of Neurosyphilis by Concurrent Infection with the Human Immunodeficiency Virus," *The New England Journal of Medicine* 316 (1987):1569-72; E. C. Tramont, "Syphilis in the AIDS Era," *The New England Journal of Medicine* 316 (1987):1600-1601; Centers for Disease Control, "Recommendations for Diagnosing and Treating Syphilis in HIV-infected Patients," *Morbidity and Mortality Weekly Report* 37 (1988):600-608; S. A. Lukehart et al., "Invasion of the Central Nervous System by Treponema Pallidum: Implications for Diagnosis and Treatment," *Annals of Internal Medicine* 109 (1988):855-62; D. M. Musher, "How Much Penicillin Cures Early Syphilis?" *Annals of Internal Medicine* 109 (1988):849-51; and E. W. Hook III, "Syphilis and HIV Infection," *The Journal of Infectious Diseases* 160 (1989):530-34.

30. M. Ho, "Cytomegalovirus," in *Principles and Practice of Infectious Disease*, 1159-72; and S. Stagno et al., "Primary Cytomegalovirus Infection in Pregnancy: Incidence, Transmission to Fetus, and Clinical Outcome," *The Journal of the American Medical Association* 256 (1986):1904-8.

31. A. C. Collier et al., "Cytomegalovirus Infection in Homosexual Men: Relationship to Sexual Practices, Antibody to Human Immunodeficiency Virus, and Cell-mediated Immunity," *The American Journal of Medicine* 82 (1987):593-601.

32. M. A. Jacobson and J. Mills, "Serious Cytomegalovirus Disease in the Acquired Immunodeficiency Syndrome (AIDS): Clinical Findings, Diagnosis, and Treatment," *Annals of Internal Medicine* 108 (1988):585-94; and W. L. Drew, "Cytomegalovirus Infection in Patients with AIDS," *The Journal of Infectious Diseases* 158 (1988):449-56.

33. E. C. Klatt and D. Shibata, "Cytomegalovirus Infection in the Acquired Immunodeficiency Syndrome: Clinical and Autopsy Findings," *Archives of Pathology and Laboratory Medicine* 112 (1988):540-44.

34. L. H. Taber et al., "Acquisition of Cytomegaloviral Infections in Families with Young Children: A Serological Study," *The Journal of Infectious Diseases* 151 (1985):948-52; R. F. Pass et al., "Increased Rate of Cytomegalovirus Infection among Parents of Children Attending Day-care Centers," *The New England Journal of Medicine* 314 (1986):1414-18; and R. F. Pass et al., "Young Children as a Probable Source of Maternal and Congenital Cytomegalovirus Infection," *The New England Journal of Medicine* 316 (1987):1366-70; S.P. Adler, "Molecular Epidemiology of Cytomegalovirus: Viral Transmission among Children Attending a Day Care Center, Their Parents, and Caretakers," *Journal of Pediactrics* 112 (1988):366-72; M.E. Dworsky et al., "Occupational Risk for Primary Cytomegalovirus Infection among Pediatric Health-Care Workers," *The New England Journal of Medicine* 309 (1983):950-53; C.L. Balfour

and H.H. Balfour, "Cytomegalovirus Is Not an Occupational Risk for Nurses in Renal Transplant and Neonatal Units: Results of a Prespective Surveillance Study," *The Journal of the American Medical Association* 256 (1986):1909-14; J.L. Gerberding et al., "Risk of Transmitting the Human Immunodeficiency Virus, Cytomegalovirus, and Hepatitis B Virus to Health Care Workers Exposed to Patients with AIDS and AIDS-related Conditions," *The Journal of Infectious Diseases* 156 (1987):1-8; and G.J. Demmler et al., "Nosocomial Cytomegalovirus Infections within Two Hospitals Caring for Infants and Children," *The Journal of Infectious Diseases* 156 (1987):9-16.

35. I. Penn, "Tumors of the Immunocompromised Patient," *Annual Review of Medicine* 39 (1988):63-73.

36. M. K. Kaplan et al., "Neoplastic Complications of HTLV-III Infection. Lymphomas and Solid Tumors," *The American Journal of Medicine* 82 (1987):389-96.

37. R. M. Selik, H. W. Haverikos, and J. W. Curran, "Acquired Immune Deficiency Syndrome (AIDS) Trends in the United States, 1978-1982," *The American Journal of Medicine* 76 (1984):493-500; and M. Marmor et al., "Kaposi's Sarcoma in Homosexual Men: A Seroepidemiologic Case-control Study," *Annals of Internal Medicine* 100 (1984):809-15.

38. B. Safai et al., "The Natural History of Kaposi's in the Acquired Immunodeficiency Syndrome," *Annals of Internal Medicine* 103 (1985):744-50.

39. D.M. Barnes, "New Clues about Kaposi's Sarcoma," *Science* 242 (1988):376-77.

40. D. M. Knowles et al., "Lymphoid Neoplasia Associated with the Acquired Immunodeficiency Syndrome (AIDS): The New York University Medical Center Experience with 105 Patients (1981-1986)," *Annals of Internal Medicine* 108 (1988):744-53; and L. D. Kaplan et al., "AIDS-associated Non-Hodgkin's Lymphoma in San Francisco," *The Journal of the American Medical Association* 261 (1989):719-24.

41. M. A. Bermudez et al., "Non-Hodgkin's Lymphoma in a Population with or at Risk for Acquired Immunodeficiency Syndrome: Indications for Intensive Chemotherapy," *The American Journal of Medicine* 86 (1989):71-76.

42. H. Hollander and J.A. Levy, "Neurologic Abnormalities and Recovery of Human Immunodeficiency Virus from Cerebrospinal Fluid," *Annals of Internal Medicine* 106 (1987):692-95; D.H. Gabuzda and M.S. Hirsch, "Neurologic Manifestations of Infection with Human Immunodeficiency Virus: Clinical Features and Pathogenesis," *Annals of Internal Medicine* 107 (1987):383-91; I. Grant et al., "Evidence for Early Central Nervous System Involvement in the Aquired Immunodeficiency Syndrome (AIDS) and Other

Human Deficiency Virus (HIV) Infections: Studies with Neuropsychologic Testing and Magnetic Resonance Imaging," *Annals of Internal Medicine* 107 (1987):828-36; R. W. Price and B. J. Brew, "The AIDS Dementia Complex," *The Journal of Infectious Diseases* 158 (1988):1079-83; and D. D. Ho et al., "The Acquired Immunodeficiency Syndrome (AIDS) Dementia Complex," *Annals of Internal Medicine* 111 (1989):400-410.

43. Centers for Disease Control, *HIV/AIDS Surveillance*, October 1989.

44. S. Pahwa, "Human Immunodeficiency Virus Infection in Children: Nature of Immunodeficiency, Clinical Spectrum and Management," *Pediatric Infectious Disease Journal* 7 (1988):S61-S71.

45. S. Blanche et al., "A Proprective Study of Infants Born to Women Seropositive for Human Immunodeficiency Virus Type 1," *The New England Journal of Medicine* 320 (1989):1643-48; and M. F. Rogers et al., "Use of the Polymerase Chain Reaction for Early Detection of the Proviral Sequences of Human Immunodeficiency Virus in Infants Born to Seropositive Mothers," *New England Journal of Medicine* 320 (1989): 1649-54.

46. A. L. Belman et al., "Pediatric Acquired Immunodeficiency Syndrome: Neurologic Syndromes," *American Journal of Diseases of Children* 142 (1988):29-35; and G. B. Scott et al., "Survival in Children with Perinatally Acquired Human Immunodeficiency Virus Type 1 Infection," *New England Journal of Medicine* 321 (1989): 1791-96.

47. Pahwa, "Human Immunodeficiency Virus Infection in Children," S61-S71.

48. Ibid.; I. M. Onorato, L. E. Markowitz, and M. J. Oxtoby, "Childhood Immunization, Vaccine-preventable Diseases and Infection with Human Immunodeficiency Virus," *Pediatric Infectious Disease Journal* 7 (1988):588-95; and Centers for Disease Control, "Immunization of Children Infection Human Immunodeficiency Virus: Supplementary ACIP Statement," *Morbidity and Mortality Weekly Report* 37 (1988):181-83.

49. N. Clumeck and P. Hermans, "Antiviral Drugs Other than Zidovudine and Immunomodulating Therapies in Human Immunodeficiency Virus Infections," *The American Journal of Medicine (Suppl. 2A)* 85 (1988):165-72; M. S. Hirsch, "Antiviral Drug Development for the Treatment of Human Immunodeficiency Virus Infections: An Overview," *The American Journal of Medicine (Suppl. 2A)* 85 (1988):182-85; R. Yarchoan, H. Mitsuya, and S. Broder, "AIDS Therapies," *Scientific American* 259 (1988):110-19; M. S. Hirsch, "The Rocky Road to Effective Treatment of Human Immunodeficiency Virus (HIV) Infection," *Annals of Internal Medicine* 110 (1989):1-3; and J. A. Oates and A. J. J. Wood, "Clinical Pharmacology of 3'-azido-2', 3'-dideoxythymidine (Zidovudine) and Related

Dideoxynucleosides," *The New England Journal of Medicine* 321 (1989):726-38.

Flee from sexual immorality. All other sins a man commits are outside his body, but he who sins sexually sins against his own body. Do you not know that your body is a temple of the Holy Spirit, who is in you, whom you have received from God? You are not your own; you were bought at a price. Therefore honor God with your body (1 Corinthians 6:18-20).

"You shall not covet your neighbor's house. You shall not covet your neighbor's wife, or his manservant or maidservant, his ox or donkey, or anything that belongs to your neighbor" (Exodus 20:17).

Therefore do not let sin reign in your mortal body so that you obey its evil desires. Do not offer the parts of your body to sin, as instruments of wickedness, but rather offer yourselves to God, as those who have been brought from death to life (Romans 6:12-13).

Who is a God like you,
    who pardons sin and forgives the transgression
    of the remnant of his inheritance?
You do not stay angry forever
    but delight to show mercy.
You will again have compassion on us;
    you will tread our sins underfoot
    and hurl all our iniquities into the depths of the sea
(Micah 7:18-19).

Chapter Eight

The Prevention of AIDS

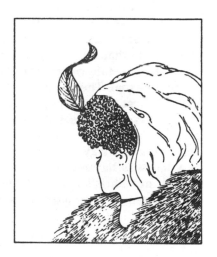

I first saw the drawing in a psychology text. If I had seen it in a kid's magazine I would have been intrigued by just another visual trick. In a psychology text I was supposed to take it more seriously. . . . Every time I looked at it I saw this hideous old woman, evil-eyed and hooked-nosed. I saw what I was conditioned to see, what my *mental set* was predisposed to see. Then suddenly she would vanish and in her place would be a sweet young thing looking coyly away from me over a fur draped on her left shoulder.

I could never look at them both at once; I had to be content with one woman or the other. The old woman was easiest for me to conjure up. Indeed she would be there immediately whenever I looked at the drawing. If I wanted to see the girl I had to do a paradigm shift to conjure her up. It became a sort of game to see first one, then the other, then the first again.

Only at times I wasn't sure who was playing the game. Was I in control? Or were they? The two of them seemed to be battling for my attention, so that now one, now the other would dominate the state of my consciousness. In fact it's still like that. The battle is not over, but at present the sweet young thing is winning.

It was the same way in real life. I didn't have one paradigm shift but many, seeing the world now one way, now another. I did not realize what was happening to me, but I bumbled through my Christian life puzzled and confused by what seemed to be happening inside me.[1]

John White

* * * * * *

This drawing is a parable of our world. Two completely different images come into view despite the same sensory input. The difference is not one of information, but one of choice.

Many dilemmas occur in the AIDS epidemic in which the same data builds a distinct view depending upon the biases of the viewer. It is why people "see" AIDS so dissimilarly. But unlike the drawing, many views offer morally right and wrong choices. If a superior choice is evident, why are people so resistant to seeing it? The preference is based upon volition, a willful alignment toward a certain position, and is often distorted by sin.

One of the most destructive judgments is the idea of "safe sex." The data available to both sides show clearly that safe sex is a misnomer, and will, in the long run, cost thousands of lives. It will most consistently sacrifice the lives of teenagers because of their immaturity, lack of foresight, and sense of invincibility. The government, media, homosexual activists, and sex educators have encouraged such suicide and will have to answer a decade hence when the grim reaper reveals the results of their senseless choice.

SAFE SEX?

Emphasizing condom usage for safety during sex began in the homosexual community. Yet "safe sex" is a semantic trick, a linguistic sedative that will kill thousands of people. Use of condoms among homosexuals or other high risk groups is hardly safe. It is safer sex in the same sense that putting one bullet in a gun chamber instead of two is safer Russian roulette. Because condoms cannot guarantee protection, it is a distortion to teach techniques that lower but do not eliminate the risk of acquiring HIV and call it safe.[2]

Laboratory studies show that latex condoms successfully block passage of HIV.[3] But tests that inflate condoms with water or mechanically simulate intercourse are scarcely comparable to sex. Condom usage was shown to decrease HIV acquisition among prostitutes and monogamous couples,[4] yet the same data also confirm that some spread of HIV to the uninfected does occur. In married couples in which one partner was HIV-infected and condoms were used, 10 percent of the healthy became infected[5] within two years (which is about the same failure rate as for pregnancy).[6] Since condoms have been routinely cited as the least effective form of contraception, that is hardly reassuring. Moreover, condom use by married couples is a best-case situation since they presumably have a higher level of education, commitment, and maturity than teens or those engaged in anonymous sex. Even married couples with complete knowledge of a partner's infection with HIV plus the benefit of extensive counseling may not utilize condoms for protection.[7]

The Problems with Condoms

HIV can be transmitted anytime. For pregnancy prevention, the first year failure rate of condoms for highly educated and motivated women thirty years and older is 4 percent or less. But among sexually active women under age twenty-five, up to one-third who use only condoms for contraception will be pregnant after one year.[8] This high failure rate occurs even though women of childbearing age are not fertile twenty-five or twenty-six days each month. No comparable safe time of the month exists for HIV spread.

Most people dislike condoms. Many men claim that condoms decrease the sensation they experience during intercourse,[9] and women do not enjoy the interruption and the anxiety of confirming proper use of the condom. If neither men nor women enjoy them, then the chances of good compliance are small. Perhaps not surprisingly, even the higher risk promiscuous heterosexuals and homosexuals still do not routinely use condoms.[10]

Using condoms requires planning ahead. The Pill became popular quickly because it divorced love-making from contraception; people prefer spontaneity in sex. Neither men nor women always plan ahead even in marriage. Dating couples may have no intention of having intercourse, but the passion of the moment overcomes their inhibitions. One partner may not want sex but is seduced or forced in the case of date rape, which has happened to one in eight college-age women.[11] Those who do plan ahead and carry condoms with them are more likely to be sexually active since few couples know of sound reasons to wait. If sex is more likely when "prepared," the high failure rate of condoms may actually increase the spread of HIV.

Women are in a vulnerable position. Within heterosexual relationships, women buy the majority of the condoms,[12] probably because they will suffer the greatest consequences from a pregnancy. But many dating women do not want to carry condoms since it makes them look "easy," and men often will refuse to use condoms since it detracts from their pleasure. Women can frequently do nothing to change this even if they know their partner is unfaithful.

Condoms are difficult to use properly. Whereas condom breakage occasionally occurs (about 1 in 140),[13] failure to use the condom at all or improper use is the likely explanation for its poor protection against HIV disease.[14] Most teenagers, the uneducated, or the immature will not use a condom correctly. Correct use requires the proper type of condom (latex), proper storage, proper timing of placement, proper positioning of the condom, proper lubrication (water-based), proper spermicide, proper anchoring during penetration, proper use during intercourse, proper timing and method of withdrawal, and proper disposal. For both partners during a time of passion to do all these tasks every time is extremely difficult.

Transmission of HIV may occur after a single encounter or may not occur despite many sexual contacts.[15] Some individuals are more infectious for HIV depending on their stage of illness, the presence of genital ulcerations, and the sexual techniques employed.[16] But on the average, one encounter in five hundred will transmit HIV if an infected and uninfected partner are involved. Few sexually active individuals go through a year with this number of encounters. But if millions of people are blithely having sex using condoms regardless of their partner's HIV status, then thousands upon thousands will discover just how false the idea of safe sex is. *According to medical studies* condoms do not lower the risk of infection nearly to the degree that the safe-sex advocates imply. Over time, sex with an HIV-infected individual while using a condom is very risky.

Why Does Safe Sex Have Such Strong Advocates?

HIV is spread even with consistent use of condoms. But the risk is like the proverbial half-empty versus half-full glass. For monogamous heterosexuals, the transmission rate of HIV with condom use is unacceptably high. We see the old hag. For those addicted to immoral sexuality with multiple partners a month, stopping sex is an unthinkable option. They see the winsome young girl and would rather risk death than stop their behavior. Those who promote safe sex are also falsely reassuring the rest of the population, against the evidence, that what they are doing is sane and safe. In essence, they are carrying others to the morgue with them.

Pseudoscientific organizations such as Planned Parenthood have made the value (as opposed to scientific) judgment that no one will stop having sex, even if his or her life depends upon it. Even scientific authors and organizations assume sexual appetites will not abate.[17] A certain fatalism exists, coupled with fuzzy thinking, that discourages dissent from the safe-sex party line. Granted, our society has become so sexualized that resisting temptation is much harder than it was in the past. That hardly means it is impossible, particularly when facing the risk of a lethal disease.

The Best Way to Avoid Sexually Transmitted HIV

Though some sexual practices are less risky than others, abstinence and intimacy with a mutually faithful, uninfected partner are the only ways to guarantee avoidance of sexually transmitted HIV. Not enough emphasis has been placed on these two biblical options. To insist that people cannot live according to these guidelines is nonsense. Throughout history, the majority of the world, both Christian and non-Christian, has held close to that standard. The rhetoric that obscures these options is not only false scientifically, it is life-threatening.

PREVENTION OF NEEDLE TRANSMISSION OF HIV DISEASE[18]

The best advice here is simple: Do not use IV drugs. If you are using drugs, obtain help to stop. If you cannot or will not stop, do not share needles. Many IV drug users are the hardest to reach because they are so estranged from the rest of society, and they do not have the educational network of the homosexual community. Their problems are so severe and seemingly beyond hope that they do not care about risking their lives. Other IV drug users belong to the middle or upper class and will probably be more affected by educational efforts. This subset of IV drug users is also more likely to have access to sterile needles and not to be so desperate.

In the past, addicts have considered AIDS a homosexual disease, and nonwhites consider it a disease of whites. In reality, AIDS is becoming as large a problem for IV drug users as it is for homosexual men. Nonwhite IV drug users are far more affected than white drug users.[19] Sharing drugs and needles involves more than simple convenience; it has cultural and ethnic importance that makes it a more difficult habit to break. Therefore the education must also be culturally and ethnically directed. If it is not, it will be as effective as speaking hillbilly to a New England blueblood.

Some moderately successful programs have reduced needle sharing in hard-hit areas such as Amsterdam and New York.[20] But even there only about half of the addicts are sterilizing their needles. Giving out clean needles is a controversial idea that has had mixed results where it has been tried. The ultimate goal should be to get addicts off drugs completely, since AIDS is only one of several ways they are likely to die.

PREVENTION OF HIV TRANSMISSION FROM BLOOD PRODUCTS

Since 1985, when the HIV antibody test and high-risk screening began, the chances of getting HIV infection through transfusions dropped precipitously to somewhere between one in 40,000 to one in 250,000.[21] Hemophiliacs can now take Factor VIII due to a new method of heat inactivation that destroys the virus.[22] Other blood products such as gamma globulin and certain vaccines never transmitted HIV.[23]

Although the risk of transmission through blood transfusions is small, work must be done to bring the risk down further. Physicians have reduced the number of transfusions over the last decade to the minimum necessary to avoid life-threatening circumstances. Family transfusions and autologous (self-stored) blood for elective surgery were originally resisted by the blood-banking industry, but are now accepted. The earlier concern that some people might not be able to get blood if some units were directed to specific people was unfounded. However, total blood donations have decreased because of latent fears that somehow giving blood can be a method of contracting AIDS.

Needle-stick injuries are an occupational hazard that most people do not face. Fortunately HIV is a difficult virus to transmit, even when a direct inoculation occurs with the small amount of blood in the tip of a needle. There is about a 1 in 250 risk for each accidental stick with an HIV-contaminated needle. The odds are still significant, and educational programs on proper use and disposal of needles are being done in hospitals across the country.[24] New auto-capping needles may help, though not eliminate injuries. All health care workers should assume that each patient is infected with HIV and exercise great care with *any* blood exposure. Even when the patient is known to be uninfected with HIV, health care workers need to be careful since other infections, particularly hepatitis B and other viruses, can be transmitted by blood exposure.

PREVENTION OF HIV TRANSMISSION FROM MOTHER TO CHILD

As HIV infection increases among heterosexuals and more women become infected, increasing numbers of infants will also be infected. Eighty percent of the children infected with HIV have acquired it from their mothers,[25] though less than one- third of the infants born to HIV-infected women become infected.[26] This is much lower than the original estimates. In 1990, most of the women in the U.S. who give HIV to their babies are either IV drug users or sexual partners of IV drug users. So drug abuse programs, whether state- or church- sponsored, will help the unborn. Women who are HIV-infected should be counseled to avoid pregnancy, since it is not clear how to keep the virus from passing through the placenta to the developing baby. However, it would be morally repugnant to recommend abortion to pregnant women who are HIV-positive, especially since 70 percent of those babies will be normal. On the other hand, some sort of support must be readied for those infants whose mothers will not live long or for those who are infected with HIV and abandoned.

Since HIV may also be transmitted from mother to child through breast-feeding,[27] it is recommended that HIV-infected women in the U.S. not breast-feed. In Africa, where good alternatives to breast-feeding are often unavailable, it is more dangerous to feed with formulas due to poor water sanitation.

PREVENTION OF HIV TRANSMISSION THROUGH ARTIFICIAL INSEMINATION

Artificial insemination with donated semen has infected several women with HIV.[28] Centers for Disease Control has recommended guidelines to virtually eliminate the possibility of transmission through semen.[29] These guidelines include exclusion of high-risk donors, screening donors with the antibody test, freezing the semen, and re-testing each donor after six months to be sure he has not recently become HIV-positive. The way the semen is stored would likely inactivate the virus even if an HIV-infected donor slipped through the screening process. Unfortunately, many donor arrangements are made privately, and adherence to these CDC guidelines is lessened substantially. For example, many lesbian couples have babies through artificial insemination from sperm donated by homosexual men.

PREVENTION OF HIV TRANSMISSION THROUGH DONATED ORGANS

Commonly donated organs such as corneas, kidneys, hearts, and livers should undergo rigorous testing beforehand to avoid a tragic second infection with HIV.[30] The number of potential infections through donated organs will be few since the number of transplants a year is much smaller than the number of blood transfusions.

CONTROVERSIAL PREVENTION METHODS

Some people have suggested more extensive measures to prevent the spread of HIV. A few of these have some merit to them; most do not.[31]

Testing everyone in America. This has little to recommend it. The chances that your eighty-seven-year-old grandmother is HIV-infected are remote, unless she had a transfusion between 1978 and 1985. To test all preteen children who have no history of transfusions, sexual abuse, or hemophilia also is unnecessary. Since AIDS strikes only restricted groups, wholesale testing is silly and expensive. It would be an administrative nightmare to test 260 million people. Because of the magnitude of the project, testing could be easily avoided by those who do not want to be tested, the very people one would most want to test. Moreover, the test would cost billions of dollars, money which could be better spent elsewhere.

Other problems exist with this widespread testing. Even though the test is good, it is not perfect. With so many people being tested, many false positives would be found with the first (ELISA) of the two-part test. Though these people would not be infected with HIV, the screening test would say they were, producing unnecessary anxiety while they waited for the confirming test (Western Blot). In addition, the larger the program, the greater the likelihood of confidentiality leaks concerning the test results.

Selective testing. Any man or woman considering marriage who has been sexually active with others previously or has used IV drugs ought to be tested on a voluntary basis to protect the uninfected partner and future children.[32] If marriage occurs even though the husband is infected, artificial insemination of his purified semen (assuming the mother remains uninfected) could prevent the spread of AIDS to the next generation.

Mandatory testing for marriage does not work well as the Illinois experience shows.[33] Only 0.011 percent of those tested in the first six months were HIV-infected and most of those had a history of high-risk behavior. About $312,000 was spent per positive test, and the total cost of testing was 1.5 times the state's total yearly expenditure on all AIDS programs. Many people who did not want to be tested simply went to neighboring states to get married. Presumably some people did not get married but began living together, since the number of marriage licenses issued by Illinois dropped by 22.5 percent from the year preceding mandatory testing. The bottom line is financial. Large funds for testing could be better used elsewhere. People who do not want to be tested can avoid it by foregoing marriage or going elsewhere (even out of the country if testing were nationally mandated). Premarital testing for syphilis, which is pointed to as the model for mandatory testing for HIV, is being dropped in many states because it is not cost effective either.[34]

Testing for HIV infection should be done at the doctor's discretion for patients entering the hospital. Pregnancy tests for unmarried women and tests for sexually transmitted diseases have been done routinely by physicians without a significant risk to confidentiality. Strict penalties should be enforced for breaches of confidentiality, except for those medical workers who unequivocally need to know test results. Laws that limit AIDS testing often hamper diagnoses and may increase the risk of accidental transmission of the AIDS virus to hospital workers who may be exposed to a patient's blood. Although health care workers are supposed to treat all patients as if they were infected with HIV, the same level of caution is seldom used on all patients as on ones known to be infected.

Other groups that would be reasonable to test are sex offenders, such as rapists and child molesters, and violent prisoners, due to the high incidence of homosexual rape and drug abuse within our prisons. The army continues to test all entering personnel to protect their own blood supply since service personnel provide battlefield transfusions. Practicing homosexuals are also excluded from the armed services, a rule which has been upheld by the judiciary.

Open reporting. People who are infected with HIV are often discriminated against when their disease becomes known to others.[35] Yet open reporting of those who are infected has no appreciable effect on curbing the spread of the disease. Since AIDS is not casually transmitted, the general population is not at risk from an HIV-infected person, making the need for open reporting negligible.

Moreover, even if open reporting were desirable, it is impractical. Those who already know they are infected or those in high-risk groups could avoid testing—or get someone to take the test using their name. Open reporting could chase people underground, which would lead to more infections, not fewer.

Selective reporting. Although it is illegal in some states, we physicians would always tell the spouse of an infected person about a positive HIV test. Since vaginal intercourse is inherently safer than homosexual sex, some women who have been sexually active with their infected husbands are not yet infected (as we saw in chapter 3). Eventually, many wives could become infected if they did not know their spouse was HIV-positive. Most people infected with HIV do not have sexual partners who are easy to contact because they are homosexual men or promiscuous heterosexuals. The only realistic way to notify these partners is to encourage voluntary notification.

Harsh penalties for deceptive transmitters of HIV. People who suspect they are infected with HIV have a moral duty not to infect others. But admitting that responsibility and deciding what to do to prevent spread to others are two different things. Many public health officials think that punitive measures for HIV spread must be discarded, since successful partner notification programs depend on voluntary information. Otherwise the person discovered with HIV likely would refuse to disclose sexual or needle-sharing partners for fear of legal reprisals.

On the other hand, some of the legal restrictions on reporting positive HIV tests have given the impression to some carriers of HIV that they can do whatever they want since their infection is no one else's business. Uninfected people who engage in sexual activity with strangers or with new acquaintances do bear a responsibility for their actions. However, that responsibility does not excuse the person with known HIV infection to sleep with whomever he or she wants.

Some legal methods to enforce responsibility, including imprisonment, should be applied to repeat offenders. Laws already in force, such as assault and battery statutes, could be invoked in cases of malicious spread of HIV disease. Others argue that the moral objection of nonchalant spread of HIV ought to be stated in a specific law to encourage a higher standard of moral behavior. For example, the Scandinavian countries and Britain already have passed punitive laws for all sexually transmitted diseases (including HIV) which state that a person who has a venereal disease and has sex without informing his or her partner can be fined or imprisoned. This is a difficult area to decide what would best prevent further spread.

Quarantine. Some have suggested that all people who are HIV-positive should be quarantined to protect the uninfected. This would make sense if AIDS were casually transmitted or if the infection only lasted a week or two like most infections. Children with chickenpox are often kept from other children for seven to ten days until they are no longer contagious. If a person were infected with bubonic plague, which can be casually transmitted, then he should be kept isolated, even against his will, until he has received antibiotics for a sufficient time to reduce the risk to others.

However, HIV infection lasts forever, so that quarantine is equivalent to life imprisonment. It would be impossible to find all the people who are infected because those who thought they might be would avoid being tested at all costs to escape lifetime estrangement from the rest of society. If they could be found, where would they be put? Texans would want them in California, and Californians would want them in New York. And how would a mass quarantine be paid for? Up to two million people would be placed in detention camps for the rest of their lives. They would have to be guarded, fed, and sheltered. Furthermore, what would be done with the HIV-infected individuals who acquired the disease through no fault of their own? Should the state quarantine a faithful husband who acquired AIDS from a blood transfusion? Who would support his family? If he is excluded from quarantine, what about the person who has the same story but has had two affairs in the last five years? Quarantine of the HIV- infected is being tried in Cuba, but the coercion and resulting loss of freedom are incompatible with a democratic society.[36]

Vaccines Protecting against HIV Infection

Some scientists have stated that a vaccine is the best way to prevent AIDS.[37] Yet vaccines are never absolutely effective or safe, and a vaccine for AIDS will be most difficult to develop. A better prevention is a change in behavior, which is safe and can start now.

Developing a vaccine is, however, a reasonable area of research. A vaccine is an intentional exposure (inoculation) of a person to an altered microorganism or organic chemicals from a microorganism that serves to protect the individual from the disease. This exposure results in immunity without having to experience the illness.[38]

Special Problems in Making an Effective HIV Vaccine[39]

A number of vaccines have been produced for various bacteria and viruses, but they vary in effectiveness and potential side-effects. An HIV vaccine, while not impossible, will be the most difficult vaccine yet made due to the following obstacles:

HIV can hide from the immune system. HIV hides from the immune system by frequent mutations, movement from cell to cell without exposure to the antibodies outside the cells, incorporation into the genetic material of the human cell, and survival inside macrophages and T-helper cells which normally assist in the destruction of foreign invaders and direct the entire immune system.

A good test animal for HIV does not exist. To produce a

vaccine, it is invaluable to have an animal that will grow the virus (as the chimpanzee does) and produce similar symptoms. But only man develops AIDS. With no test animal, vaccines must be tested in human subjects, a frightening concern if the vaccine proves ineffective. Vaccines can be partially tested after they have been administered by measuring antibodies produced, but an exposure of the person to the actual virus is the best way to know if it is protective. Although antibodies have been induced by experimental vaccines in chimpanzees, when challenged with HIV those antibodies were not protective against HIV infection.

HIV has a long incubation period. HIV infection takes an average of ten years from the time of exposure to the appearance of the first symptoms. It will take fifteen years or longer to manifest itself in some people. How long should an effective vaccine be tested to know if it is truly safe? Virtually all current vaccines are directed against viruses or bacteria with incubation periods of days to weeks, rather than years.

HIV causes cancer. It is not clear how HIV causes cancer, but there is a significant risk that a live but weakened HIV vaccine (as in the oral polio vaccine) could also cause Kaposi's sarcoma or lymphoma, just as very rarely the oral polio vaccine causes paralytic polio.

One way to test an AIDS vaccine may be to give the vaccine early in the infection when the immune system is still operational, boosting the immune system and either eradicating the virus or prolonging the life of the patient. Although several vaccines have been developed and introduced into humans to test for side effects, ultimate protection through vaccines is unlikely for many years.

CHRIST AND THE PREVENTION OF AIDS

Some Christians have questioned the desire for a vaccine at all. Jesus would not have questioned the hope for a vaccine as long as it is not used to enable a person to continue a hedonistic life-style. The longer people stay alive physically, the longer the Holy Spirit has to show them they are dead spiritually. Jesus healed many people physically, not because physical affliction was their main problem (although they thought it was), but to show them that he was the answer to their bigger problem of spiritual taintedness and alienation from God.

If Christians lack compassion toward AIDS sufferers, then homosexual men and promiscuous heterosexuals will continue to view "safe sex" as attractive, and the epidemic will spread further. If we act lovingly toward these outcasts, then they are more likely to listen and see the wrongness and danger in "safe sex." Our love will help prevent the spread of HIV.

Moreover, all of Christ's teachings can be thought of as a form of vaccination against the serious problems of life. When he taught that lust was adultery of the mind, he was deterring adultery. When he taught that those who would be first shall be last, he was averting spiritual pride. When Jesus said that one cannot serve God and money, he was deflecting materialism. Jesus, the compassionate Good Physician, was most willing to attempt preventative care. As his followers and fellow healers, we should willingly do the same.

Chapter 8, Notes

1. John White in *Power Encounters*, ed. Kevin Springer (San Francisco: Harper and Row, 1988), 69-70. Illustration taken from E.G. Boring, "A New Amiguous Figure," *American Journal of Psychology* 42 (3): 444-45. It was originally presented under the title "My Wife and My Mother-in-Law" by cartoonist W.E. Hill in *Puck*, 6 November 1915.

2. E. J. Emanuel and L. L. Emanuel, "Is Our AIDS Policy Ethical?" *The American Journal of Medicine* 83 (1987):519-20; and Centers for Disease Control, "Condoms for Prevention of Sexually Transmitted Diseases," *Morbidity and Mortality Weekly Report* 37 (1988):133-37.

3. Centers for Disease Control, "Condoms for Prevention," 133-37; C. A. M. Rietmeijer et al., "Condoms as Physical and Chemical Barriers against Human Immunodeficiency Virus," *The Journal of the American Medical Association* 259 (1988):1851-53; and "Can You Rely on Condoms?" *Consumer Reports*, March 1989, 135-41.

4. J. Mann et al., "Condom Use and HIV Infection among

Prostitutes in Zaire (letter)," *The New England Journal of Medicine* 316 (1987):345; M. A. Fischl et al., "Evaluation of Heterosexual Partners, Children, and Household Contacts of Adults with AIDS," *The Journal of the American Medical Association* 257 (1987):640-44; and M. A. Fischl and G. M. Dickinson, "Heterosexual Transmission of Acquired Immunodeficiency Syndrome (letter)," *The Journal of the American Medical Association* 257 (1987):2288-89.

5. Fischl et al., "Adults with AIDS," 640-44.

6. D. R. Mishell, "Contraception," *The New England Journal of Medicine* 320 (1989):777-87.

7. M. V. Ragni and P. Nimorwicz, "Human Immunodeficiency Virus Transmission and Hemophilia," *Archives of Internal Medicine* 149 (1989):1379-80.

8. Mishell, "Contraception," 777-87.

9. "Can You Rely on Condoms?" 135-41; and C. Sonnex et al., "Condom Use by Heterosexuals Attending a Department of GUM: Attitudes and Behavior in the Light of HIV Infection," *Genitourinary Medicine* 65 (1989):248-51.

10. K. Henry, M. T. Osterholm, and K. L. MacDonald, "Reduction of HIV Transmission by Use of Condoms (letter)," *American Journal of Public Health* 78 (1988):1244; C. Hooykaas et al., "Heterosexuals at Risk for HIV: Differences between Private and Commercial Partners in Sexual Behavior and Condom Use," *AIDS* 3 (1989):525-32.

11. Josh McDowell and Dick Day, *Why Wait?* (San Bernardino, Calif.: Here's Life Publishers, 1987), 22.

12. "Can You Rely on Condoms?" 135-41.

13. Ibid., 135.

14. Centers for Disease Control, "Condoms for Prevention of Sexually Transmitted Diseases," *Morbidity and Mortality Weekly Report* 37 (1988):133-37.

15. S. D. Holmberg et al., "Biologic Factors in the Sexual Transmission of Human Immunodeficiency Virus," *The Journal of Infectious Disease* 160 (1989):116-25.

16. Ibid.

17. N. Hearst and S. B. Hulley, "Preventing the Heterosexual Spread of AIDS: Are We Giving Our Patients the Best Advice?" *The Journal of the American Medical Association* 259 (1988):2428-32; J. J. Goedert, "What Is Safe Sex? Suggested Standards Linked to Testing for Human Immunodeficiency Virus," *The New England Journal of Medicine* 316 (1987):1339-42; M. F. Goldsmith, "Sex in the Age of AIDS Calls for Common Sense and 'Condom Sense,' " *The Journal of the American Medical Association* 257 (1987):2261-66; and J. Whyte, "Teaching Safe Sex," *The New England Journal of Medicine* 318 (1988):387.

18. D. C. Des Jarlais, S. R. Friedman, and W. Hopkins, "Risk Reduction for the Acquired Immunodeficiency Syndrome among

Intravenous Drug Users," *Annals of Internal Medicine* 103 (1985):755-59; D. C. Des Jarlais, S. R. Friedman, and R. L. Stoneburner, "HIV Infection and Intravenous Drug Use: Critical Issues in Transmission Dynamics, Infection Outcomes, and Prevention," *Reviews of Infectious Diseases* 10 (1988):151-58; W. Booth, "AIDS and Drug Abuse: No Quick Fix (News & Comment)," *Science* 239 (1988):717-19; R. A. Hahn et al., "Prevalence of HIV Infection among Intravenous Drug Users in the United States," *The Journal of the American Medical Association* 261 (1989):2677-84; P. W. Brickner et al., "Recommendations for Control and Prevention of Human Immunodeficiency Virus (HIV) Infection in Intravenous Drug Users," *Annals of Internal Medicine* 110 (1989):833-37; J. R. Cooper, "Methadone Treatment and Acquired Immunodeficiency Syndrome," *The Journal of the American Medical Association* 262 (1989):1664-67; V. P. Dole, "Methadone Treatment and Acquired Immunodeficiency Syndrome Epidemic," *The Journal of the American Medical Association* 262 (1989):1681-82; E. E. Schoenbaum et al., "Risk Factors for Human Immunodeficiency Virus Infection in Intravenous Drug Users," *The New England Journal of Medicine* 321 (1989):874-79; and Centers for Disease Control, "Update: Acquired Immunodeficiency Syndrome Associated with Intravenous-drug Use: United States, 1988," *Morbidity and Mortality Weekly Report* 38 (1989):165-70.

19. Des Jarlais, Friedman, and Stoneburner, "HIV Infection and Intravenous Drug Use," 151-58; and Centers for Disease Control, "HIV/AIDS Surveillance," December 1989.

20. G. V. Stimson, "Syringe-exchange Programmes for Infecting Drug Users," *AIDS* 3 (1989):253-60; and H. M. Ginzburg, "Needle Exchange Programs: A Medical or a Policy Dilemma?" *American Journal of Public Health* 79 (1989):1350-51.

21. J. W. Ward et al., "Transmission of Human Immunodeficiency Virus (HIV) by Blood Transfusions Screened as Negative for HIV Antibody," *The New England Journal of Medicine* 318 (1988):473-78; T. F. Zuck, "Transfusion-transmitted AIDS Reassessed," *The New England Journal of Medicine* 318 (1988):511-12; P. D. Cumming et al., "Exposure of Patients to Human Immunodeficiency Virus through the Transfusion of Blood Components that Test Antibody-Negative," *The New England Journal of Medicine* 321 (1989):941-46; J. E. Menitove, "The Decreasing Risk of Transfusion-associated AIDS," *The New England Journal of Medicine* 321 (1989):966-968; and M. J. Hughes et al., "Prevalence of HIV Antibody among Blood Donors in California," *The New England Journal of Medicine* 321 (1989):974-75.

22. Centers for Disease Control, "Safety of Therapeutic Products Used for Hemophilia Patients," *Morbidity and Mortality Weekly Report* 37 (1988):441-50.

23. "Safety of Immune Globulins in Relation to HTLV-III," *FDA*

Drug Bulletin 16 (1986):3; and D. P. Francis et al., "The Safety of the Hepatitis B Vaccine: Inactivation of the AIDS Virus during Routine Vaccine Manufacture," *The Journal of the American Medical Association* 256 (1986):869-72.

24. Centers for Disease Control, "Recommendations for Prevention of HIV Transmission in Health-Care Settings," *Morbidity and Mortality Weekly Report* 36 (1987, suppl 2S):1-18; and Centers for Disease Control, "Guideline for Prevention of Human Immunodeficiency Virus and Hepatitis B Virus to Health-Care and Public-Safety Workers," *Morbidity and Mortality Weekly Report* 38 (1989, suppl S-6):1-37.

25. Centers for Disease Control, "HIV/AIDS Surveillance."

26. The European Collaborative Study, "Mother-to-Child Transmission of HIV Infection," *Lancet* 2 (1988):1039-43; Task Force on Pediatric AIDS, "Perinatal Human Immunodeficiency Virus Infection," *Pediatrics* 82 (1988):941-44; S. W. Nicholas et al., "Human Immunodeficiency Virus Infection in Childhood, Adolescence, and Pregnancy: A Status Report and National Research Agenda," *Pediatrics* 83 (1989):293-307; and S. Blanche et al., "A Prospective Study of Infants Born to Women Seropositive for Human Immunodeficiency Virus Type 1," *The New England Journal of Medicine* 320 (1989):1643-48.

27. Nicholas et al., "Infection in Childhood, Adolescence, and Pregnancy," 293-307.

28. G. J. Stewart et al., "Transmission of Human T-cell Lymphotropic Virus Type III (HTLV-III) by Artificial Insemination by Donor," *Lancet* 1 (1985):581-84.

29. Centers for Disease Control, "Semen Banking, Organ and Tissue Transplantation, and HIV Antibody Testing," *Morbidity and Mortality Weekly Report* 37 (1988):57-58, 63.

30. Centers for Disease Control, "Transmission of HIV through Bone Transplantation: Case Report and Public Health Recommendations," *Morbidity and Mortality Weekly Report* 37 (1988):597-99.

31. F. N. Judson, "What Do We Really Know about AIDS Control?" *American Journal of Public Health* 79 (1989):878-82.

32. P. D. Cleary et al., "Compulsory Premarital Screening for the Human Immunodeficiency Virus: Technical and Public Health Considerations," *The Journal of the American Medical Association* 258 (1987):1757-62.

33. B. J. Turnock and C. J. Kelly, "Mandatory Premarital Testing for Human Immunodeficiency Virus: The Illinois Experience," *The Journal of the American Medical Association* 261 (1989):3415-55.

34. A. M. Brandt, "AIDS in Historical Perspective: Four Lessons from the History of Sexually Transmitted Diseases," *American Journal of Public Health* 78 (1988):367-71.

35. R. J. Blendon and K. Donelan, "Discrimination against People with AIDS: The Public's Perspective," *The New England Journal of Medicine* 314 (1988):1022-26.

36. R. Bayer and C. Healton, "Controlling AIDS in Cuba," *The New England Journal of Medicine* 320 (1989):1022-24.

37. T. J. Mathews and D. P. Bolognesi, "AIDS Vaccines," *Scientific American* 259 (1988):120-27.

38. A. R. Hinman et al., "Immunization," in *Principles and Practice of Infectious Disease*, 3d ed., ed. G. L. Mandell, R. G. Douglas, and J. E. Bennett (New York: Churchill Livingstone, 1989), 2320-22.

39. P. J. Fischinger, "Strategies for the Development of Vaccines to Prevent AIDS," in *AIDS: Etiology, Diagnosis, Treatment, and Prevention*, 2d ed., ed. V. T. Devita, S. Hellman, and S. A. Rosenberg (New York: J.B. Lippincott, 1988), 87-104; D. M. Barnes, "Obstacles to an AIDS Vaccine," *Science* 240 (1988):719-21; W. C. Koff and D. F. Hoth, "Development and Testing of the AIDS Vaccines," *Science* 241 (1988):426-32; A. S. Fauci, moderator, "Development and Evaluation of a Vaccine for Human Immunodeficiency Virus Infection," *Annals of Internal Medicine* 110 (1989):373-85; and M. L. Clements, "AIDS Vaccines," in *Principles and Practice of Infectious Disease*, 1112-21.

"The person with such an infectious disease must wear torn clothes, let his hair be unkempt, cover the lower part of his face and cry out, 'Unclean! Unclean!' As long as he has the infection he remains unclean. He must live alone; he must live outside the camp" (Leviticus 13:45-46).

"'Or if [a person] touches human uncleanness—anything that would make him unclean—even though he is unaware of it, when he learns of it he will be guilty'" (Leviticus 5:3).

While Jesus was in one of the towns, a man came along who was covered with leprosy. When he saw Jesus, he fell with his face to the ground and begged him, "Lord, if you are willing, you can make me clean."

Jesus reached out his hand and touched the man. "I am willing," he said. "Be clean!" And immediately the leprosy left him (Luke 5:12-13).

"Ah, Sovereign LORD, you have made the heavens and the earth by your great power and outstretched arm. Nothing is too hard for you" (Jeremiah 32:17).

Chapter Nine

The Air-tight Case against Casual Contagiousness

S tephanie, a woman at our church, wanted to talk with me privately. She and her husband, Charlie, are two special people who are always working behind the scenes to keep the church running smoothly. When she said it concerned the book I was writing, I knew this would not be the routine type of question doctors get in the hallways from friends. She told me her brother is a homosexual and lives in Houston in the midst of the homosexual community. Stephanie's brother recently watched his best friend die of AIDS and has discovered that he is infected with HIV as well. Currently he is healthy, although his doctor is giving him medication to try to slow the deterioration of his immune system.

Stephanie loves her brother and is sad about his physical and spiritual state. Accordingly, she and her family visit him frequently. But her last visit had a chilling effect on her because of new anxieties about her brother's disease. Her brother has always cared deeply for her four children and is affectionate with them. He is careful to avoid kissing them on the mouth, and he would never allow them to come in contact with an open wound. But the scene she described as we spoke was quite frightening for her. She recounted having a meal with her brother while one of the children sat in his lap. He was feeding her child with a fork, and he was eating with the same utensil as well.

Stephanie and Charlie desire to show this young man the love of Christ; they do not want to treat him as an outcast, as the rest of the heterosexual world has. But it is one thing to minister to him personally; it is another to directly involve her children. Stephanie asks, how is it possible to minister freely to a person with AIDS when you fear for your life or the life of a family member?

* * * * * *

Many Christian writers claim that HIV is spread by casual contact. The various stated or implied methods of casual spread are through coughing;[1] contact with saliva,[2] sweat,[3] tears,[4] or urine[5] from toilet seats or towels;[6] from food handlers;[7] and from mosquito[8] and bedbug bites.[9] These writers have not given hard evidence to back up their claims. Rather, they have made mistakes in logic and interpretation of data in devising these supposed methods of transmission. To be fair, secular writers also raise the issue of casual contagiousness, but Christian writers seem to have a fixation with it. In this chapter we will demonstrate that the chances of acquiring AIDS in these ways is virtually nil.

Invoking fears about casual contagiousness in this epidemic is disturbing because it inhibits ministry to AIDS patients. Christians historically have had a strong witness in their ministry to the sick, even during easily spread epidemics such as the plague. As historian William H. McNeill has said:

> One advantage Christians had over their pagan contemporaries was that the care of the sick, even in time of pestilence, was for them a recognized religious duty. . . . The effect of disastrous epidemics, therefore, was to strengthen Christian churches at a time when most other institutions were being discredited.[10]

Christians should not fear death in the same way non-believers do. Our lives are in the hands of the sovereign Lord, and death will not come before its appointed time. If we are called to care for the sick, we should take precautions, pray for safety, and then serve joyfully as unto the Lord. Even if AIDS were casually spread, many Christians should be involved in service to AIDS patients and their families. However, by God's grace, we have little to fear since AIDS is *not* casually spread. We can comfortably visit patients in the hospital, allow children infected with the virus into our Sunday schools, minister in the homosexual community, and help in drug-rehabilitation programs.

We know beyond a reasonable doubt that AIDS is not a casually spread disease. The reasons include careful study of who acquires AIDS and who does not, comparison with other viral and sexually transmitted diseases, and specific laboratory research.[11]

EVIDENCE AGAINST THE CASUAL SPREAD OF HIV

1. There are no documented cases of casual spread from HIV-infected patients to household members.

If AIDS were casually spread, the people most likely to acquire it would be the parents, children, and siblings of AIDS patients. Children are prone to casual contagions since they eat and drink using the same utensils or cups after others, chew on the same toys as siblings, kiss on the mouth abundantly, and even share toothbrushes. Yet no cases exist where family members of AIDS patients acquired the AIDS virus, except through the usual methods of sex and childbirth.[12]

Consider the number of times an HIV-infected child's saliva, tears, runny nose, and sweat would touch a brother or sister, yet there is no spread of the virus. Conversely, think how often a normal child brings home colds, flu, diarrhea, and sore throats from school or day-care and then spreads them to other family members. The difference is these are casually spread diseases, not sexually spread ones such as

AIDS, syphilis, gonorrhea, or genital herpes. No one worries about acquiring syphilis apart from sexual contact. We should not worry about AIDS either.

Studies in various parts of the world concur: AIDS is spread only by significant mixing of blood, sexual intercourse, or through childbirth.[13]

The proponents of the casual spread theory have relied on unqualified statistics to support their contention. One statistic quoted by Gene Antonio suggests that in central Africa, persons in the same household as an AIDS patient have three times the likelihood of becoming infected as someone in the general population.[14] At first glance that statistic seems to imply casual contagiousness, but it actually does nothing of the sort. Clustering of HIV-infected adults and children is not the same as casual spread from a household contact. If a young man catches the virus from visiting prostitutes, both his wife and subsequent children are likely to become infected. However, they all will have contracted the infection in the usual ways (through sexual intercourse and childbirth).[15] Moreover, severe anemia from malaria in African children is treated with blood not screened for HIV. Because family members are often the donors of that blood, spread from one infected adult member to the children is common.[16]

A similar misuse of numbers occurs when James McKeever says, "17% of the housemates of AIDS victims came down with AIDS, even though there was no sexual contact."[17] Babies born to infected mothers are at high risk. The 17 percent are simply the babies who contracted the virus during childbirth. By not qualifying the statement, McKeever leaves the reader with the impression that AIDS is casually transmitted. Citing statistics without explanations heightens fear unnecessarily.

2. HIV is transmitted to health care workers only through blood.

Physicians, nurses, and lab technicians who care for people with AIDS are more intensely exposed to HIV than almost any other group. Doctors examine the patients for signs of cancers and infections. Nurses change dressings, start IVs, and wash incontinent patients too weak to make it to the toilet. Technicians draw blood from AIDS patients numerous times a day. Other than family members no group of people would be more likely to acquire HIV infection casually than the health care workers who have close, non-sexual contact with AIDS patients.

Prior to the discovery of HIV and the ability to test for the infection, many health care workers (including one of this book's authors) were extremely cautious when working with AIDS patients. Though many methods of disproving casual contagiousness existed (listed in this chapter), no one could prove it until an actual test for the infection was available.[18] Since 1985, health care workers across the world have been tested for HIV, and the tests have all been negative except in cases involving direct blood exposure.[19] Even when accidental inoculation of blood contaminated with HIV occurred, less than 0.5 percent became infected.[20] Thus a definite but very low risk exists for occupational spread of the virus—all of it related to exposure to blood.[21]

Three women became infected with HIV after direct exposure to contaminated blood.[22] In two of these exposures the nurses had open wounds (cracked skin and dermatitis) exposed to blood, while the third had contaminated blood splashed on her face and in her mouth. These unfortunate infections confirm that gloves and special precautions must be used when exposure to blood or body fluids is anticipated. Health care workers are routinely exposed to blood and should be careful, but out of tens of thousands of exposures to blood during surgery, in the emergency room, and during deliveries of babies, only three workers have been reported infected with HIV through non-needle-stick incidents. In most jobs and social settings, people do not come in contact with the blood of other individuals at all.

Neither of us has any concern about shaking hands, talking, hugging, or having dinner with an AIDS patient. And we have far more exposure to HIV than the average person. We are careful when we draw blood, assist in surgery, or help deliver a baby, but these are occupational hazards to which only a few people are exposed. With proper training and care, even risk from these can be greatly minimized. If the risk for doctors and nurses is almost solely from HIV-contaminated blood in needle-stick injuries, then the average person need not fear normal social interaction with an AIDS patient.

3. *Dentists have low risk for occupational infection with HIV.*

Dentists, dental hygienists, and assistants are exposed to a number of viruses during their day-to-day activities. Most of these are casually transmitted viruses such as cold, flu, and oral herpes viruses, but on occasion would include HIV. Because of sporadic low numbers of HIV in the saliva, and dental procedures that result in bleeding, splattering, and aerosolizing of oral fluids, dentists would be at high risk for contracting HIV if it is casually spread. But only two dentists have become HIV-positive without the usual methods of spread, although few dentists follow the Centers for Disease Control guidelines for avoiding contact with blood.[23] The two dentists who contracted HIV were presumed to be infected by contaminated blood from a patient coming in direct contact with an open sore or by blood being splattered into their eyes or mouths. If the spread of HIV occurred by coughing or by exposure to saliva, dentists would be the primary risk group for acquiring AIDS, and many more cases of infection would have been identified.

4. *The demographics of AIDS are completely different from those of casually spread diseases.*

In the U.S. about 90 percent of the AIDS patients are male, and the vast majority of these are in the sexually active group between 20-49 years of age.[24] The demographics of AIDS are virtually identical to every other sexually transmitted disease and are unlike casually spread diseases such as colds, flu, diarrhea, and sore throats. The people with AIDS are the least likely to get casually spread diseases because young adults are normally the most healthy age group.

Those in the age range from two to fourteen are the

most susceptible to casual contagions. Two year olds are with other children more often than they were as infants and so get sick frequently with colds, fevers, vomiting, and diarrhea. As they are exposed to various infectious agents and develop immunities, their frequency of illness drops off and is much lower by the teenage years. The only patients who are HIV-positive in the two- to fourteen-year-old range are ones who contracted the disease from sex, transfusions, or during birth. Moreover, the elderly, who are more likely to be sexually monogamous or to have ceased sexual activity altogether, have no chance of getting HIV except through transfusions. Yet their likelihood of getting colds, the flu, and other casually spread illnesses increases as their immune systems weaken with aging.

The comparison of age groups on a graph is particularly impressive in disproving casual contagiousness of AIDS. The line representing HIV infection is highest at the ages where casually contracted diseases are lowest. Conversely, where casual contagiousness is highest, the chance of contracting AIDS is lowest.[25]

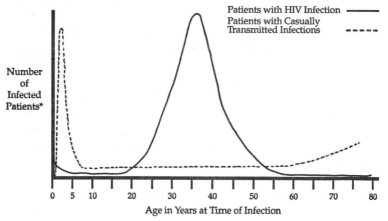

**Ages of Patients with HIV Infection
Compared with Ages of Patients
with Casually Transmitted Infections**

* This graph shows age distribution at onset of infection (not actual numbers of cases) of casually transmitted illnesses, such as colds, influenza, and chickenpox, versus HIV infection (see note 25, page 205).

5. The spread of (serum) hepatitis B is similar to the spread of AIDS.

Epidemiologists at the Centers for Disease Control were virtually certain how AIDS was spread only six months after the first cases were reported.[26] This is because the spread of AIDS in the U.S. followed the same pattern as another viral illness, hepatitis B, which is spread by sex and transfusions. Hepatitis B was originally identified in blood transfusion recipients in the 1960s. It was later shown to be a sexually transmitted disease in the 1970s, mainly as a problem in homosexual men. The AIDS epidemic followed by five to ten years the epidemic of hepatitis B in homosexuals.

Further research and experience with the disease and testing for the virus have only strengthened the early conclusion. Hepatitis B is actually twelve to sixty times more easily spread by accidental needle-sticks and blood contact than is HIV.[27] Yet few people worry about casual spread of serum hepatitis, even though it can be a debilitating and lethal disease. The battle about casual contagiousness for HIV continues only because authors are inciting fears without any substantiation for their claims.

6. Doctors who treat AIDS patients say it is not casually spread.

No reputable physician studying the AIDS epidemic doubts how HIV is spread. All agree it is spread only by the transfer of body fluids, especially blood and semen, through birth, sex, and sharing needles. No reason exists to doubt what the experts say since they will gain no advantage by lying or falsifying data. They also have abundant experimental and epidemiologic evidence to support their claims.

Despite the agreement of the experts, Antonio claims the medical community knows AIDS *is* spread casually, but is not telling the public to avoid alarm. He says health workers are waging a "consistent campaign of disinformation" about AIDS.[28] This is false and shows a complete lack of understanding of how the medical community works. In medicine, unlike in the media or government, it would be virtually impossible to cover up the possibility of casual spread. Not that physicians are less biased or prone to sin than people in other professions, but the manner in which medical research is conducted—independently and in many parts of the world—make a cover-up very unlikely.

Suppose I am doing research on the use of a new drug against a resistant form of malaria. I know that if the drug works well, I will have articles published, obtain tenure at the university, be a major speaker at seminars, and become internationally known. I hope against hope that the drug works well, but alas, it is a failure in the laboratory. With all the potential benefits for my career if it were to work, why am I not tempted to lie about the results? If I claimed a major breakthrough in treatment, a dozen laboratories across the world would try to confirm my studies. When all of them failed to reproduce my results, at best I would appear to be a fool, at worst a liar. If it were discovered that I altered test results, I would be fired from the university and disgraced before my colleagues.

If the early articles in this epidemic were wrong in saying that AIDS was spread only by sex or transfusions, many papers would have been produced showing otherwise. That did not occur. From the beginning of the epidemic to the present, all articles in respected medical journals confirmed that the disease is not casually spread.[29] True, mistakes can occur in medical research, but they are usually in areas more diffi cult to prove. How a disease is spread is one of the easiest things to demonstrate, and a major mistake here by all the experts in the field is not a reasonable possibility.[30]

7. *AIDS patients who have no identified risk factors do not suggest alternate modes of transmission.*

Anywhere from 3 to 5 percent of the patients with AIDS have no identifiable risk factor when their diagnosis is first reported. Some writers suggest this confirms casual spread, but no evidence exists for such an assertion. Many of the unidentified cases simply were unable to be investigated because the patient died suddenly, refused to cooperate, or disappeared. Many of the patients classified with no risk factors are there temporarily until investigators can conduct personal interviews, check medical backgrounds, and obtain supplemental blood tests on other members of the family. Of the few for whom no definitive risk factors can be confirmed even after investigation, many have a history of sexually transmitted diseases or exposure to prostitutes and so are presumed to have contracted the disease through sexual transmission. A number of others may have lied about past IV drug use. (See chapter 6 for a detailed breakdown of these patients without known risk.)

8. The disparity of HIV infection in Haiti and the Dominican Republic argues against casual contagiousness.

Haiti occupies the western third of the island of Hispaniola. The only other country on this large island is the Dominican Republic, which shares a two-hundred-mile border, the same topography, the same climate, and similar insect-borne and casually transmitted diseases. However, colonial history, language, religion, ethnic composition, and political systems distinguish the two countries. Another distinguishing feature is the extent of HIV infection.

HIV infection appeared six years earlier in Haiti than it did in the Dominican Republic, and Haiti has twice as many cases to date, even though both countries have the same population. As of December 1986, no children in the Dominican Republic had been infected with HIV, even though children are the most readily exposed to insect-borne illnesses. HIV infection is not spread uniformly through all ages throughout the island as is the case with tuberculosis (which is spread through respiration) or malaria (which is spread by mosquito bites). Moreover, 10 percent of the Haitian laborers working in the Dominican Republic sugar cane fields have HIV, while a much lower portion of the Dominican workers are infected. If two groups of men are working side-by-side and one group has a 10 percent level of infection and the other has only 1 percent, that eliminates the possibility of casual spread since the men are in the same location, doing the same job, with the same exposure. The only sound explanation is the men act differently off the job, visiting prostitutes, homosexual bars, or using IV drugs.[31]

9. HIV is not spread by mosquitoes.

Some suggest that mosquitoes spread HIV since insects can ingest infected blood, and some of the highest concentrations of AIDS are in mosquito-infested areas of Florida and central Africa.[32] A region in Florida has the highest AIDS rate per capita in the U.S., and this area has been thoroughly investigated by epidemiologists from the CDC. The researchers identified each available HIV-positive subject in the area and determined that all contracted the virus by the usual channels of IV drug use, sexual promiscuity, or childbirth.[33] Although these subjects were exposed to prevalent viruses transmitted by insect bites, no relation was found between *HIV infection* and insect exposure. Also, those infected with HIV were not clustered in households nor were there infections in children between the ages of two and ten or in adults older than sixty, lending further evidence against casual or insect spread.

In Africa, it is merely coincidence that the area of the continent with the highest concentration of AIDS is also the area with the most mosquitoes. Central Africa also has the densest population areas and the most sexually active peoples on the continent because more young adults are there.[34] These factors, not mosquitoes, are the reasons AIDS is there. It is just as spurious to say mosquitoes cause the spread of AIDS in these African locations as it is to say mosquitoes cause the poverty, malnutrition, and war that are also widespread there.

Moreover, if HIV were transmitted by mosquitoes, the two- to fourteen-year-olds would be most at risk because they play outside, wear the least clothing, and are the least likely to be concerned about insect bites. AIDS in Africa has a similar age distribution as in the U.S., although many more women are involved because the disease is more often heterosexually transmitted there. Children are not infected with HIV either in the United States or Africa unless they have had a transfusion, have been sexually abused, or have contracted the virus before or during birth.

It is true that mosquitoes can harbor the virus if they

bite an AIDS patient. However, as Dr. Robert Gallo, the best known U.S. researcher on AIDS has said:

> Mosquitoes bite. They take blood and virus particles. It shouldn't surprise anybody that they can harbor the virus. But we have no indication that the virus replicates inside the mosquito and no evidence to show that mosquitoes can transmit AIDS.[35]

People may think that a mosquito is like a tiny syringe and needle—that it can take in contaminated blood and inject it into its next victim. But for a mosquito, bedbug, or other biting insect to transmit a disease, the infectious agent must almost always thrive inside the insect. The ingested blood is the insect's food; it is taken into the stomach and digested there. Before the insect can pass on the disease, the organism must incubate a certain amount of time inside the insect. For the mosquito, it takes nine to twelve days after biting an infected person for it to spread yellow fever and three to five days for malaria. With the tsetse fly, it takes three to four days before it can spread the parasite for African sleeping sickness.[36] No scientific evidence suggests that, once ingested by an insect, HIV reproduces, migrates, and concentrates in the insect's salivary glands, ready to infect subsequent hosts.[37] Likewise, the vast majority of infectious diseases such as flu, colds, pneumonia, and impetigo are not spread this way because the infectious agent does not live inside biting insects.

Mechanical spread by insects is a speculative concern. Suppose a feeding insect is interrupted and goes on to its next victim carrying HIV in its mouth or body parts. Theoretically, it might be able to spread HIV. Some factors that have to be considered include the quantity of infected blood in the insect, the time between feedings, how long HIV could survive in this abnormal circumstance, and how many viruses are required to cause infection in the new host. Less than 0.5 percent of needle injuries which inject blood contaminated with HIV result in transmission of the infection, and these involve much larger quantities of blood than in an insect bite. Considering all factors, one entomologist estimates that the risk of transmission of HIV by insects is virtually nonexistent.[38] None of the first 100,000 cases of AIDS in the U.S. has been spread in this manner, and it is unlikely that any of the next hundred thousand will be either.

10. AIDS is not spread by coughing.

The spread of infectious diseases by coughing is common, and the distance infectious particles travel by coughing determines who gets infected. Some writers propose coughing as a form of transmission of AIDS and use as evidence the fact that AIDS patients have transmitted tuberculosis to health care workers.[39] Yet to say that an AIDS patient can transmit tuberculosis, an airborne infection, and imply that this same patient might be able to transmit HIV by the same route is poor logic and is medically inaccurate. No evidence exists that proximity to a coughing AIDS patient places one at risk for contracting AIDS.

11. HIV is not spread through saliva.

Research suggests that HIV is contained in the saliva of some HIV-infected people.[40] This finding is cited frequently by some to suggest casual contagiousness.[41] However, these writers do not explain the findings in this research that make the reports look less ominous. Only one in seventy-one AIDS patients had the virus in his saliva, and always in small concentrations. Epidemiologic studies of dentists and dental hygienists do not demonstrate increased risk for HIV infection, nor do studies show an increased risk of nonsexual spread to household members of an HIV-infected person despite the normal sharing of items contaminated with saliva such as food, eating utensils, and toys. One AIDS patient who bit seven hospital workers failed to transmit the virus.[42] Eight children bitten by HIV-infected children showed no evidence of spread.[43]

Our mouths are sometimes contaminated with blood from brushing or flossing of teeth, gingivitis, or trauma. Under most circumstances the small amount of blood in the mouth of an AIDS patient would be markedly diluted and insufficient to spread the disease even if the patient were to bite another person. If a tiny amount of infected blood were swallowed while kissing, the low numbers of virus particles would be quickly destroyed by the stomach acids. Furthermore, no cases have been proven of the spread of AIDS to health care workers or household members exposed only to the saliva of an AIDS patient. Some evidence exists that saliva actually inactivates the virus.[44] It is possible, though yet unproven, that if a significant amount of blood and virus were in the mouth, bites or deep kissing might convey some risk. For this reason, the CDC recommends that HIV-positive people refrain from deep kissing.

12. *HIV is fragile outside the body.*

Some writers cite the ability of the virus to survive prolonged periods of drying (up to ten days), and strongly imply that the virus is much more dangerous than if it lived only for minutes.[45] But to argue that the virus's long survival outside the body leads to the probability of casual spread is a giant logical leap with several fallacies.

First, these experiments of prolonged drying were done under ideal conditions for the virus (in protected petri dishes). Allowing the growth media to dry was the only potentially destructive action taken. Under normal circumstances, drying would be only one of several destructive events for the virus. Normally, HIV would be exposed to ultraviolet light, which would destroy the virus. Many scavenger insects and bacteria would ingest the blood that contained HIV. In someone's home, blood or sputum containing the virus is not likely to be left on the kitchen table or floor for long. In short, HIV would not have the opportunity to survive for nearly as long under normal conditions.

Also, the concentration of HIV in the samples for the experiment was 100,000 times higher than would be contained in a normal sample of blood.[46] Even with these concentrated samples, the rate of viral inactivation was rapid; the vast majority of the viruses died from simple drying. If the concentrations were more realistic, then the surviving viruses would be too few to infect anyone unless the solution was injected.

The virus is fragile. Virtually any household cleaning agent (such as diluted household bleach, hydrogen peroxide, Lysol, and alcohol) or sunlight will destroy it.[47] The chances of HIV surviving for ten days is virtually zero, unless it were protected in a scientific laboratory. Many bacteria are much hardier and just as lethal as HIV, but only rarely cause disease. For example, the botulism, gas gangrene, tetanus, and anthrax bacteria, which cause lethal diseases in humans, form spores that allow them to survive indefinitely. Yet in the United States one rarely hears of deaths from these even though they are more difficult to destroy and kill humans much more rapidly than HIV. The reason is that in a sanitary, modern country, these bacteria seldom have the opportunity to enter our bodies.

Even if the virus survived in dried blood, to cause disease it would need to penetrate several layers of skin, be in sufficient numbers to overcome the body's initial defenses, and adhere to the specific white blood cells in the body that it infects. HIV is harmless outside of the body. Despite some writers' concern about the survival of HIV, no patient has acquired AIDS from dried blood or sputum.

13. No risk exists in ministering to AIDS patients.

It might be helpful to put the risk of AIDS in proper perspective. Suppose a sixty-year-old pastor goes to the hospital to comfort a man who has AIDS. The patient also has a severe case of cold sores (oral herpes), has active tuberculosis, and has recently contracted the flu. If the pastor has a proper perspective, what should he be most concerned about?

There is about a one in one million chance he will die in a car wreck on the way to the hospital. There is a one in seventy-five thousand chance this sixty-year-old man will die of a heart attack on the day he visits the AIDS patient. If the pastor contracts herpes, tuberculosis, or the flu from inhaling infectious microscopic droplets, he has a small but real chance of dying of one of those diseases. Influenza would probably be the most serious since it can be particularly dangerous for older people. Tuberculosis is a much more treatable disease than it used to be, but even today thousands die from it every year (although most of these are people who do not care for themselves, such as chronic alcoholics). Herpes (cold sores) is a common disease that affects millions of Americans. For the most part cold sores are more of a nuisance than anything else, but a small number of Americans die every year from the herpes virus invading the brain to cause herpes encephalitis. Therefore, the pastor would be irrational to be concerned about HIV. He should be far more concerned about the drive to the hospital or about contracting the flu, in which case he should be equally concerned about visiting anyone in the hospital.

14. *HIV is unlikely to be spread even through non*casual *means not involving sex or transfusions.*

It is conceivable that a person could acquire AIDS outside of the regular ways. For example, a two-year-old girl has AIDS acquired through a blood transfusion. Another child strikes her on the face, and she begins bleeding inside her mouth. In retaliation, she bites the boy who struck her and draws blood. It is possible, although extremely unlikely, for the bitten child to become HIV positive.[48]

After having a blood sample taken, a hospitalized AIDS patient has two drops of blood fall on his bedside tray. A visitor with an open wound could be exposed to the virus should the wound come in contact with the blood on the tray. AIDS has never been transmitted that way, nor have we seen any disease conveyed that way, but it is theoretically possible. One could even imagine bizarre circumstances where someone could catch AIDS off a toilet seat. None of these would be considered casual transmission.

15. *HIV is unlikely to mutate into a more contagious organism.*

It is well known that HIV is capable of a large degree of mutation or antigenic drift, causing variation from one virus strain to another. Already a second HIV has been discovered in western Africa with a sufficiently different genetic make-up to call it HIV-2. Undoubtedly, more strains will be forthcoming. Because of these viral changes, lay people are

concerned that new AIDS viruses could have casually contagious transmission routes. Although such a change is theoretically possible, we are unaware of any virus that changed
principle routes of spread as it changed genetic structure.[49] It
is unlikely that the AIDS virus will be the first.

If we are worried about HIV mutations, we should be
just as concerned about mutations elsewhere. The viral feline
leukemia could mutate and become contagious for humans.
The herpes virus could mutate and cause the lethal brain
infection commonly instead of rarely. Chickenpox, an easily
contracted illness, could mutate to become lethal to all children. We could worry about many events that are unlikely to
occur. Or we could follow the sound advice of Christ, who
said, "Do not worry about tomorrow, for tomorrow will
worry about itself. Each day has enough trouble of its own"
(Matthew 6:34).

16. *The AIDS virus has yet to be spread casually, and it is
not reasonable to expect casual spread in the future.*

The book that pushes the idea of casual spread hardest
actually states that there are no cases in which the disease
has been spread casually. However, the writer chooses
against the evidence to believe that a real threat of casual
spread exists: "[The] lack of evidence concerning non-sexual,
non-blood transfusion related means of transmission is not a
firm guarantee of actual or potential lack of risk."[50]

This is the "Yes, but" objection. No matter how much
evidence is given against casual spread, one can always say,
"Yes, but . . ." and create scenarios in which a person could
possibly get the disease casually. It is impossible to prove
absolutely that AIDS cannot be spread casually because the
person who objects can always claim that the *next* case might
be casually spread, even though the first two million cases
were not. But this objection is not based on reason; it is an
illogical choice given the evidence. Some Christians want
absolute guarantees for a comfortable life, but that is not
what Christ told us to expect in his Sermon on the Mount.
We will be persecuted. We ought to love our enemies. We are
to give to the needy even if it means we make do with less.

SUMMARY

There is no evidence of casual contagiousness of HIV, and it is irresponsible for writers to raise the issue without any substantiation. In this chapter we discussed at length the following arguments against casual spread:

1. No person living with an AIDS victim has ever contracted the disease unless that person had sexual contact or shared needles with the infected person, or was born to a mother with HIV infection.

2. No health care worker has ever contracted AIDS from his interaction with AIDS patients except from a needle-stick or a significant mixing of blood.

3. Dentists, who are at high risk for contracting casually spread illnesses, do not acquire AIDS casually.

4. AIDS has spread through the population the way sexually transmitted and transfusion-spread diseases do and completely differently from casually spread diseases.

5. AIDS is spread most similarly to hepatitis B, which is not spread through casual contact.

6. Health care professionals who work with AIDS all concur that AIDS is not spread through casual contact.

7. Patients with AIDS who have no identified risk factor do not suggest alternate modes of transmission.

8. The different percentages of HIV-infected persons in Haiti and the Dominican Republic show that spread by insects and casual contact is extremely unlikely.

9. Mosquitoes do not spread AIDS.

10. AIDS has never been spread by coughing.

11. AIDS has never been spread through saliva.

12. HIV is fragile outside of a person's body, and is not likely to infect someone apart from person-to-person contact.

13. No one has ever acquired AIDS through casual contact, so the possibility of getting it while ministering to others is virtually zero.

14. Noncasual spread other than by sex and transfusions is possible but extremely remote.

15. HIV is not likely to mutate into a casually spread virus because no other virus has ever done so.

16. Although it cannot be absolutely proven that there will never be a case of the AIDS virus spread casually, it has yet to occur and it is not reasonable to expect it to occur in the future.

Chapter 9, Notes

1. David Chilton, *Power in the Blood* (Brentwood, Tenn.: Wolgemuth & Hyatt Publishers, 1987), 13; Gene Antonio, *The AIDS Cover-Up? The Real and Alarming Facts about AIDS* (San Francisco: Ignatius Press, 1987), 119; James M. McKeever, *The AIDS Plague* (Medford, Ore.: Omega Publications, 1987), 30; and David R. Reagan and Thomas Baker, *What the Bible Says about AIDS* (McKinney, Tex.: Lamb and Lion Ministries, 1988), 24.
2. Chilton, *Power in the Blood*, 27; and Antonio, *AIDS Cover-Up?*, 97.
3. Antonio, *AIDS Cover-Up?*, 8.
4. Ibid., 97; and McKeever, *AIDS Plague*, 35.
5. Antonio, *AIDS Cover-Up?*, 7; and Reagan and Baker, *What the Bible Says*, 4.
6. Chilton, *Power in the Blood*, 33; and Patrick Dixon, *The Truth about AIDS* (East Sussex, U.K.: Kingsway Publications Ltd., 1987), 103.
7. Antonio, *AIDS Cover-Up?*, 51; McKeever, *AIDS Plague*, 36; and Reagan and Baker, *What the Bible Says*, 24.
8. Chilton, *Power in the Blood*, 13; and Antonio, *AIDS Cover-Up?*, 72.
9. Dixon, *Truth about AIDS*, 95.
10. William H. McNeill, *Plagues and Peoples* (Garden City, N.Y.: Anchor Press, 1976), 121.
11. M. A. Sande, "Transmission of AIDS: The Case against Casual Contagion," *The New England Journal of Medicine* 314 (1986):380-82; G. H. Friedland and R. S. Klein, "Transmission of the Human Immunodeficiency Virus," *The New England Journal of Medicine* 317 (1987):1125-35; A. R. Lifson, "Do Alternate Modes for Transmission of Human Immunodeficiency Virus Exist?" *The Journal of the American Medical Association* 259 (1988):1353-56; and M. E. Chamberland and J. W. Curran, "Epidemiology and Prevention of AIDS and HIV Infection," in *Principles and Practice of Infectious Diseases*, 3d ed., ed. G. L. Mandell, R. G. Douglas, and J. R. Bennett (New York: Churchill Livingstone, 1989), 1038.
12. J. R. Kaplan et al., "Evidence against Spread of Human T-Lymphotropic Virus/Lymphadenopathy-associated Virus (HTLV-III/LAV) in Families of Children with the Acquired Immunodeficiency Syndrome," *Pediatric Infectious Diseases* 4

(1985):468-71; R. R. Redfield et al., "Frequent Transmission of HTLV-III among Spouses of Patients with AIDS-related Complex and AIDS," *The Journal of the American Medical Association* 253 (1985):1571-73; J. M. Jason et al., "HTLV-III/LAV Antibody and Immune Status of Household Contacts and Sexual Partners of Persons with Hemophilia," *The Journal of the American Medical Association* 255 (1986):212-15; G. H. Friedland et al., "Lack of Transmission of HTLV-III/LAV Infection to Household Contacts of Patients with AIDS or AIDS-related Complex with Oral Candidiasis," *New England Journal of Medicine* 317 (1986):344-49; J. M. Mann et al., "Prevalence of HTLV-III/LAV in Household Contacts of Patients with Confirmed AIDS and Controls in Kinshasa, Zaire," *Journal of the American Medical Association* 256 (1986):721-24; M. A. Fischl et al., "Evaluation of Heterosexual Partners, Children, and Household Contacts of Adults with AIDS," *Journal of the American Medical Association* 257 (1987):640-44; T. A. Peterman et al., "Risk of Human Immunodeficiency Virus Transmission from Heterosexual Adults with Transfusion-associated Infections," *The Journal of the American Medical Association* 259 (1988):55-58; and D. B. Brettler et al., "Human Immunodeficiency Virus Isolation Studies and Antibody Testing: Household Contacts and Sexual Partners of Persons with Hemophilia," *Archives of Internal Medicine* 148 (1988):1299-1301.

13. Friedland and Klein, "Transmission of the Human Immunodeficiency Virus," 1125-35.

14. Antonio, *AIDS Cover-Up?*, 101.

15. T. C. Quinn et al., "AIDS in Africa: An Epidemiologic Paradigm, *Science* 234 (1986):955-63.

16. A. E. Greenberg et al., "The Association between Malaria, Blood Transfusions, and HIV Seropositivity in a Pediatric Population in Kinshasha, Zaire," *The Journal of the American Medical Association* 259 (1988):545-49.

17. McKeever, *AIDS Plague*, 86.

18. M. S. Hirsch et al., "Risk of Nosocomial Infection with Human T-cell Lymphotropic Virus III (HTLV-III)," *The New England Journal of Medicine* 312 (1985):1-4; and S. H. Weiss et al., "HTLV-III Infection among Health Care Workers: Association with Needle-stick Injuries," *The Journal of the American Medical Association* 254 (1985):2089-96.

19. Centers for Disease Control, "Update: Human Immunodeficiency Virus Infections in Health-Care Workers Exposed to Blood of Infected Patients," *Morbidity and Mortality Weekly Report* 36 (1987):285-89; J. M. Mann et al., "HIV Seroprevalence among Hospital Workers in Kinshasha, Zaire: Lack of Association with Occupational Exposure," *The Journal of the American Medical Association* 256 (1986):3099-102; and B. N'Galy et

al., "Human Immunodeficiency Virus Infection among Employees in an African Hospital," *The New England Journal of Medicine* 319 (1988):1123-27.

20. R. Marcus and the CDC Cooperative Needlestick Surveillance Group, "Surveillance of Health Care Workers Exposed to Blood from Patients Infected with Human Immunodeficiency Virus," *The New England Journal of Medicine* 319 (1988):1118-23.

21. D. K. Henderson et al., "Risk of Nosocomial Infection with Human T-cell Lymphotropic Virus Type III/Lymphadenopathy-associated Virus in a Large Cohort of Intensively Exposed Health Care Workers," *Annals of Internal Medicine* 104 (1986):644-47; Centers for Disease Control, "Update: Acquired Immunodeficiency Syndrome and Human Immunodeficiency Virus Infection among Health Care Workers," *Morbidity and Mortality Weekly Report* 37 (1988):229-39; and C. E. Becker, J. E. Cone, and J. Gerberding, "Occupational Infection with Human Immunodeficiency Virus (HIV)," *Annals of Internal Medicine* 110 (1989):653-56.

22. Centers for Disease Control, "Health-Care Workers Exposed to Blood of Infected Patients," 285-89.

23. Centers for Disease Control, "Recommended Infection-control Practices for Dentistry," *Morbidity and Mortality Weekly Report* 35 (1986):237-41; D. D. Ho et al., "Infrequency of Isolation of HTLV-III Virus from Saliva in AIDS (letter)," *The New England Journal of Medicine* 313 (1985):1606; R. S. Klein et al., "Low Occupational Risk of Human Immunodeficiency Virus Infection among Dental Professionals," *The New England Journal of Medicine* 318 (1988):86-90; C. Siew, S. E. Gruninger, S. A. Hojvat, "Screening Dentists for HIV and Hepatitis B (letter)," *The New England Journal of Medicine* 318 (1988):1400-1401; and R. S. Klein et al., "Dentists and Risk of HIV (letter)," *The New England Journal of Medicine* 319 (1988):113-14.

24. Centers for Disease Control, "HIV/AIDS Surveillance," December 1989.

25. W. L. Heyward and J. W. Curran, "The Epidemiology of AIDS in the U.S.," *Scientific American* 259 (1988):72-81. The part of the graph depicting casually transmitted illnesses is a combination of all casually transmitted diseases and is common knowledge among physicians. A graph depicting risk would depend on many factors such as the actual illness involved, cause of the casual spread, ethnic susceptibilities, and frequency of contact with other people.

26. Randy Shilts, *And the Band Played On: Politics, People, and the AIDS Epidemic* (New York: St. Martin's Press, 1987), 107; and D. P. Francis, J. W. Curran, and M. Essex, "Epidemic Acquired Immune Deficiency Syndrome: Epidemiologic Evidence for a Transmissable Agent," *Journal of the National Cancer Institute* 71 (1983):1-4.

27. As noted, less than 0.5 percent of accidental needle-sticks contaminated with HIV-infected blood result in HIV infection, while 6 to 30 percent of accidental needle-sticks tainted with hepatitis B blood result in hepatitis B infection in the victim. Centers for Disease Control, "Recommendations for Preventing Transmission of Infection with Human T-Lymphotropic Virus Type III/Lymphadenopathy-Associated Virus in the Workplace," *Morbidity and Mortality Weekly Report* 34 (1985):682-95.

28. Antonio, *AIDS Cover-Up?*, xii.

29. M. S. Gottlieb et al., "*Pneumocystis Carinii* Pneumonia and Mucosal Candidiasis in Previously Healthy Homosexual Men: Evidence of a Newly Acquired Cellular Immunodeficiency," *The New England Journal of Medicine* 305 (1981):1425-31; Centers for Disease Control Task Force on Kaposi's Sarcoma and Opportunistic Infections, "Epidemiologic Aspects of the Current Outbreak of Kaposi's Sarcoma and Opportunistic Infections," *The New England Journal of Medicine* 306 (1982):248-52; H. W. Jaffe, "Acquired Immune Deficiency Syndrome in the United States: The First 1,000 Cases," *The Journal of Infectious Diseases* 148 (1983):339-45; A. S. Fauci, "Epidemiology," in "Acquired Immunodeficiency Syndrome: Epidemiologic, Clinical, Immunologic, and Therapeutic Considerations," *Annals of Internal Medicine* 100 (1984):92-94; R. M. Selik and H. W. Haverkos, "Acquired Immune Deficiency Syndrome (AIDS) Trends in the United States, 1978-1982," *The American Journal of Medicine* 76 (1984):493-500; H. W. Curran et al., "The Epidmiology of AIDS: Current Status and Future Prospects," *Science* 229 (1985):1352-57; G. H. Friedland and R. S. Klein, "Transmission of the Human Immunodeficiency Virus," *The New England Journal of Medicine* 317 (1987):1125-35; H. W. Haverlos and R. Edellman, "The Epidemiology of Acquired Immunodeficiency Syndrome among Heterosexuals," *The Journal of the American Medical Association* 260 (1988):1922-29; R. L. Berkelaman et al., "Epidemiology of Human Immunodeficiency Virus Infection and Acquired Immunodeficiency Syndrome," *The American Journal of Medicine* 86 (1989):761-70; and Chamberland and Curran, "Epidemiology and Prevention," 1038.

30. From time to time research has been fabricated and the investigators caught due to the reasons given. These have always been isolated events. There has never been a concerted effort by the medical community to hoodwink the public on any medical issue.

31. Centers for Disease Control, "Opportunistic Infections and Kaposi's Sarcoma among Haitians in the United States," *Morbidity and Mortality Weekly Report* 31 (1982):353-61; J. Vieira et al., "Acquired Immunodeficiency in Haitians: Opportunistic Infections in Previously Healthy Haitian Immigrants," *The New England Journal of Medicine* 308 (1983):125-29; A. E. Pitchenik et al.,

"Opportunistic Infections and Kaposi's Sarcoma among Haitians: Evidence of a New Acquired Immune Deficiency State," *Annals of Internal Medicine* 98 (1983):277-84; J. W. Pape et al., "Characteristics of the Acquired Immunodeficiency Syndrome (AIDS) in Haiti," *The New England Journal of Medicine* 309 (1983):945-50; J. W. Pape et al., "The Acquired Immunodeficiency Syndrome in Haiti," *Annals of Internal Medicine* 103 (1985):674-78; The Collaborative Study Group of AIDS in Haitian-Americans, "Risk Factors for AIDS among Haitians Residing in the United States: Evidence of Heterosexual Transmission," *The Journal of the American Medical Association* 257 (1987):635-39; R. E. Koenig et al., "Prevalence of Antibodies to the Human Immunodeficiency Virus in Dominicans and Haitians in the Dominican Republic," *The Journal of the American Medical Association* 257 (1987):631-34; and Pan American Health Organization, Washington, D.C.

32. Talk given by the chief of the Health Department of the State of Mississippi at a seminar on AIDS, Dallas, Texas, October 1987.

33. K. G. Castro et al., "Transmission of HIV in Belle Glade, Florida: Lessons for Other Communities in the United States," *Science* 239 (1987):193-97.

34. Norman Miller and Richard C. Rockwell, eds., *AIDS in Africa: The Social and Policy Impact* (Lewiston, N.Y.: The Edwin Mellen Press, 1988), 31 ff.

35. W. Booth, "News & Comment: AIDS and Insects," *Science* 237 (1987):355-56.

36. V. C. Vaughan, R. J. McKay, and R. E. Behrman, eds., *Nelson's Textbook of Pediatrics* (Philadelphia: W. B. Saunders Co., 1979), 938, 995, 1004.

37. Examples of this biological spread of first replicating and then completing an essential life cycle in an insect include malaria, African sleeping sickness, Chagas' disease, yellow fever, and dengue fever.

38. Charles Bailey, an entomologist with the U.S. Army Medical Research Institute of Infectious Disease in Fort Detrick, Maryland, estimated the chances of a single unit of virus being introduced by an insect, given the above factors, "would be one in ten million." Booth, "News & Comment," 355-56. (It would take hundreds of particles to have any likelihood of producing the disease.)

39. Talk given by Gene Antonio, author of *The AIDS Cover-Up?*, to the Citizens against Pornography, Austin, Texas, November 1987.

40. J. E. Groopman et al., "HTLV-III in Saliva of People with AIDS-related Complex and Healthy Homosexual Men at Risk for AIDS," *Science* 226 (1984):447-49; and D. Ho et al., "Risk of Transmission of HTLV-III Virus from Saliva in AIDS," *New England Journal of Medicine* 313 (1985):1606.

41. Antonio, *AIDS Cover-Up?*, 107-8; and Reagan and Baker, *What the Bible Says*, 4.

42. C. Tsoukas et al., "Risk of Transmission of HTLV-III/LAV from Human Bites" (paper presented at the Second International Conference on AIDS, Paris, 23-25 June 1986).

43. M. F. Rogers, C. R. White, and R. Sanders, "Can Children Transmit HTLV-III/LAV?" (paper presented at the Twenty-sixth Interscience Conference on Antimicrobial Agents and Chemotherapy, New Orleans, 1 October 1986).

44. P. N. Fultz, "Components of Saliva Inactivate Human Immunodeficiency Virus," *Lancet* 2 (1986):1215.

45. Reagan and Baker, *What the Bible Says*, 4; Antonio, *AIDS Cover-Up?*, 112; and Chilton, *Power in the Blood*, 21.

46. L. Resnick et al., "Stability and Inactivation of HTLV-III/LAV under Clinical and Laboratory Environments," *Journal of the American Medical Association* 255 (1986):1887-91.

47. L. S. Martin, J. S. McDougal, and S. L. Loskoski, "Disinfection and Inactivation of Human T Lymphotropic Type III/Lymphadeopathy-associated Virus," *Journal of Infectious Diseases* 152 (1985):400-3.

48. Rogers, White, and Sanders, "Can Children Transmit HTLV-III/LAV?"; and Tsoukas et al., "Transmission of HTLV-III/LAV from Human Bites."

49. There is a subtle but vitally important difference between changes in route of transmission of a virus as it changes composition and the type or severity of disease that often occurs with changes in genetic structure. A classical example is influenza. While each winter may bring new flu epidemics affecting the general population to a greater or lesser degree (depending on vaccination status, amount of antigenic change, and previous exposure to influenza over the life of the individual), note that the route of transmission never changes—influenza is always spread by close contact and respiratory droplet. Measles can be devastating to a population that has never been exposed to it before (such as occurred with the American Indians) but the route of transmission has remained the same. Syphilis seems to cause less severe disease in the twentieth century compared to the 1500s and 1600s, but it has always been a sexually transmitted disease.

50. Antonio, *AIDS Cover-Up?*, 12.

Part 3

THE CHURCH AND AIDS

*The path of the righteous is like the first gleam of
    dawn,
    shining ever brighter till the full light of day*
(Proverbs 4:18).

*"You are the light of the world. A city on a hill can-
not be hidden. Neither do people light a lamp and put
it under a bowl. Instead they put it on its stand, and it
gives light to everyone in the house. In the same way,
let your light shine before men, that they may see your
good deeds and praise your Father in heaven"*
(Matthew 5:14-16).

*For it is by grace you have been saved, through
faith—and this not from yourselves, it is the gift of
God—not by works, so that no one can boast. For we
are God's workmanship, created in Christ Jesus to do
good works, which God prepared in advance for us to
do* (Ephesians 2:8-10).

*Live such good lives among the pagans that, though
they accuse you of doing wrong, they may see your
good deeds and glorify God on the day he visits us* (1
Peter 2:12).

Chapter Ten

The Need for a New Direction

"**I** know men; and I tell you that Jesus Christ is no mere man. Between Him and every other person in the world there is no possible term of comparison. Alexander, Caesar, Charlemagne, and myself have found empires; but upon what do these creations of our genius depend? Upon force. Jesus alone found His empire upon love; and to this very day millions would die for Him."

Napoleon Bonaparte

Napoleon saw something modern Christians have either forgotten or failed to practice: the kingdom of Christ is a kingdom of love. Although he saw the truth, Napoleon did not act upon it, having already been seduced by ambition and power. Christians also fall before the enticements of the world, while giving lip service to the love of Christ. This is the main reason people see little difference between the world and the church. It is time for a new direction.

Love should be our first principle to follow, but it is not the only one. Scripture also gives boundaries in moral areas, such as, "Flee fornication," "Do not lie with a man as one lies with a woman," and "You shall not commit adultery." To say, "I love you; do whatever you want," like some senile grandfather, is hardly loving. But neither is it loving to say, "You brood of vipers! Who warned you to flee from the coming wrath?" like a self-appointed John the Baptist. A place exists for such harsh words, but they had best be the result of a direct call from God. Too often such latter-day prophets have been seduced by the power Napoleon experienced and are not following the call of the Spirit. Once love has been actively demonstrated, then God may prompt one to address the sin in another person's life.

Many mistakes have been made in the name of Christ in this epidemic. We will discuss some of these errors, both scientific and biblical. Over the next several chapters, we will develop a Christian response to the AIDS epidemic based on the life of Christ. This response does not ignore sin, but neither does it use the truth of Scripture to pummel opponents.

INTEGRATION OF MEDICINE AND SCRIPTURE

Understanding the medical characteristics of AIDS is foundational to making policy decisions. While doctors often make moral choices affecting their patients, they are not inherently qualified to solve ethical dilemmas. Any lay person, once he understands the medical factors surrounding an ethical question, is just as qualified as the physician to present a course of action. However, if that medical information is in error, so likely will be the moral decision on which it is based.

Since all technology is amoral, medical decisions are subservient to spiritual values. Therefore, for the Christian, decisions in medicine and public health come under the authority of Scripture. Medical and biblical truth must be integrated to avoid decisions that are medically unsound or morally deficient. Christians are in a unique position to make the difficult choices necessary for the public good while still guaranteeing the protection of the individual created in God's image.

Two broad categories of mistakes have been made. Medical errors primarily lead to fears for self and family. Theological errors lead to self-righteousness and complacency toward a dying world. Both are equally harmful since they make Christians appear unloving and primarily interested in personal peace and prosperity. Since it is impossible to describe every error, we will describe broad types of mistakes, illustrated by specific examples, and then advise how to identify these kinds of errors in the future.

Factual Errors

Factual lapses might appear the least grievous of errors, particularly when lay writers make statements on medical issues. However, they are the easiest to avoid since abundant, accurate information is readily available on AIDS. Moreover, because basic facts are the foundation upon which other thinking is built, these errors can lead to mistaken conclusions, even if the reasoning is reliable.

Medicine is a complicated discipline requiring a minimum of seven years of post-graduate study before one is competent to practice it. Its vocabulary and methods of problem solving are unique. This does not make it above other disciplines, nor does it exclude nonmedical people from writing about it. But it does require more preparatory work to be qualified to understand and criticize the field. Factual errors indicate the writer has not done his homework and cast doubt on his work as a whole.

The habitat of the virus has been falsely described. British author Patrick Dixon says the AIDS virus is common in many animals. He also claims a cat died of AIDS in San Francisco.[1] Gene Antonio twice states that HIV has been found in green monkeys in Africa. Later he suggests that it had crossed over to man from diseased sheep.[2] These are false ideas. Human immunodeficiency virus is well named since it causes disease only in humans. It reproduces in chimpanzees but causes no illness. HIV has not been found in other mammals, which is unfortunate since it is hard to study vaccines and drugs if they cannot be tested on a sick animal. Simian immunodeficiency virus causes an AIDS-like disease in monkeys, but it is only distantly related genetically to HIV.

Other false claims about the virus include David Reagan's statement that this is the first retroviral infection in humans; it is actually the third. Also, he and others claim that the virus is exceptionally hardy.[3] However, HIV is easily destroyed by household cleaners and sunlight. Many viruses and bacteria are much more difficult to destroy. Antonio suggests that one AIDS virus introduced into the body will likely cause infection.[4] This is unlikely since large numbers of people have engaged in risky behavior with infected individuals without acquiring HIV. Even with direct injection, the immune system is able to destroy many viral particles. The number of viruses necessary to cause infection depends upon the virulence of the strain of HIV and the immune strength and genetic factors of the person exposed. David Chilton also says that "we are all equally at risk" to acquire HIV.[5] This is an absurd idea, and particularly odd coming from Chilton, since he goes to great lengths to claim that AIDS is a homosexual disease.

Christian writers have also distorted the treatments for AIDS. Dixon claims that medical technology has failed to produce a single drug to destroy viruses.[6] But in the last two decades, a number of effective anti-viral drugs have been developed. Antonio states twice that no vaccines have been made against RNA-type viruses, such as HIV.[7] This is patently false. Most vaccines have been directed against RNA viruses, including rabies, polio, measles, mumps, rubella, and influenza. Although many problems exist in perfecting a vaccine (as we enumerated in chapter 8), the fact that HIV is an RNA virus is not a difficulty as Antonio implies. Antonio later suggests that a vaccine is theoretically impossible.[8] Developing an effective vaccine will be very difficult, but not impossible.

Antonio discusses the "abysmal lack of understanding regarding this complex and fatal disease," yet in less than ten years scientists have learned more about this virus and the disease it causes than almost any other viral infection. This information includes the structure, biochemistry, method of cellular destruction, manner of spread, and therapy for treatment. This wealth of information existed when Antonio penned those words. Many details of this disease have yet to be understood, but that is true of all illnesses.

Medical Authorities Quoted Out of Context

This common mistake often leads to heightened fear because the citations usually exaggerate the situation as being worse than it is. One author claims that forty different AIDS viruses exist according to the National Cancer Institute and the Pasteur Institute, the two most famous centers for AIDS research. However, these two centers claim that only two different viruses have been isolated.[9] The forty viruses claimed are actually slight variations on the same virus, the equivalent of different hair color or body size in human beings. Most viruses and bacteria have dozens of different strains, so the HIV is not unique in this regard. The two viruses, HIV-1 and HIV-2, have distinctive proteins and genetic material and almost surely will require different vaccines. This is not true for the forty strains.

James McKeever claims that Robert Gallo, the most famous American AIDS researcher, has said that a cure for AIDS was impossible in anyone's lifetime.[10] Although Gallo realizes the task is difficult, he does not say it is impossible. He has actually expressed some optimism about treatments being developed that will enhance life, if not completely cure AIDS. Paul Cameron strongly implies that Gallo had seen convincing evidence that mosquitoes could transmit AIDS,[11] a position Gallo has taken a strong stand against. (See our more complete discussion of this in chapter 9.) McKeever quotes Max Essex of Harvard out of context when the latter said the blood supply is not absolutely safe.[12] No reputable scientist has ever suggested the blood supply is utterly safe. Even before the AIDS epidemic, transfusions carried the risk of potentially life threatening viral infections and allergic reactions. Essex was not saying anything frightening or novel as McKeever implies. Essex was also quoted by Antonio as saying that 20 to 30 percent of college-age women were going to acquire HIV.[13] Although that is theoretically possible (if all college women receive lobotomies), it is unlikely except under the absolute worst scenario, a fact of which Essex is keenly aware.

Authors have misquoted research in the same manner that people misquote Scripture. Either the writer misunderstands the source he is quoting or he has preconceived notions he is trying to prove. With a fixed bias, the writer goes to medical sources looking for a quote that will support his contention, when it actually does not. In the process, error is committed twice: the author is unfair to his sources, drawing them into his mistake, and the author is unfair to his readers, generating unnecessary anxiety with his false conclusions.

Perpetuation of Unfounded Ideas

Ideas that have been proven false are sometimes resurrected to support unwarranted conclusions. Two claims repeatedly emphasized by Christian authors well illustrate this mistake.

"AIDS can be spread casually or by insect bites." This assertion has been made dozens of times, and we showed clearly in chapter 9 that it has been disproven. The second mistake is related to the first: "AIDS is the deadliest epidemic since the Black Plague." Although AIDS is a terrible disease that will cause more death in the industrialized countries than any other *infectious* disease of the last fifty years, it is not in the same category as bubonic plague. The only way it could be so severe is if it were transmitted casually or by insect bites, which it is not.

A report from the Centers for Disease Control in early 1990 showed that the number of AIDS cases had risen only 9 percent over the previous year.[14] Yet most Christian books on

AIDS emphasize the annual doubling of the number of victims and make claims such as the following:

- By 1991 sixty-four million in the U.S. will be infected with HIV;[15]

- By 1997 fifty million in the U.S. will be infected;[16]

- By 1998 20 percent of the U.S. will be dead or dying of AIDS.[17]

These figures are so skewed they are ludicrous. For example, this simplistic doubling each year of U.S. casualties never goes beyond 64 million. The reason is obvious—if you carry the calculations out two more years, 128 million will be infected by 1992 and 256 million by 1993. The entire population of the United States would be infected before the middle of the 1990s. Not even casually contracted lethal illnesses such as smallpox or plague came close to that rate of spread. And AIDS is a simple epidemic to stop compared to lethal illnesses of the past: start practicing biblical principles about sex and IV drug abuse.

AIDS needs to be put in perspective. Heart disease and cancer cause more death in the U.S. each year than AIDS likely ever will. And the one million annual deaths from heart disease and the one-half million deaths from cancer are several times the number of deaths from AIDS in its entire first decade. Moreover, in underdeveloped countries, diseases such as dysentery, malaria, measles, and whooping cough already cause millions of deaths yearly, and developed countries have shown little concern. We are concerned about the AIDS epidemic only because it directly affects us.

Mistakes of Emotional Manipulation

We often respond more readily to appeals targeted at our emotions rather than our intellects when important areas of our lives such as health, children, or livelihood are threatened. This type of appeal is common in the AIDS epidemic.

Many authors appeal to our aversion to the homosexual life-style when they claim that homosexuals are a serious threat to our families and health. Two authors vividly describe the extreme practices of a minority of homosexual males.[18] Describing homosexual practices, other than anal sex and promiscuity, is not relevant to the discussion since they do not contribute to the epidemic. The only purpose in discussing them is to repel the reader, which drives a wedge between Christians and male homosexuals, most of whom are also disgusted by these extreme practices. Scripture states that homosexual acts are wrong regardless of how "clean" or "unclean" they are. Two lesbians sensuously kissing are committing sin just as surely as the homosexual male involved in sadomasochistic sex. It is natural for the Christian to be offended by these practices, but that does not lessen our call to minister to homosexuals. The drunk passed out on the ground, the prostitute petitioning on the street corner, and the drug addict lost in a chemical high will not make us comfortable either, but that is the nature of our fallen world. Jesus did not avoid uncomfortable situations; he slept in the house of sinners, conversed with prostitutes, and touched lepers.

Medical economics is another area of emotional manipulation. Several authors claim that AIDS will bankrupt the insurance companies,[19] destroy our medical-care system,[20] and wreck the national economy.[21] Chilton even claims that if the epidemic continues to be only mild, then "productivity will have plummeted to a third-world level."[22] These authors support their contentions by multiplying the initial cost estimate for the care of the average AIDS patient, which was forty-seven thousand dollars per patient from time of diagnosis to death, by the inflated number of victims discussed above. The errors made here are two-fold. First, the number of victims will not be nearly as many as they claim. Second, the cost of care per patient will undoubtedly come down, as it already has. (Most recent estimates make the cost per patient about twenty-five thousand dollars.) The current costs are not out of range for other chronic diseases such as cancer, renal disease, and heart disease.[23] Virtually any new disease or type of therapy costs more initially. Although the authors' claims are deceptive, it is true that we do not have unlimited funds for medical care. Hard choices will have to be made about expenditures for HIV and other illnesses.

Mistakes of Logic

A number of times authors quote medical information accurately, but then leap to untenable conclusions. Antonio quotes an article citing 6 percent of AIDS patients with unknown transmission, and then strongly implies that this confirms casual contagiousness or spread through mosquitoes.[24] That 6 percent is now down to less than one-half of 1 percent (see chapter 6), and most of those have a history of sexually transmitted diseases and are presumed to have caught HIV by sexual contact. Antonio should have been aware that many people lie about their immoral behavior, but he fails to qualify the information and thereby gives a false impression. He also tries to establish respiratory spread of AIDS by linking it to tuberculosis, which is spread by coughing.[25] Just because AIDS patients may spread TB through coughing does not mean they can spread HIV the same way. It is illogical and irresponsible to make such a connection.

Another fallacious maneuver described in the previous chapter is the use of unqualified statistics to suggest casual contagiousness, such as the 300 percent increase in AIDS risk if one lives under the same roof with a person with AIDS or that 17 percent of housemates contract AIDS by nonsexual means. These statistics are easily explained by the routine methods of spread through sexual intercourse and childbirth.

Accusations of Deception

The claims of intentional cover-up are outlandish. One author implies that public health officials are not being honest with the public, another says they are knowingly being dishonest, and another claims that a "consistent campaign of disinformation" has occurred.[26] As we showed in chapter 9, these are serious charges that are not supported with substantive data. We are not saying the medical community has not made mistakes—we point out some errors ourselves. But the mistakes made usually have involved policy matters rather than some nefarious attempt to deceive the public. The medical information may be clear; how to implement changes in society to slow the spread of HIV disease usually are not.

Judging Written Material about AIDS

These criticisms of Christian writings on AIDS could continue for some time. Many more examples exist. But rather than dwell on these criticisms, we want to give guidelines so that you will be able to evaluate inaccuracies. Here are some questions you should ask:

Does the quoted material accurately depict what the original author said, or is there a discrepancy between the quote and the interpretation of the quote? Is the quoted information from a respected source, such as a medical journal, or is it from second-hand sources, as in a newspaper or magazine? A major difference exists between quotes from the *New England Journal of Medicine* and the *National Enquirer*.

Is the author logical in going from facts to conclusions? Are the conclusions more excessive than the quotes from which they were derived?

Is the author deviating in the extreme from what objective experts are saying? Are there supporting statements from other doctors? What do experts you trust in your community say?

Is the author suggesting some application that goes beyond the implications of the facts or examples given? Do the applications appear to be self-serving or lacking in compassion?

Is the author taking one or two cases that may be untrue or at least rare exceptions and trying to enforce generalized actions for society based on them?

When the Christian author and publisher place a work in circulation that is inflammatory and untrue, it not only discredits them, it also discredits our Lord. Authors and publishers need to be responsible for what they print.

THEOLOGICAL MISTAKES

Most of the errors mentioned thus far were addressed in the medical section of this book. Although these mistakes are important, they are not as serious as the errors we will cover in the rest of this chapter. As the epidemic continues, most of the medical errors will become manifestly false. It will be obvious by the middle of the 1990s that sixty-four million Americans do not have HIV disease. Also, as the epidemic becomes an accepted part of American life, like cancer or heart disease, it will be apparent that people who visit or eat with AIDS patients do not become ill. In other words, the books we have criticized will not only become obsolete, they will also stand as a testimony to the hysteria of their time.

On the other hand, the ways in which Christians are to respond are based on Scripture and do not depend on the medical developments of the epidemic. The Christian community has a solid basis for making decisions on AIDS (or any other disease) right now. No better method exists for deciding actions than to mimic our Lord when he walked with men. The rock that is our foundation for action is Christ. We have abundant examples in his life of the proper response to sin, disease, suffering, and death. Yet the Christian community has often responded incorrectly to this epidemic because of the following mistakes.

Ignoring the Sin

This position is represented by a number of liberal churches and church leaders who prefer to believe modern psychological dogma rather than the Word of God. They claim that homosexuals are a persecuted minority who must be accepted regardless of their practices. Several books on AIDS written by people who claim a Christian faith take this position.[27] Many more are bound to follow. Yet no reference to homosexuality in Scripture presents it in a favorable light. It is always referred to as sin, which is destructive personally and repugnant to the Lord. Too often what is called love is modern American sentimentalism borne out of the concept of absolute freedom for all people to do whatever they desire. It deifies a warped idea of love while ignoring truth and character.

Misunderstanding the Sin of Immoral Sexuality

Some pastors believe that no more serious sin exists than homosexuality. This idea helps energize the belief that AIDS is a judgment on homosexuals. This mistake is the opposite extreme of the previous one. Active homosexuality is a terrible sin deserving of spiritual death, but it is not worse than murder, rape, or unrepentant blasphemy, which are also deserving of death.

We are called upon as Christians to love others in spite of their sin. The Great Commission is a command to spread the good news to all people, not just to non-sinners. To show compassion toward the spiritually sick is not to condone their sin. Jesus was criticized by the Pharisees for his desire to minister to sinners. If we do not reach out as Christ did, then we are acting like the Pharisees, whom Jesus strongly rebuked.

The claim that homosexuals are being judged by God, while he excludes adulterers, perpetrators of incest, and murderers, has to do with cultural, not scriptural influences. Only one passage (Romans 1) gives the suggestion that homosexual acts are more severe than other sexual sins, yet even there the verses do not state that homosexual acts are the most dreadful. (This mistaken impression of the severity of homosexuality will be thoroughly developed in the next three chapters.)

The Secularization of Evangelical Christianity

Christians often act like non-Christians, and one of secular man's most basic concerns is death. Since secular man thinks his existence ends when he dies, he may have an inordinate desire to extend life. This desire may be manifested in various ways, such as an exercise craze, attempts to appear young, midlife crises, and avoidance of death and suffering in society. It would be morbid to say that one should look forward to possible suffering prior to death. But for the Christian, death has lost its sting. Or has it? Most of the books that suggest casual contagiousness for AIDS give little emphasis to ministering to AIDS patients in spite of the supposed danger. Yet our heritage as Christians has been to proclaim the good news as God leads regardless of the cost. In some situations that might mean imprisonment; in others, loss of job or prestige; in others, loss of life from illness or martyrdom. We have been purchased with a great price and our lives are not our own. Thankfully, in the case of AIDS, our lives are not at risk.

Even more odious is the concern that the AIDS epidemic will affect our standard of living. We are warned repeatedly in various Christian books that the medical costs of the epidemic will cause major repercussions in our economy. Although some concern should be voiced, an inordinate concern for our pocketbooks when many are dying is reprehensible.

Another theological error that is harder to depict is the tendency for the Christian community to rejoice that God's laws on sexuality have been vindicated by this epidemic. Although God's good purposes for restricting the expressions of our sexuality have become clearer, why do we have to exult in that? We should not need the confirmation of dying people to know that Scripture is true.

Self-righteousness

Placing ourselves above others is a terrible theological error. Jesus responded to it with anger, more so than with any other sin, because self-righteousness is a way of making oneself a god. Since no one except the Lord knows the hearts of others, we will not overtly accuse anyone of this sin. However, we have seen actions and read works by Christians that show signs of self-righteousness, such as degrading others, boasting of personal accomplishments, and showing a limited tendency to love the unlovely.

All of these run counter to the clear example of Christ who, though equal to God, chose the lowly position of a servant to reach a lost world. Jesus as God Incarnate was willing to eat with sinners, talk with the prostitutes, and sleep in the houses of immoral businessmen. Jesus did not ignore the sin he saw around him; rather, he reached out to the sinners because, as the Great Physician, he had come to heal the sick. Jesus understood the terrible consequences of sexual sin, but he refused to write these people off as unworthy of his compassion.

TIME FOR A NEW DIRECTION

Ecclesiastes gives us wise instruction for our current circumstances. It is a study of life lived under the sun, life without God. Life under the sun is trivial, discouraging, and full of pain. We, who have Christ, may have forgotten what it means to be "under the sun." Charles Swindoll said it well in his introductory remarks on Ecclesiastes:

> One of the reasons we are so boring as a people is that we read our immortality message into every single scene. It is also the reason that we don't have too many real answers for the real problems in life. We are too quick with the ultimate answers to feel the horror of the present pain.[28]

Life "under the sun" is full of pain. Dying slowly of a debilitating disease, whether self-caused or not, is horrible. Salvation answers do not ring true to an unsaved man unless accompanied by the sacrificial compassion of Christ.

It is time for us who have been reborn through the Spirit to remember what it is like to be "under the sun." Until we are willing to remember and to share the hurt, our answers will seem other-worldly. Jesus is the example. He was willing to sacrifice his high place and to have no place to rest his head. He was willing to be scourged, to carry the cross for his execution, and to feel the violation of his body by nails and a sword. Jesus did all this and more and asks us to do the same—for those "under the sun."

Chapter 10, Notes

---

1. Patrick Dixon, *The Truth about AIDS* (Eastbourne, U.K.: Kingsway Publications, 1987), 62, 94.

2. Gene Antonio, *The AIDS Cover-Up?* (San Francisco: Ignatius Press, 1987), 1, 26, 43.

3. David Reagan and Thomas Baker, *What the Bible Says about AIDS* (McKinney, Tex.: Lamb and Lion Ministries, 1988), 3-4.

4. Antonio, *AIDS Cover-Up?*, 7.

5. David Chilton, *Power in the Blood* (Brentwood, Tenn.: Wolgemuth and Hyatt, 1987), 14.

6. Dixon, *Truth about AIDS*, 48.

7. Antonio, *AIDS Cover-Up?*, 126.

8. Ibid., 129.

9. Chilton, *Power in the Blood*, 48.

10. James McKeever, *The AIDS Plague* (Medford, Ore.: Omega Publications, 1986), 38.

11. Paul Cameron, *Exposing the AIDS Scandal* (Lafayette, La.: Huntington House, 1988), 59.

12. McKeever, *AIDS Plague*, 79.

13. Antonio, *AIDS Cover-Up?*, 241.

14. Centers for Disease Control update on AIDS in Associated Press report, "Spread of AIDS Cases Slowing for Most Groups," *Austin American-Statesman*, 9 February 1990.

15. Ibid., 133; and Reagan and Baker, *What the Bible Says*, 6.

16. McKeever, *AIDS Plague*, 46.

17. Ibid., 11.

18. Chilton, *Power in the Blood*, 31-45; and Antonio, *AIDS Cover-Up?*, 33-65.

19. Chilton, *Power in the Blood*, 24; and McKeever, *AIDS Plague*, 93.

20. Antonio, *AIDS Cover-Up?*, 240; and Chilton, *Power in the Blood*, 24.

21. Antonio, *AIDS Cover-Up?*, 138.

22. Chilton, *Power in the Blood*, 24.

23. H. Fineberg, "The Social Dimensions of AIDS," *Scientific American* 259 (1988):133.

24. Antonio, *AIDS Cover-Up?*, 106-7.

25. Ibid., 120-21.

26. Chilton, *Power in the Blood*, 28; Cameron, *AIDS Scandal*, 48; and Antonio, *AIDS Cover-Up?*, xii.

27. Eileen Flynn, *AIDS: A Catholic Call for Compassion* (Kansas City, Mo.: Sheed and Ward, 1985); Earl Shelp and Ronald Sunderland, *AIDS and the Church* (Philadelphia: Westminister Press, 1987); and Elisabeth Kubler-Ross, *AIDS: The Ultimate Challenge* (New York: Macmillan Publishing Co., 1987).

28. From Charles Swindoll, "Living on the Ragged Edge," a series of taped sermons on Ecclesiastes (1983). In 1984 the sermons were aired on the radio program, "Insight for Living." These sermons were later developed into the book *Living on the Ragged Edge* (Waco, Tex.: Word Books, 1985), but the quote was not included.

Do you not know that the wicked will not inherit the kingdom of God? Do not be deceived: Neither the sexually immoral nor idolaters nor adulterers nor male prostitutes nor homosexual offenders nor thieves nor the greedy nor drunkards nor slanderers nor swindlers will inherit the kingdom of God. And that is what some of you were. But you were washed, you were sanctified, you were justified in the name of the Lord Jesus Christ and by the Spirit of our God (1 Corinthians 6:9-11).

If a man is found sleeping with another man's wife, both the man who slept with her and the woman must die. You must purge the evil from Israel (Deuteronomy 22:22).

"'Do not lie with a man as one lies with a woman; that is detestable.
"'Do not have sexual relations with an animal and defile yourself with it'" (Leviticus 18:22-23).

We know that the law is good if one uses it properly (1 Timothy 1:8).

Chapter Eleven

Homosexuality and Sins against the Body

The Ecstasy

The San Francisco Gay Freedom Day Marching Band blared the opening notes to "California Here I Come," and the parade started its two-mile trek down Market Street toward City Hall. More than 30,000 people, grouped in 240 contingents, marched in the parade past 200,000 spectators. The parade was the best show in town, revealing the diversity of gay life. Clusters of gay Catholics and Episcopalians, Mormons and atheists, organized for years in the city, marched proudly beneath their banners. Career-designated contingents of gays included lawyers and labor officials, dentists and doctors, accountants and the ubiquitous gay phone-company employees. There were lesbian moms, gay dads, and homosexual teenagers with their heterosexual parents. Gay blacks, Latinos, Asian-Americans, and American Indians marched beneath banners proclaiming their dual pride. The campy Gays Against Brunch formed their own marching unit. A group of drag queens, dressed as nuns and calling themselves the Sisters of Perpetual Indulgence, had picked the day for their debut.

Gay tourists streamed to this homophile mecca from all over the world for the high holy day of homosexual life. Floats came from Phoenix and Denver; gay cowboys from the Reno Gay Rodeo pranced their horses down Market Street, waving the flags of Nevada and California, as well as the rainbow flag that had become the standard of California gays.[1]

* * * * * *

The Agony
    The fight against venereal diseases was proving to be a Sisyphean task. Ostrow was director of the Howard Brown Memorial Clinic, which provided a sensitive alternative for gay men who wanted to avoid the sneers of staffers at the Chicago Public Health clinics. The screening in Ostrow's clinic had revealed that one in ten patients had walked in the door with hepatitis B. In San Francisco, two-thirds of gay men had suffered the debilitating disease. It was now proven statistically that a gay man had one chance in five of being infected with hepatitis B virus within 12 months of stepping off the bus into a typical urban gay scene. Within five years, infection was a virtual certainty.
    Another problem was enteric diseases, like amebiasis and giardiasis, caused by organisms that lodge themselves in the intestinal tracts of gay men with alarming frequency. At the New York Gay Men's Health Project, where Dan William was medical director, 30 percent of the patients suffered from gastrointestinal parasites. In San Francisco, incidence of "Gay Bowel Syndrome," as it was called in the medical journals, had increased by 8,000 percent after 1973. Infection with these parasites was a likely effect of anal intercourse, which was apt to put a man in contact with his partner's fecal matter, and was virtually a certainty through the then-popular practice of rimming, which medical journals politely called oral-anal intercourse.
    What was so troubling was that nobody in the gay community seemed to care about these waves of infection.[2]

* * * * * *

*T*hese words, written by a homosexual, recount the homosexual climate in some of the tolerant cities in the late seventies and early eighties. Even then a virus, as yet undescribed, was slowly depleting the T-helper cells of many of these marchers. AIDS is one more demonstration that sexual immorality of all types is intrinsically harmful. Not only is immorality a sin against God, it also leads to problems such as sexually transmitted diseases, frequent divorces, children born to single parents, and over one million abortions a year. In sex, as in religion, when it is good (biblical) it is very, very good; and when it is bad, it is horrid.

SEXUAL PERVERSION

John and I have committed sexual perversions. So have you, the reader. Each of us has perverted the good gift of sexuality, at least within our own mind. We lust after another person's spouse; we use sex to gain power over our husband or wife; we dwell on the attractiveness of a movie star; we become obsessed with being married if we are single or we want to be with someone else if we are married; we fantasize about homosexual affairs. In secular society, sin has been dismissed as nonexistent. In Christian circles, it has been minimized so as not to trouble us. Anyone who thinks he has not sinned sexually has either defined sin as overt action, which neither the Old Testament ("You shall not covet your neighbor's wife") nor Jesus does ("Anyone who looks at a woman lustfully has already committed adultery with her in his heart"), or he has discounted his errant desires as insignificant, forgetting that all sin is significant to God. We write this not to bring despair, because all sin is forgivable, but to bring reality to the discussion of sexual sin. None of us is so blameless that we can self-righteously condemn the homosexual or promiscuous heterosexual for his or her sins.

All have sinned and fall short of God's glory; all have also been sinned against. Consider the slightly built teenage boy who prefers reading novels to battering bodies in football. This is "unforgivable" for a fifteen year old. The other boys do not let him forget it; the girls tease him without mercy. The "in" crowd calls him "homo" and "fag" and after a while he may start believing it. His father is distant, giving no approval to his talents or his person. He goes to college and meets an affirming, middle-aged man who celebrates his gifts, treats him with the respect he has craved, and teaches him a new form of sexuality.

All have sinned; all have been sinned against. Consider the fourteen-year-old girl who has a normal childhood until her stepfather begins showing a lot of interest in her when she enters puberty. She tries to resist his advances but is confused by her desire to be close to her dad and his sexual desire for her. She explains her anxiety to her mother, who reassures her that men are like that and she might as well get used to it. After being abused a number of times over several months, she decides she can never get used to it and becomes one of the million runaways a year. Her $87 runs out by the second week, and she becomes hungry. She meets other boys and girls "turning tricks" on the street and thinks she would never do that. She gets hungrier. She cannot get a job because she's too young, has no identification, and no clean clothes. A pimp sees her innocence and says he can buy her clothes, food, and shelter. You'll get used to it, he claims. And this time she has to—at least with the help of drugs.

All have sinned; all have been sinned against. Consider the twenty-six-year-old woman with three young kids abandoned by her husband of eight years. She has no skills, so she goes on welfare and Medicaid. If she works as an unskilled laborer, she cannot work enough to get ahead because she loses her government assistance. She does not have the money or energy with three preschool children to finish vocational training. Friends and family help a little, but her dependence on government and family helps destroy her self-esteem. Along comes a man who says she is pretty, who seems good with the kids, and who will support her. He moves in, and she feels better for a while, until his drinking starts. After several beatings, she has the police forcibly evict him. Along comes another man, who says she is pretty and that he'll help with the bills. She feels better until he tires of her and disappears one day. Along comes another man . . .

All have sinned; all have been sinned against. These situations are far more common than most of us are aware. Sexual immorality is always sin, but the story behind the sin often makes it more understandable. That which we would never do becomes possible under the right circumstances. Our society has created a sexually inhumane culture that is light-years away from the fulfillment promised by the high priests of "free love." The reality is ugly, exploitive, and particularly detrimental to the weak. As the family continues to deteriorate, more children and teens will see drugs and sex as the only highs that make life worth continuing. Until the church does more to help these people in a tangible way, we have no right to denounce them as subhuman. Christ never berated any person he met, no matter how lascivious that person's life. On the other hand, neither should we blithely accept justifications for sin. As a church we must stand against sin but with genuine tears and sadness for the sinner.

HETEROSEXUAL PROMISCUITY

Promiscuity of any sort is a perversion. The heterosexual variety is causing HIV disease to make slow inroads into the general population. AIDS will likely increase, since in our hypersexualized society, sexual union with many others is not only given tacit acceptance, it is encouraged. The "safe sex" campaign, which wrongly implies that condoms are completely protective, encourages sexual experience even in our teenagers. Promiscuous behavior eventually becomes either addictive or numbing. As with drug addiction, sexual addiction produces a compulsion toward increased frequency and more exotic experiences. Sex quickly becomes boring if there is no depth to the relationship between the partners. The promiscuous individual then looks for a novel experience with others, wrongly assuming there is something inadequate about his partner rather than with his expectations for sex. As Ecclesiastes says, "It is like chasing the wind." One cannot catch the wind no matter how many partners, how many positions, or how exotic the sexual practices.

Promiscuous sex can also be numbing, especially for women. Sex is given liberally to achieve secondary gains such as security, companionship, money, or drugs. The lonely woman frequently does not enjoy the act itself, but has sex to gain intimacy. Companionship and security could be provided by Christians to the millions of single mothers, but the church has not adapted to the changing times. These women need the love of Christ desperately, but few new programs have been initiated to minister to them. Instead of Christ's love, women often turn in desperation to the exploitive "love" of men who use them for a while and then discard them. Moreover, Christians should be aware of the ease of falling into sexual sin, since we have seen many Christian leaders commit immorality. If reborn men and women succumb to the seduction of the time, how much more forgiving should we be of the lonely man or woman who yields, hoping for some meaning and intimacy in life.

HOMOSEXUALITY JUSTIFIED?

A growing theological trend to justify homosexual acts has occurred over the last thirty years. Yet nowhere does the Old or New Testament declare homosexuality to be good. Not one single story, not one single verse. Eight passages condemn it outright including: "Do not lie with a man as one lies with a woman; that is detestable" (Leviticus 18:22); "Men committed indecent acts with other men, and received in themselves the due penalty for their perversion" (Romans 1:27b); "Neither the sexually immoral . . . nor homosexual offenders . . . will inherit the kingdom of God" (1 Corinthians 6:9-10). Many additional verses denounce homosexuality implicitly, such as verses about Sodom and Gomorrah or the tendency of some to go after "strange flesh." On the other hand, neither does Scripture overemphasize homosexuality and suggest it is the worst of all sins. Materialism, self-righteousness, and heterosexual sins are condemned far more often.

It is impossible to legitimize homosexuality from

Scripture without misinterpreting some verses and disregarding others. As one New Testament Greek scholar put it, "The fact is that an ancient Greek, or a modern scholar of ancient Greek, even if he were reading the New Testament for the first time . . . would have not the slightest difficulty in understanding [that the New Testament condemns homosexuality]."[3] Nevertheless, homosexuals who want religious involvement attempt this reinterpretation. For example, the Metropolitan Church is a national denomination composed largely of homosexual men. They attempt to justify their behavior in the following ways:

1. *Love is the overriding emphasis in Scripture; therefore, any love between people is acceptable.*

This is the sort of theology emphasized in Bishop Robinson's *Honest to God* and Joseph Fletcher's *Situation Ethics*, both published in the 1960s. Many other works since then suggest the same ideas. But the love spoken of in the New Testament is self-sacrificing *agape*, not the grasping for self-desire evident in the free-love culture. Agape love can be expressed toward everyone without measure, except in a sexual sense, which is reserved solely for heterosexual marriage. Moreover, although love is the greatest commandment, it is not the only one. Love does not eliminate our responsibility to obey other commandments, including those on sexual purity, laid down by God.

2. *Jesus never directly condemned homosexuality.*

Although Jesus does not mention homosexuality by name, he does say that any form of sexuality outside of heterosexual marriage is sinful, since it is man and woman who are to be joined (Matthew 19:4-5).[4] The only alternative to marriage between a man and a woman that Jesus offered was celibacy (Matthew 19:11-12). Arguments from silence are weak and can be used to justify many other sins. Christ did not say anything specifically against wife-beating, incest, or bestiality, but few would say these are therefore acceptable.

Many say that the Old Testament laws, including those condemning homosexuality, are obsolete, but Paul, Peter,

and Jude in the New Testament specifically condemn homosexual acts, and most all the New Testament writers emphasize that marriage is heterosexual. None of the old moral law
was eliminated; it was strengthened by Jesus when he said
that not only immoral action was sinful, but also immoral
thought. Jesus said he came to fulfill the Law, not to overturn it. Some rituals of the Old Testament are no longer necessary because they were mere shadows of what was to
come, that is, Christ.

3. *The church has misunderstood the meaning of passages
that appear to condemn homosexuality.*

Derrick Bailey in 1955 (*Homosexuality in the Western
Christian Tradition*) was the first serious theologian to suggest
that no condemnation of homosexuality occurs in the Bible.
Many others have followed.[5] By linguistic twisting, the sin of
Sodom and Gomorrah becomes homosexual rape and lack of
hospitality. The condemnation against unnatural sin in
Romans 1:26-27 is distorted to condemn only heterosexuals
who go against their nature and practice homosexuality. (By
this reasoning a "true" homosexual would be sinning if he
married a woman since that would be acting against his
nature.) First Corinthians 6:9 is said to refer not to homosexuality in general but to homosexual prostitution or pederasty.[6]

So claim some homosexual apologists. These modern
theologians have not discovered some ancient text that gives
clear reasons to reinterpret these passages. The only situation that has changed is the way our society thinks about
homosexuality. It is not a coincidence that Bailey's book
came out just a few years after the flawed Kinsey report on
male sexuality, which dramatically overemphasized the
amount of homosexuality in America (see chapter 4).

Passages condemning homosexuality have been uniformly interpreted since their writing. All of the church
fathers, the medieval scholastics, and biblical scholars until
the twentieth century asserted that the New Testament condemned homosexuality.[7] Also Jewish commentators until
modern times unvaryingly said that the sins of Sodom and

Gomorrah included homosexuality (there were others as listed in Ezekiel 16:49-50). The standard for all modern studies of biblical Greek is Bauer, Arndt, and Gingrich's *A Greek-English Lexicon of the New Testament*, which is used by liberal and conservative theologians alike. According to this lexicon, our modern translations of the Bible accurately reflect what the Greek states: homosexuality is condemned.[8] To change what has been the clear understanding of Scripture through the ages without new discoveries is to impose one's beliefs on Scripture. If these people want to accept homosexuality as normal, that is their option, but they do so against the indisputable teaching of the Bible.

Dispelling Other Arguments
for the Validity of Homosexuality

Proponents of homosexuality offer many other arguments for the validity of their behavior, but these arguments are faulty as well and are easily answered. We need to remind ourselves, however, that our response should be given in the spirit of reconciliation demonstrated in 1 Peter 3:15: "Always be prepared to give an answer to everyone who asks you to give the reason for the hope that you have. But do this with *gentleness and respect.* . . ." The attractiveness of God in our lives is what entices people to Christianity, coupled with reasonable answers to their objections.

1. Homosexuality is not a choice.

If no choice is involved, then how can an individual be condemned for being a homosexual?

Historical transformations. Prior to "scientific" psychology, homosexuality was not considered a permanent state. Psychologist Stanton Jones says that homosexuality as a lifelong desire virtually never exists in preindustrial societies.[9] French philosopher Michel Foucault, a homosexual who died of AIDS, admitted that before Victorian times people considered homosexuality to be immoral actions, not a definitive orientation. Not until nineteenth-century England did it begin to be thought of as a disease of consistent desire.[10] Freudian psychotherapy added that homosexuality was due to arrested development in childhood.[11] Earlier in the twentieth century, many argued that genetics or hormones caused a man or woman to be attracted to the same sex. This notion has fallen out of favor for lack of scientific evidence. Over the last two centuries, the perception of homosexuality has changed from sexual sin to abnormal orientation to genetic or hormonal determinism to something entirely normal. None of these alterations occurred because of new scientific knowledge, just a new outlook or "faith."

Genes or hormones? Pro-homosexual scientists such as Evelyn Hooker,[12] Masters and Johnson,[13] and sex researcher John Money[14] all deny that genes or hormones cause homosexuality. Money postulates that embryonic hormonal exposure may influence outcome, but it is not determinative. Moreover, studies on identical twins, the facile movement of many between homosexual and heterosexual activity, and the virtual nonexistence of permanent homosexual orientation in third-world societies strongly refute genetic or hormonal determination of homosexuality.

Is homosexuality changeable? Homosexuals say they cannot change, yet the vast majority of psychologists until recent times have stated that homosexuals can change, albeit with some difficulty. Alfred Kinsey, in his 1948 report on male sexuality, documented how fluid the movement is from homosexuality into heterosexuality and vice versa.[15] Studies showing that 65 percent of homosexual men have had sex with a woman in the past few years strongly suggest the flux of homosexual desire.[16]

Masters and Johnson report successful cures in 50 to 60 percent of their homosexual patients.[17] Numerous other professionals report similar success by various means (individual psychotherapy, group therapy, behavior modification, aversion therapy, and positive reinforcement).[18] Despite the rhetoric of homosexual activists, *all* studies which have attempted conversions from homosexuality to heterosexuality have had significant success.[19] Moreover, Christian therapists such as Rekers and Wilson have had even greater success with Christians in the homosexual life-style who became committed to change.[20]

Homosexual activists argue that these people either were never truly homosexuals or they did not truly change. But this is circular reasoning. There is no blood test or sign that someone is "truly homosexual" or that one is "truly changed" because those are not valid categories. A homosexual act is a sin, not a state of being. Therefore one can look only at behavior to validate change. As one author said, "I have never met a former white, former black, or former Hispanic. But I do know a number of former homosexuals."[21] So do we. Change is not easy because sexual addictions have usually occurred for some time and to escape them requires lots of love, therapy, and support. But there is no sinful behavior that the power of Christ cannot overcome. Many men and women can testify that Christ has changed their desire for the same sex into normal heterosexual desire.

2. *Homosexuality is entirely natural.*

No difference in physiology. Since no physiologic differences exist between avowed homosexuals and heterosexuals, militant homosexuals now assert that their behavior is normal. They claim that to prefer same-gender sex is analogous to a heterosexual man preferring to have sex with a blonde. Homosexual activists originally said homosexuality was normal because it was determined by genes or hormones. When there was no evidence for this, the activists did a reversal and said homosexuality was normal because there was no difference between their biological makeup and that of heterosexuals. Consistency in reasoning is lacking; consistent belief against the evidence is not. Studies of murderers, pederasts, thieves, and liars would also not show a physiological difference from other people because these actions involve sinful choices, not biological differences.

Homosexuality is obviously a nonnatural phenomenon in other ways. The rectum is not designed for the penetration that occurs during anal sex, a common sexual practice among homosexual men, and lesbians often use artificial apparatuses during their sexual activity. Most couples desire children, yet reproduction for the homosexual couple is impossible without artificial insemination or "womb borrowing."

Moreover, an imbalance exists in same-sex unions. Men and women are different, not just physically but emotionally, behaviorally, psychologically, intellectually, and spiritually.[22] These differences complement each other in normal heterosexual relationships, but in same-sex relationships that balance is lost. Men, who are more naturally promiscuous, have a hard time finding committed homosexual relationships; most homosexual men do not desire monogamy, but have been forced to be less promiscuous because of AIDS.[23] Lesbians tend toward longer term relationships than do homosexual men. This is in keeping with women in general, who are more relational and security conscious than men.

Lesbians have been studied much less than homosexual men, in part because the numbers are significantly lower. Although they are less promiscuous than homosexual men, their relationships are more likely to be disturbed by misunderstanding, insecurity, and jealousy. Instability is common.[24] Some studies show a rate of alcoholism and drug abuse twenty times as frequent as in the general population.[25]

Psychiatrists say homosexuality is normal. As we saw in a previous chapter, the American Psychiatric Association (APA) voted in 1973 to remove homosexuality from its list of disorders. But the vote was tainted. Evelyn Hooker, who chaired the committee that made the pro-homosexual recommendation, had studied homosexuality in the 1950s at the urging of several close homosexual friends. She was also intimately involved with several early homosexual liberation groups, giving talks to encourage and to inform them of other pro-homosexual psychologists. She came to the conclusion, not surprisingly, that homosexuality was not abnormal.[26] Since the committee was slanted with her as chairman, a pro-homosexual outcome was expected. A slim majority of the general assembly affirmed the committee's recommendation.[27]

Despite the APA vote, controversy surrounded the decision among psychiatrists in part because the National

Gay and Lesbian Task Force had conducted intense lobbying to influence the vote, including threats to disrupt APA meetings and research.[28] (Modern "science" is now conducted by ballots, lobbying, and threats; so much for scientific objectivity.) Despite the APA's stance, 69 percent of its members continue to view homosexuality as aberrant,[29] and treatments for conversion from homosexuality are routinely discussed in journals.[30] Three out of four Americans are still convinced homosexuality is wrong in all circumstances, despite a steady diet of propaganda from the media.[31] Part of the problem in this whole debate is that homosexuals are usually no more sick than adulterers, liars, or people who shortchange the IRS. They are sinners, and that does not routinely show up on tests.

Homosexuals feel normal. Feelings are notoriously poor ways of gauging what is right and wrong. We can convince ourselves that something is right regardless of the havoc it may cause. Nonetheless this line of reasoning is common among homosexuals and their supporters: "The fact that you are sexually and, even more important, emotionally drawn to someone of the same sex *cannot* be wrong, as nothing you *feel* deeply within yourself can be wrong."[32] We wonder how that author would respond if we substituted murder, rape, child abuse, or bestiality for homosexuality. Fortunately, our society has laws that keep people from acting on these types of feelings.

3. *Homosexuality hurts no one, so what happens between consenting adults should be all right.*

The Bible emphasizes that what people do sexually dramatically affects society. In our time of multitudes of abortions, venereal diseases, divorces, and AIDS deaths, the empirical evidence is conclusively in agreement with Scripture. The same type of fallacious arguments have been advanced for the use of recreational drugs, orgies, and pornography. What we do in private does affect society.

Society's outward acceptance of homosexuality removes one of the main restraints on this aberrant activity. Since it is unhealthy psychologically and physically, the barriers should remain in place. Moreover, in the case of homosexual men, a large medical bill was created to pay for their rampant sexually transmitted diseases even before AIDS. The effect on children in an age of crumbling family values is further cause for concern. A sexual identity crisis is being seen increasingly in children, and increasing openness of society towards homosexuality will only make matters worse.[33]

The attempt by homosexual radicals to move homosexuality into mainstream America shows that they do not accept their own rhetoric. If this were only an issue between consenting adults, then it could have been kept in the closet. Their strong desire to get it out in the open is an attempt to gain acceptance from everyone. In no sense are we suggesting that homosexuals should be denied constitutional rights that everyone in the U.S. enjoys, but the Christian community can be consistent in demonstrating love and acceptance of the homosexual as a lost individual while opposing statutes to legalize same-sex liaisons.[34]

4. *Many of the great men and women of history have been homosexuals.*

This argument suggests that since many of the great people in history have been homosexuals, homosexuality cannot be all bad. The implicit suggestion is that homosexuals are more sensitive and artistic than others, and we should value their great contribution to society. But studies indicate that homosexuals are no more creative on the average than heterosexuals, even if Oscar Wilde, Walt Whitman, Henry James, Willa Cather, and Gertrude Stein were homosexual.[35] We are sure other lists could demonstrate that murderers, child molesters, and wife beaters have produced great artistic achievements. That hardly makes their aberrant behavior right.

HOMOSEXUALITY—THE WORST SIN?

Although the Bible clearly calls homosexuality sin, some Christians in America have made it the most perverse of all sins. This is manifested in evangelical churches by a tendency toward sorrow and righteous anger over adultery, but revulsion and hatred in cases of homosexual sin. But homosexuality is not the worst of all sins, and we agree with one evangelical scholar that "too often [Scripture verses have] been as tools of a homophobic polemic which has claimed too much."[36] Homosexuality is a severe sin, being one of the few sins in the Old Testament punishable by death. Other sins that warranted the death penalty included murder, adultery, and rape, all of which were direct attacks on the family as ordained by God. In the Sermon on the Mount, Jesus did not lessen the severity of such sins, but intensified them by teaching that they begin in the mind.

Sexual sins are destructive because they are sins against one's own body and not simply against God and others. "All other sins a man commits are outside his body, but he who sins sexually sins against his own body" (1 Corinthians 6:18). But nowhere in Scripture is it suggested that homosexuality is worse than other sexual sins. Even Romans 1:18-32 is a general condemnation of mankind rather than a polemic against homosexuals. None of the standard commentaries suggest that the passage says that homosexuality is the worst of sins, only the most unnatural.

Homosexuality never occurs in a vacuum. Other sins will always occur with it because the basic sin is rebellion against God, not sexual immorality. Even in Sodom, the most famous example of homosexuality, the sins went far beyond lusting after the same sex. In Ezekiel, God accuses Sodom of being "arrogant, overfed and unconcerned; they did not help the poor and needy. They were haughty and did detestable things before me" (16:49-50).

Paul, the writer of Romans, at no other point states or implies that homosexuality is a more severe sin. In Galatians, prior to listing the fruit of the Spirit, Paul lists the acts of the sinful nature, beginning with sexual immorality (Galatians 5:19-21). If sodomy were a worse sin than other forms of sexual immorality, Paul would have singled it out for special condemnation. In another of Paul's lists of sins, homosexuality is located in the middle of the list after idolatry and adultery; no unique denunciation is given (1 Corinthians 6:9-11). In addition, this list ends with Paul's joy that although some of the Corinthians had been involved with these sins, including homosexuality, they were now cleansed and forgiven in Christ.

Jesus also said Sodom and Gomorrah would come under less severe judgment than the cities of Israel that rejected the gospel. After giving instructions to his disciples to go to the "lost sheep of Israel", Jesus says, "If anyone will not welcome you or listen to your words, shake the dust off your feet when you leave that home or town. I tell you the truth, it will be more bearable for Sodom and Gomorrah on the day of judgment than for that town" (Matthew 10:14-15). In a similar passage, Jesus claims that Sodom would have more likely repented of her sins than the cities of the Galilee region, including his adult home town of Capernaum (Matthew 11:20-24).

No evidence can be found in Scripture that homosexuality is the most decadent sin. All sin ultimately comes down to rebellion against the loving Creator, and homosexuality is just one of many manifestations of this rebellion.

CULTURAL PREJUDICE

Since homosexuality is not the most horrible of sins, why do Christians in the U.S. often treat it as such? In part, the problem involves cultural prejudice arising from uniquely American distinctives unrelated to scriptural authority. Two broad areas are apparent. First, a pervasive myth exists in America concerning our ideals of maleness, which are often based on a simplistic and idealized view of American history. The colonists carved a new nation out of the eastern seaboard. The pioneers who went West continued the tradition by being rugged, self-reliant, and independent. Twentieth-century America is the "can-do" society that rescued Europe from two major wars and effected economic domination over the world by our strength of character.

Nothing is beyond our capabilities. Clint Eastwood, Humphrey Bogart, and Sylvester Stallone epitomize the hard, silent, powerful male who has little room for tears, friends, weakness, or relationships.

The stereotype of the homosexual male is the antithesis of this American archetype. Therefore, we react against homosexuality not because it is sinful but because it is unmanly. Homosexuality was not pointed out for special condemnation in the early church, even though it was much in evidence in the pagan cultures. Nor is there a tendency now in Europe to denounce homosexual activities, although that is largely due to Europe having been in a post-Christian era longer than the States.

A second problem is more legitimate and understandable. The homosexual community is a different culture from the rest of society and is built on two strong foundations: intense sexual involvement often with multiple partners, and the strong cohesiveness of a segregated, maligned community. These two foundations are foreign to evangelicals, who reside in the conservative mainstream. We feel more comfortable in our own social and ethnic groups, but the divide between evangelicals and homosexuals is huge compared to most cultural partitions. The level of sexual activity among homosexual men is enormous, especially before the AIDS epidemic. In the famous Bell and Weinberg study of the seventies, 28 percent of homosexual men had participated in sex with more than one thousand men. Only rarely were men in absolutely monogamous relationships.[37] Moreover, the varieties of sexual techniques, including anal sex, sadomasochism, cross-dressing, contact with fecal material and urine, are so bizarre for most people that aversion is natural. Twenty years of "gay liberation" and homosexual activists' celebration of their sin have also caused revulsion in middle-class America. "Gay is beautiful" hardly rings true when one considers the reality of anonymous sex with hundreds of partners, sadistic beatings, multiple venereal diseases, and high levels of depression, suicide attempts, and substance abuse among homosexual men.[38] The level of promiscuity and the aggressiveness of homosexual activism in the U.S. appears to be higher than that in Europe, causing a larger rift here between homosexual men and society at large.[39]

Outside of their sexuality and their subculture, homosexuals are like most everyone else. Consequently, reaching out to the homosexual requires love in action to touch him where he feels the need. Although his true need lies in the spiritual arena (as with heterosexuals), the homosexual man is worried about his job, how he appears to others, whether other people truly care for him, and so on. Since he is created in the image of God, we should have no trouble seeing his significance even while recognizing his sin.

However, the Christian community has treated homosexual sin in a different fashion from most other sins. If an alcoholic becomes interested in Christianity, he must admit his sin, accept Christ, and be willing to change. The same is true of those involved with pornography, workaholism, materialism, or most any other sin. It is our impression, and the impression of most redeemed homosexuals, that the church's attitude toward the unredeemed homosexual is that he must change *completely* before becoming a Christian and a member of a church. Most of us did not come to Christ under those conditions and too many of us have changed little since accepting Christ. Yet we not only expect the homosexual to deny the life-style, friends, and beliefs he has accepted, perhaps for years, but we also expect him to do it on his own. It is a new form of legalism.

The two foundations of the homosexual community do make for special problems in ministry. First, because of the tight-knit community, it is notoriously ineffective to attack a homosexual's "gayness." That only confirms in his mind the need for homosexuals to be unified against the condemnation of the straight community. Christ's love and sacrifice for him as a person must be the primary emphasis. All people realize they are sinners in the broad sense, and homosexuals are no different. When we allow them to see their need for Christ, then they will be convicted by the Spirit of God and their reading of Scripture.

The other problem is that the intensity of the sexual activity of many homosexuals leads to a form of sexual addiction that is difficult to break. Like most addictions, counseling, group therapy, and help from those who have broken away are needed. Ultimately, the best person to reach out to the homosexual is the one who has himself escaped that life-style. Regrettably, these men are often caught in between, not truly accepted by the Christian community and cut loose from their old life and friends. In the end the most efficacious way of reaching homosexuals may be to provide a loving community for those who leave the homosexual life and to send missionaries into the culture supported by prayers, love, and finances.

Many sexual perversions existed in the days of Christ, including homosexuality. We have no record that Jesus had contact with homosexuals or taught on the subject specifically, but he did clearly teach that marriage binds together one man and one woman for a lifetime. This is the only legitimate and healthy form of sexual expression. The tragic results of the sexual revolution are a bitter confirmation to our society that Christ was correct.

However, it is just as true that Jesus, while not legitimizing sexual expression outside of marriage, reached out with compassion to sexual sinners. He would not have tolerated any form of mean-spirited gay-bashing. Adultery, prostitution, and lust were the sexual sins of Jesus' day, and he reached out to those caught in them because he saw the imprint of God on every person despite the muck they had dragged the image through. Does anyone doubt that Jesus would reach out to the suffering AIDS patients, to the morose men who are HIV positive, and to the men who have watched numerous friends succumb to these diseases? If we have no doubts what he would do were he here on earth, how can we do anything less?

Chapter 11, Notes

1. Randy Shilts, *And the Band Played On: Politics, People, and the AIDS Epidemic* (New York: St. Martin's Press, 1987), 14.

2. Ibid., 18-19.

3. J. Harold Greenlee, "The New Testament and Homosexuality," in *What You Should Know about Homosexuality*, ed. Charles Keysor (Grand Rapids, Mich.: Zondervan Publishing House, 1981), 102.

4. The Greek words used specifically indicate male and female, not husband and wife, so there is no validity for same-sex marriage. Ibid., 82.

5. John Oswalt, "The Old Testament and Homosexuality," in *What You Should Know about Homosexuality*, 71.

6. Letha Scanzoni and Virginia Mollenkott, *Is the Homosexual My Neighbor?* (San Francisco: Harper and Row, 1978), 67.

7. That is not to say that Christians have always maintained purity in this area, for sexual sins of all types have been committed through the centuries. Homosexual sin would have been a temptation in monasteries and convents, for example.

8. Walter Bauer, William F. Arndt, F. Wilbur Gingrich, *A Greek-English Lexicon of the New Testament and Other Early Christian Literature*, 2d ed. (Chicago: University of Chicago Press, 1979), 109.

9. Stanton Jones, "Homosexuality According to Science," *Christianity Today*, 18 August 1989, 29.

10. Tim Stafford, *The Sexual Christian* (Wheaton, Ill.: Victor Books, 1989), 134.

11. William P. Wilson, "Medical and Psychological Evidence on Homosexuality," in *Answers to Your Questions about Homosexuality*, ed. Cynthia Lanning (Wilmore, Ky.: Bristol Books, 1988), 134.

12. William H. McKain, Jr., "Ministry and Homosexuality," in *What You Should Know about Homosexuality*, 203.

13. Frank Worthen, *Steps Out of Homosexuality* (San Rafael, Calif.: Love in Action, 1984), 3.

14. John Money quoted in Constance Holden, "Doctor of Sexology," *Psychology Today*, May 1988, 46.

15. Margaret White, *AIDS and the Positive Alternatives* (Basingstoke, U.K.: Marshall Pickering, 1987), 22.

16. David Chilton, *Power in the Blood* (Brentwood, Tenn.: Wolgemuth and Hyatt, 1987), 16.

17. Stafford, *Sexual Christian*, 141.

18. William P. Wilson, "Biology, Psychology, and Homosexu-

ality," in *What You Should Know About Homosexuality*, 163-64; and Wilson, "Medical and Psychological Evidence," in *Answers to Your Questions about Homosexuality*, 152-54.

19. Jones, "Homosexuality According to Science," 29.

20. Wilson, "Medical and Psychological Evidence," in *Answers to Your Questions about Homosexuality*, 154.

21. Randy Alcorn, *Christians in the Wake of the Sexual Revolution* (Portland, Ore.: Multnomah Press, 1985), 282.

22. Wilson, "Medical and Psychological Evidence," in *Answers to Your Questions about Homosexuality*, 133.

23. Randy Shilts, *And the Band Played On* (New York: St. Martin's Press, 1987). The entire book chronicles the resistance of most homosexual men to change their activities even in the face of the deadly virus.

24. Stafford, quoting a Blumstein and Schwartz study, *Sexual Christian*, 139.

25. Wilson, "Medical and Psychological Evidence," in *Answers to Your Questions about Homosexuality*, 148.

26. John D'Emilio, *Sexual Politics, Sexual Communities* (Chicago: University of Chicago Press, 1983), 73-74, 117; Scanzoni and Mollenkott, *Homosexual My Neighbor?*, 82-83.

27. Alcorn, *Christians in the Wake*, 142.

28. Jones, "Homosexuality According to Science," 26.

29. Ibid.

30. Wilson, "Medical and Psychological Evidence," in *Answers to Your Questions about Homosexuality*, 151.

31. Jones, "Homosexuality According to Science," 27.

32. Nick Bamforth, *AIDS and the Healer Within* (New York: Amethyst Books, 1987), 66.

33. George Alan Rekers, *Shaping Your Child's Sexual Identity* (Grand Rapids, Mich.: Baker Book House, 1982), 3.

34. For a helpful resource on gay rights laws, see Roger Magnuson, *Are Gay Rights Right?* (Portland, Ore.: Multnomah Press, 1990).

35. Scanzoni and Mollenkott, *Homosexual My Neighbor?*, 33.

36. D. H. Field, "Homosexuality," in *The New Bible Dictionary*, 2d ed., ed. J. D. Douglas et al. (Leicester, U.K.: Inter-Varsity Press, 1982), 488.

37. Jones, "Homosexuality According to Science," 27.

38. Ibid., 26.

39. See Shilts, *And the Band Played On*, to confirm the increased promiscuity in America. This is also indirectly confirmed by the delayed onset of AIDS in Europe compared with the U.S., despite European proximity to Africa and close cultural ties to the U.S. and Canada. We have also talked to a number of homosexual men and redeemed homosexuals, who anecdotally confirmed these ideas.

Has not the LORD made them one? In flesh and spirit they are his. And why one? Because he was seeking godly offspring. So guard yourself in your spirit, and do not break faith with the wife of your youth (Malachi 2:15).

"Haven't you read," [Jesus] replied, "that at the beginning the Creator 'made them male and female,' and said, 'For this reason a man will leave his father and mother and be united to his wife, and the two will become one flesh'? So they are no longer two, but one. Therefore what God has joined together, let man not separate" (Matthew 19:4-6).

The man and his wife were both naked, and they felt no shame (Genesis 2:25).

Marriage should be honored by all, and the marriage bed kept pure, for God will judge the adulterer and all the sexually immoral (Hebrews 13:4).

Chapter Twelve

Christians and Sexuality

L isa is a young parent I met while taking care of her first child, a beautiful little boy named Cody. When I first met Lisa I felt quite paternal toward her because of her vulnerability and openness. I did not realize there was more to it.

The larger picture became evident later when I discovered that Lisa had done a remarkable thing: she had given up her child for adoption to a Christian couple. This couple continued to come to me as their pediatrician, and I thought they would make excellent parents. But I was surprised by the turn of events and intrigued as to why Lisa would be willing to give up her son, who was the joy of her life. I called her and asked if she would come to the office to talk with me, to which she consented.

The story she told me was depressing, but I had heard similar ones many times before. She had been sexually abused as a child by her stepfather and had left her home when she was sixteen to move in with her boyfriend, with whom she later broke up. Lisa had been trained by her abuser that men want childlike, compliant women, and she played the part. Consequently, she dressed provocatively; spoke in a high, childlike voice; and acted totally dependent with me and presumably with any man she was around. She went out with men she did not like simply because they asked her. She slept with them because they wanted her, whether she cared for them or not. Lisa never enjoyed the sex and always despised herself afterwards.

I asked her what she wanted in life. She smiled and pointed over my shoulder and said, "I want that!" I turned to see the smiling faces of my wife, children, and myself in a family portrait. "I want that and I'll do anything to get it," she repeated. We talked for a while longer, and I emphasized to her that she was God's child and explained why she had come to act the way she did. I told her she had to learn to see herself as God did—as someone worth great value and not some plaything for men. We prayed together for her and her decision to give up Cody while she attended to her chaotic life.

The next time she came in to talk with me, I was amazed at the transformation. She was a different person. God had turned on a light of understanding for her, and she had started saying no to all the men who had previously taken advantage of her vulnerability. Lisa had started dressing more chastely. She also was speaking in a deeper, womanly voice, something she was unaware of until I pointed it out to her. By God's grace Lisa realized she was created in the image of God and had great worth, and so she began to treat herself with dignity. Her change in voice and dress had occurred, not because I counseled her directly about them, for I had said nothing on these issues previously, but because she realized that a person who has dignity does not parade that which is too valuable to give away.

Lisa continues to have many areas in her life that need modifying. She did not come to her position in life overnight, and despite some sudden, positive changes, she is unlikely to attain purity and maturity without a long struggle, prayer from friends, and consistent seeking after God. But God has already blessed her with some substantial changes, and if she is faithful to him, he will continue those blessings.

* * * * * *

Lisa's story could be told by many other women, who have become the primary victims of the sexual revolution. Because women bear children, they are more vulnerable in a sexually "free" culture. Moreover, the tendency for women to be more security and relational oriented goes counter to the lack of commitment in the singles' scene. Yet despite those factors, many women feel compelled to surrender their bodies in hopes of gaining the intimacy they desire. For the most part they have been sorely disappointed.

The AIDS epidemic does not stand isolated. Many changes in society allowed the arrival of the epidemic, foremost being the sexual revolution. However, the church, which overtly tried to counter the sexual revolution, has accepted too many of its premises and so has gradually assumed a similar mindset. The Bible's teaching on sexuality and marriage gives not only proscriptions ("Thou shalt not!"), but also sets up an ideal we are to follow. We will explore the biblical teaching on sexuality and see how that differs from the church's emphasis today.

SEX AS SACRED IN SOCIETY

A society spends the most time and energy, once the basic necessities of life are satisfied, on what it deems most important. In ancient Hebrew and American Puritan writings, one can hardly read a single paragraph without encountering a reference to God Almighty. What items have replaced God in our communications media? Only sex, money, and self-love satisfy the time and energy requirements for what is sacred in our culture. These are the gods of a new age.

Consider how many times a day we are violated by encroaching sexuality. The morning newspaper contains sexually titillating stories, provocative advertisements for movies, and scantily clothed models showing how minuscule the newest swimsuits have become. If we turn on the radio, we might hear disc jockeys asking housewives to describe their biggest sexual fantasy or their most exotic sexual experience. Turn on a morning talk show and we can catch an interview with prostitutes who practice sadomasochism on their clients. Leave the TV on to watch the latest soap opera and find out how exciting immoral sex can be. The commercials use sex to sell, yet sexuality has little correlation with the quality of blue jeans the models squeeze into or the taste of the chewing gum with which the bikini-clad women "double their pleasure."

If you go for a drive to escape the sexuality, you are likely to see bumper stickers that suggest certain professions do "it" better or at least in unusual places or positions. The billboards give us no respite. Nor do the people we meet when we stop for a walk in the park. The women dress in clothes two sizes too small, two inches too short, or two grades too thin. Little is left to the imagination. The men open their shirts to the midriff, drive sporty cars for sex appeal, and act as if they are God's gift to women everywhere.

If you see the latest movie, you are likely to hear sexual innuendos that once came only from the mouths of sailors, see nudity once restricted to the gynecologist's office, and watch sexual intercourse once limited to X-rated movies in the seamy section of town. And this "progress" has happened with hardly a peep from middle America or the church. Sadly, our children are exposed to almost as much lasciviousness as we are. Worse, they are taught by the advertisements they see and the fashion displays they examine that they need to act sexually like little adults by the time they are twelve years old.

THE FALSE PREMISES OF THE SEXUAL REVOLUTION

The sexual revolution was bound for failure. The victims were inevitable because the authors of the revolution rebelled against the teachings of God. Those in the free-love culture held certain premises that should have forecast its inevitable failure even to the non-Christian. Let's briefly look at those false premises.

People are basically good and will not abuse the power of sexuality. Unbelievably, some still naively assert the basic goodness of man despite the barbarism in the twentieth century and all the abuses of the sexual revolution. As G. K. Chesterton suggested, the Fall is the one Christian doctrine that has overwhelming empirical support.[1]

Our first and foremost priority is to please our own sexual desires. However, in a fallen world, personal fulfillment virtually always becomes selfishness and exploitation. Consider the homosexual going to the baths or the promiscuous heterosexual going to a singles' bar. They do not arrive there with a heartfelt desire to serve other people. They are there to satisfy their personal urges—period.

Good sex is the goal rather than a deep relationship with another human being. This promise of personal fulfillment from physical sexuality is far more than sex can deliver and is confirmed by the revolving-door relationships and marriages common in our culture. This lie led directly to the AIDS crisis in the U.S. as homosexual men tried to find fulfillment in frenetic sexual activity.

Sex can be enjoyed indiscriminately without affecting the individual. However, recreational sex, just as recreational drug use, is a lie. The post-sixties' culture is littered with people who have been abused, depressed, and exploited by casual sexuality. Casual sex becomes addictive because it is enjoyable, available, and counterfeits true intimacy. But after the high of intercourse comes the depressing realization of the triteness of a relationship based solely on sex.

Immediate pleasure is much preferred over delayed gratification. Our culture tells us we are to enjoy things immediately, whether it be easy credit, easy job, or easy sex. But we can actually have only a little of what life offers, and that with great difficulty, work, and sacrifice. The important aspects of life involve relationships with other people and with our Creator. But these take sacrifice, time, and commitment, which are antithetical to the world.

Good sex leads to a good relationship with one's lover—so the reasoning goes for those who want to live together before marriage to establish "sexual compatibility." Studies have shown conclusively that premarital sex and cohabitation, even among older couples, are much more likely to lead to separation or divorce if marriage does occur.[2] Any good marriage demonstrates that the converse is true: good sex comes out of a good relationship.

Not every "liberated" person holds to all these premises, but most do, whether they have thought through them or not. They are all clearly false to anyone who has experienced the real world and its disappointments.

THE FAILURE OF THE CHURCH

Christians have faltered in the area of sexuality, accepting much of the folly of the world. Although the church thinks more traditionally than the world, our behavior is only a little better. Adultery, homosexuality, and premarital sex are also found in the church.[3]

The church has failed substantially in several areas affecting sexuality:

The church has failed to see the historical roots of the sexual revolution and how deeply ingrained it is in our society (see chapter 4). Our response has been unrealistic, failing to shield our own children from the dangers of the worldly ethos.

The church has adopted the world's premises about sexuality (though with a Christian twist) rather than offering a biblical view. This has had destructive results. Although few Christians accept the basic goodness of man, we do worse and accept the basic goodness of ourselves. We are vulnerable to the sins of the flesh as we have seen repeatedly among Christian leaders and laity alike.

We compete with the world's hypersexuality, saying that good sex will make a good marriage, when it is commitment, communication, and sacrifice that come first. By implying that sex is the key to marriage, we teach our unmarried youth to focus on the physical in their relationships with the opposite gender, we encourage technique instead of commitment, and we prepare all for disappointment in marriage because sex is not meant to be the ultimate satisfaction. Marriage is two lumpish people joining together with all their faults. How can we expect total bliss from that?[4]

We have embraced eros *instead of* agape *love.* No Greek word could better describe the sexual revolution than *eros.* The advocates of this sexual "freedom" would unashamedly agree. This is the heart of the problem, because eros is love that desires to have or possess and so is basically self-centered. A person controlled by eros enters a relationship (if there is a relationship at all) to seize what he desires.[5] The Christian version of this is the adoption of self-actualizing psychology, which demands self-fulfillment in marriage in place of sacrifice.

We have failed by telling our youth and others to "Just Say No!" as if yelling it loudly and often enough will transfer mystical help to stay pure. How can they possibly hear us when all the world is exclaiming, "Just Say Yes!"[6] and throwing in the instruction manuals with graphic pictures to boot? We must aggressively underscore the heartache wrought by "free love."

We have made the unmarried Christian feel less than complete, by overemphasizing the joys of marriage. We do not see Jesus, Paul, or the myriad of other Christians who have never married as somehow incomplete. By our unbiblical emphasis we hamstring our singles, who remain in a holding pattern until they are supposedly fulfilled through marriage.

We have failed to demonstrate that sexuality means much more than sexual intimacy. Men and women are created in God's image, yet are unalike. Each gender has inherent weaknesses and strengths that go beyond the obvious physical differences. Sexuality is involved in all interactions between men and women, especially as we celebrate the distinctions. Too often we confine women to narrowly defined ministries, sacrificing their talents as teachers, counselors, and administrators. We limit men by asking them to lead our churches without enough balancing counsel from our equal-but-different co-laborers.

THE BIBLICAL VIEW OF SEXUALITY

The AIDS epidemic involves a specific disease; it is also a symptom of a society that has abandoned godly ideas and behavior. Insofar as the church has failed to proclaim biblical guidelines, we share in the sin that has led to the deaths of tens of thousands of people. It is time for the church to take the commandments of God seriously instead of flowing with the trends of the world. Scripture gives limited teaching on sexuality, but what is said should be taken to heart. We turn our attention now to some of those significant passages.

> *The LORD God said, "It is not good for the man to be alone. I will make a helper suitable for him" (Genesis 2:18).*

This is the first statement in Scripture where something is described as not good. Aloneness is not the preferred state for humans. We were made to relate to God and to other people. No wonder so much sadness is apparent in our post-Christian world which tries to live as if God were dead and our fellow beings were unnecessary. When independence is so highly treasured, marriages become matters of convenience. Most spouses use their mates to gain sex, possessions, and children. Christian marriages are also joined together with such flimsy glue. True intimacy is lacking, yet the need for relationships remains more compelling than sexual needs.

This verse also tells us that the suitability of the helper is important and accentuates the complementary nature of men and women as partners. By God's design, men and women were made to be two parts of a whole, and this makes the marriage of same-sex couples intrinsically unsuitable. We are simply created with basic characteristics that make male and female "fit." Therefore, since we were created to complement each other, the intrinsic differences between genders is very good.

> *"Haven't you read," [Jesus] replied, "that at the beginning the Creator 'made them male and female,' and said, 'For this reason a man will leave his father*

*and mother and be united to his wife, and the two will
become one flesh'? So they are no longer two, but one.
Therefore what God has joined together, let man not
separate" (Matthew 19:4-6).*

Jesus states that men and women are to be joined
together in a permanent bond, declaring both homosexuality
and heterosexual promiscuity aberrant. Moreover, he further
emphasizes the necessity of human relationships in that the
man and the woman first come from the nurturing of their
individual families into the nurturing of a new family.
Scripture is antithetical to the independence and self-sufficiency of modern society. We are much more fragile alone
than we think.

God himself joins and sanctifies every marriage; such
is its overwhelming importance. Frivolous divorce, the trend
of the modern church following the world's lead, is anathema to God. Becoming one flesh means a permanent bond
has been made and to separate is to cause one's own flesh to
tear. Nowhere in Scripture does it say that marriage is easy.
On the contrary, joining together two sinful people is a guarantee of trouble. But God's word does say that marriage is
an inviolable commitment to be protected and nurtured. It
should be looked after like a great treasure, for indeed it is.
The world has despised this gem, and great heartache has
resulted. Anything short of great honor to marriage is dis-
honoring to God.

*The man and his wife were both naked, and they felt
no shame (Genesis 2:25).*

When the man first saw the woman, he exclaimed with
obvious delight, "This is now bone of my bones and flesh of
my flesh!" He delighted in her physically as she did in him;
they experienced no shame in their nakedness with each
other. This God-given blessing was to be shared with only
one other—the one joined to oneself in marriage. The church
is not to despise sexuality within marriage. It should be
taught openly that sex is a gift from God. The physical joy
between husband and wife should be celebrated, and

children ought to see the delight of parents for each other as they kiss, hold hands, or express affection for each other. Children can then model this behavior at the proper time as they begin their own families.

Flee from sexual immorality. All other sins a man commits are outside his body, but he who sins sexually sins against his own body (1 Corinthians 6:18).

Christians have ignored this command and fallen into sexual sins nearly as often as nonbelievers. Granted, it is hard to escape from all temptations given the nature of the world, but most Christians make no effort. When we watch the same movies and television programs as the world, listen to the same jokes, and put ourselves in compromising positions, we are being foolish. When Paul exhorted Timothy to teach the older women who would then teach the younger, he was not being old-fashioned, he was being sensible. When he told Timothy to treat the younger women with absolute purity, he was not being overly cautious, he was being realistic. How much more should we be careful in our modern world where men and women rub shoulders daily, our senses are titillated at every opportunity, and leisure time and resources make immorality much easier.

All Christians, pastors and elders included, need to consider themselves vulnerable to sexual immorality. Placing ourselves in compromising situations is nothing short of tempting God. Pastors counseling women should do so in monitored settings and probably for a limited time before referring them to mature women in the church. Single Christians ought to date under monitored circumstances so that temptation is lessened and the Lord is glorified. Opportunities for group dating under the auspices of the church should be available. Our failure to maintain sexual purity in the church will not be reversed until the Lord's honor is more important to us than our own freedom to do what we want.

Now to the unmarried and the widows I say: It is good for them to stay unmarried, as I am (1 Corinthians 7:8).

Scripture clearly states that marriage is good; it also clearly states that singleness is good. They are equal conditions and should be equally esteemed by the church. In either condition, all purity must be observed.

What about the aloneness mentioned so prominently in Genesis? That need is satisfied by our relationship to Christ and our fellowship with other believers. "For in [Christ] all the fulness of Deity dwells in bodily form, and in Him you have been made complete" (Colossians 2:9-10, NASB). All of the fullness of agape love can be enjoyed with others outside of marriage.

Singleness is not an illness to be cured; it is a blessing to be enjoyed as it offers greater freedom, mobility, flexibility, and lower financial and time commitments. In addition to a number of celibate people in the Bible, many latter-day Christians have had victorious lives in part due to their singleness. Saint Francis, Mother Teresa, Corrie Ten Boom, and C.S. Lewis (celibate nearly all his life) excelled in their Christian walk. For many it is difficult to forego marriage, sexual intimacy, and children, but for each drawback of the celibate life, a positive alternative exists. The greater freedom, mobility, and flexibility allow the single person to acquire extra schooling, go into missions, pursue a career, and travel. The time required for children and family can be turned to the family of God in ministry, counseling, and teaching. The unmarried are complete in Christ regardless of what the world may say.

There is neither Jew nor Greek, slave nor free, male nor female, for you are all one in Christ Jesus (Galatians 3:28).

Feminists are gravely mistaken in declaring the differences between the genders insignificant. However, the church has gone too far and made the distinctions rigid, denying women their full abilities to minister within the church. Our God displays both male and female attributes: He is our protector and husband while desiring to nurture us like a mother hen nurtures her young. In a similar manner, God has made men and women complementary to assist each other in a hostile world. The sexes perceive, feel, and react differently, which is to our corporate benefit. Though some offices in the church are reserved for men, a woman, submissive to her husband or church leaders, should have many opportunities for service. In the Bible women served as judges, were heroes of entire books, supported Christ financially, stood by the Savior when he was crucified, acted as prophets, and recognized the risen Lord before his male disciples did. God utilized women in important times in history; so should the church today.

If we exalt only the physical differences between men and women, we minimize God's balance in human creation. Sexuality means much more than physical intimacy. When a man comforts a woman who is weeping for a sick child, he is acting as a sexual being. As a woman shows a man how to nurture his own children, she is acting as a sexual being. As a male leader in the church talks to husbands about marital problems, he is acting as a sexual being. As a woman leader in the church counsels other women scarred by childhood abuse, she is acting as a sexual being. As children are attracted during play to their own gender, they are acting as sexual beings.

> *Submit to one another out of reverence for Christ.*
> *Wives, submit to your husbands as to the Lord. For the husband is the head of the wife as Christ is the head of the church, his body, of which he is the Savior. Now as the church submits to Christ, so also wives should submit to their husbands in everything.*
> *Husbands, love your wives, just as Christ loved the church and gave himself up for her. . . . In this same way, husbands ought to love their wives as their own bodies. He who loves his wife loves himself (Ephesians 5:21-25, 28).*

Marriage partners are to voluntarily serve each other, just as our Lord took the lowly position of foot washer. It is out of this servanthood that mature sexuality within marriage comes. The husband is not to lord it over his wife or demand submission from her nor is she to usurp his authority. Indeed, they are to serve each other selflessly in the same manner that Christ served the church. Loving one's mate in a Christlike fashion leaves no room for exercising dominion.

This agape love seeks the best for the person loved and never treats the other as an object. Relationship, commitment, and sacrifice are its characteristics. God's love for us is the archetype we are to mimic, including love for our enemies. Agape is epitomized in 1 Corinthians 13 as being patient, kind, not envious, not boastful, rejoicing in truth, sacrificing, protecting, trusting, hopeful, and persevering. The contrast between this godly love and the impoverished "love" promoted by the sexual revolution is striking.

This is not simply word play. It underscores the foundational difference between sexuality within a Christian context and that found in the world, for agape love governs even the physical expression of love in marriage. Agape may be seen in non-Christians, who bear God's image and retain some nobility. So too can the grasping love of eros be manifested by Christians, especially if we have drunk deeply of our self-indulgent culture. To understand the richness of agape, our children must see it fleshed out in our lives.

"Just Say Yes!" to commitment and striving for the best for one's partner. "Just Say Yes!" to being pure before God, "naked and unashamed" on one's wedding night. "Just Say Yes!" to mutual love, encouragement, physical joy, creation of children, and loving sacrifice for a dying world. Yes, we will gladly compare the Christian experience of marriage with the Playboy philosophy, for Christian sexuality is good, better than what the sexual revolution offers.

THE CROSS AND SEXUALITY

Jesus is the church's bridegroom; in a spiritual sense we are all married. But our earthly marriages are a witness to the heavenly marriage with our Savior. In this age of sexual perversity which has culminated in the AIDS epidemic, Christian marriages have failed to be the "city on a hill" that beckons to the lost. Our marriages are more than isolated relationships between one man and one woman, and their failure reverberates throughout society. If the sacredness of marriage is squandered by immorality or instability, the lost may come to ridicule or doubt our professed devotion to our Bridegroom. But if Christians will strive for agape love which echoes God's commitment to us, our family life becomes a tangible witness to our faith.

Chapter 12, Notes

1. G. K. Chesterton, *Orthodoxy* (Garden City, N.Y.: Image Books, 1959), 15.

2. Tim Stafford, *The Sexual Christian* (Wheaton, Ill.: Victor Books, 1989), 114, 122.

3. Ibid., 12, 192; Randy Alcorn, *Christians in the Wake of the Sexual Revolution* (Portland, Ore.: Multnomah Press, 1985), 24; Josh McDowell and Dick Day, *Why Wait?* (San Bernardino, Calif.: Here's Life Publishers, 1987), 24; and John White, *Flirting with the World* (Wheaton, Ill.: Harold Shaw Publishers, 1982), 75.

4. Stafford, *Sexual Christian*, 69.

5. *The New International Dictionary of New Testament Theology*, s.v. "Love."

6. Stafford, *Sexual Christian*, 130.

Now there were some present at that time who told Jesus about the Galileans whose blood Pilate had mixed with their sacrifices. Jesus answered, "Do you think that these Galileans were worse sinners than all the other Galileans because they suffered this way? I tell you, no! But unless you repent, you too will all perish. Or those eighteen who died when the tower in Siloam fell on them—do you think they were more guilty than all the others living in Jerusalem? I tell you, no! But unless you repent, you too will all perish" (Luke 13:1-5).

Be imitators of God, therefore, as dearly loved children and live a life of love, just as Christ loved us and gave himself up for us as a fragrant offering and sacrifice to God (Ephesians 5:1-2).

"But I tell you: Love your enemies and pray for those who persecute you, that you may be sons of your Father in heaven. . . . If you love those who love you, what reward will you get? Are not even the tax collectors doing that? And if you greet only your brothers, what are you doing more than others? Do not even pagans do that?" (Matthew 5:44-47).

When we are cursed, we bless; when we are persecuted, we endure it; when we are slandered, we answer kindly (1 Corinthians 4:12-13).

Chapter Thirteen

Is AIDS the Judgment of God?

J ohn and I had an eye-opening experience one evening in the fall of 1987. A Christian author of a bestselling book on AIDS was about to speak to a large, diverse audience of several hundred people in our hometown. The local pastor and activist who preceded the main speaker finished his introduction with a startling comment: Anyone who interrupted the proceedings with even a question would be escorted from the room. He then pointed to various security officers strategically placed around the auditorium. The events that followed seemed to warrant his blunt warning.

As the main speaker approached the podium, a local homosexual activist stood up and began to voice objections to the author's position. Previously notified local news cameras began to record the drama. The security officers hurried across the room to carry out the outspoken critic. Quickly, a number of other men began to speak out. In all, about a third of the audience was composed of male homosexuals who were there to harass the speaker. Although there were insufficient numbers of security officers to escort them all out, the hecklers eventually decided to leave together as they chanted, "Shame! Shame!" and "Nazis! Nazis!" Then they held a rally and news conference just outside the door.

Many of the Christians in the audience shouted back during these events, some of them angrily. The main speaker, finally able to begin his talk, laced it with sarcastic remarks directed toward these homosexuals, some of whom were dying of AIDS. At one point he even did a caricature of the limp-wristed stereotype of a homosexual male. His talk also contained many medical inaccuracies that served to heighten the audience's fears about AIDS.

Several homosexuals remained behind to hear the speech. Occasionally, one would interrupt with a question or objection and would be escorted from the room. Sometimes there would be a quiet exchange between the speaker and a homosexual, the latter pleading for the speaker to be fair or less sarcastic. Peppered throughout the talk were derogatory comments about the homosexuals from the apparently Christian portion of the audience. There was no discernible difference in attitude between the two groups. Would Christ have responded differently in that setting?

We, and many others there, felt uncomfortable with either faction. Certainly, we are not ideal Christians in thought or deed, but it did seem that many of the Christians were acting against their Master's wishes. Jesus commanded us to love our enemies, to turn the other cheek, and to rejoice when we are persecuted for his sake. Had these commandments been forgotten, or was there something else clouding the thinking and therefore the actions of these Christians? We knew some of the men and women in the audience and knew they genuinely loved the Lord, so carnality was not the only problem. But, as we will see, the way one views the AIDS epidemic affects how one responds to it.

* * * * * *

JUDGMENT DEFINED

A recurring theme among evangelicals is that AIDS is a judgment of God directed at homosexuals.[1] This is an important idea to examine, because the way we think about the epidemic will determine the way we act toward its victims.

Does the idea of AIDS being God's judgment on homosexuals stand up to critical biblical analysis? If it does (or does not), what implications does this have?

Initially, it is important to define what we mean by judgment. We are not talking about God's discernment that something is good or evil, but rather the actions God takes or the events he allows to discipline or destroy a person or people. In this sense there are three levels of judgment in the Bible, and people may be confused about the relationship between judgment and AIDS because they do not take these different levels into account.

Universal Judgment

The first and most basic form of judgment is what we will call *universal judgment*. The world and all who are in it are under judgment because of sin. As a result, the world is no longer a Garden of Eden: women bring forth children in pain, work is a struggle, and everyone ages and dies (Genesis 3; Romans 5:12-21, 8:20-23). In this life none can escape universal judgment completely, even Christians; we all become ill, we all think and reason imperfectly, and we are all tainted by sin (1 John 1:8-10). By God's grace we can partly escape this judgment in this life, since he can heal us of infirmities, sanctify our thinking and actions, and draw us closer to himself through the work of Christ and the indwelling of the Holy Spirit.

Because we all live under universal judgment, we must accept the reality that death or disease could strike at any time, whether we deserve it or not. Even if we live righteous lives, we still suffer because of the sin in the world. Although substantially innocent of wrongdoing, we could be killed by a drunk driver, be murdered in a robbery attempt, injured in an earthquake, or die of cancer. We cannot eliminate this uncertainty no matter how much we try to shield ourselves with wealth or armies or the best doctors in the world. This is the judgment about which Christ taught in the parable of the rich fool—no man knows the time of his death (Luke 12:16-21). This aspect of life keeps us all humble beneath the sovereign hand of God.

Cause-and-Effect Judgment

A second form of judgment is what we will call *cause-and-effect judgment*. This judgment has two branches, one that is understood by all people, the other that is seen clearly only by those who hold to traditional Judeo-Christian morality.

The first branch acknowledges that there are certain physical laws in effect that have irreducible consequences if we violate them. We die if we jump off a tall building, drink a lethal amount of alcohol, or get trapped under water. The consequences of our actions are quick and sure. We do not have to go to school to learn this truth about living in the world; we begin learning about it as children the first time we fall and scrape our knee.

The second branch of cause-and-effect judgment is in the moral and spiritual realm. This form of judgment involves God's cause-and-effect rules of morality. It wasn't necessary for the Creator to tell us about the physical laws—these we soon discovered on our own—but because we are fallen and live in a fallen world, the moral aspect of judgment had to be spelled out for us in Scripture.

> Do not be deceived: God cannot be mocked. A man reaps what he sows. The one who sows to please his sinful nature, from that nature will reap destruction; the one who sows to please the Spirit, from the Spirit will reap eternal life (Galatians 6:7-8).

This form of judgment shows up in the Ten Commandments and in prohibitions on drunkenness, rape, and homosexuality, among many others. If we do not follow these wise directives given by our Maker, then negative consequences will result in our person and in our society. Cause-and-effect judgment also includes positive effects resulting from loving one another, obeying parents, and generally living righteously. Deuteronomy 28 records a covenant God made with Israel by which he promises to bless the nation if they obey his laws and curse them if they disobey. Although this is not a contract between God and Gentile Christians today, it is a good model for seeing that consequences follow obeying and disobeying God's commands.

These consequences do not seem as obviously binding as those associated with the physical laws, but they are pervasive nonetheless. They are particularly evident as a whole society tends to obey or disobey them. A particular husband might "get away" with adultery, but as a whole nation becomes adulterous, the family disintegrates, causing severe repercussions. A teenager may seem to "get away" with premarital sex, but as a whole society becomes licentious, millions of teenage pregnancies and broken youthful marriages are the results. Of course, even the ones who don't get caught reap consequences, though not as clearly as when a whole society disobeys God. Even if no one else knows, the sin will result in separation from God, stress between the people involved, and guilt or depression in the individual sinner.

Mankind has rebelled against God throughout history. We have seen this rebellion clearly in the Western world in the last twenty years, particularly in the area of sexual mores, as people have questioned and gone against many of the commands and principles given in Scripture. Some have claimed sex is good in all its possibilities,[2] adultery is good to help a marriage grow,[3] homosexuality is normal,[4] and children should experiment at any age with sex.[5] To all these and to their related deviations from God's moral law, he gives a resounding "No!" Moreover, God has not given us these rules because he wants to stop us from enjoying life. Rather, our wise Father has given his immature and rebellious children boundaries so that we will not harm ourselves. (Immorality is wrong because God says it is. However, it helps us to accept his rules if we know they are given for our benefit.)

The effect caused by adultery is not a fuller marriage, but a broken one. The results of self-centeredness in parents are alienated children. The whirlwind reaped by lack of boundaries on sexuality are millions of abortions, teenage pregnancies, childhood sexual abuse, and masses of people with sexually transmitted diseases.

Specific Divine Judgment

The third type of judgment is what we will call *specific divine judgment*, the type most Christians have in mind when they say AIDS is God's judgment on homosexuals. Specific divine judgment in the Bible occurs when God directly intervenes to punish a specific group of people. This can be as broad as the worldwide flood or as narrow as the stoning of Achan and his family for disobedience. God can use as his instrument of judgment supernatural events, such as the fire and brimstone that rained on Sodom and Gomorrah, or man, as when Joshua's armies destroyed Canaanite cities (Joshua 8). Judgment can be conditional, depending for its occurrence on the number of righteous people in Sodom and Gomorrah (Genesis 18), or on the repentance of the wicked in Nineveh (Jonah 3); or it can be unconditional, as when God told David that his child conceived through adultery with Bathsheba must die (2 Samuel 12). It can be as short in duration as the earthquake that destroyed Korah and his followers (Numbers 16), or it can take a long time, as in the forty years of judgment that Israel suffered while wandering in the desert (Numbers 14).

How does specific divine judgment differ from the universal and cause-and-effect judgments? First, specific divine judgment is directed toward a specific group of people at a specific time for a specific act of rebellion against God or for their innate wickedness. For example, at the time of the flood, "The LORD saw how great man's wickedness on the earth had become, and that every inclination of the thoughts of his heart was only evil all the time" (Genesis 6:5). God told Abraham that he would not inherit the land of Canaan because "the sin of the [inhabitants] has not yet reached its full measure" (Genesis 15:16). Their evil had become full by the time of Joshua, when those living in Canaan routinely practiced religious ceremonies that included prostitution and child sacrifice (Leviticus 18:21, 20:1-5; 2 Kings 23:10). God judged them using the armies of Israel as his instrument.

God chooses when he will judge. The sins occurring at the time of the flood have occurred subsequently, but there has been only one flood. Prostitution and child sacrifice as part of religious observances have occurred at many other times in other cultures, yet not all these nations were destroyed. God chooses if and when specific divine judgment occurs.

Second, specific divine judgment is announced by God himself or by his prophets. In one sense every general commandment in Scripture is an announcement by God of a cause-and-effect judgment. However, these judgments are applicable to all, unlike specific divine judgment. It is always and for everyone wrong to be an active homosexual, and there are consequences if one practices homosexuality. But fire and brimstone will not rain on every homosexual as it did on Sodom and Gomorrah, because that was a specific divine judgment announced by God.

Moreover, all specific divine judgments are announced before the judgment begins. The judgment might last for an extended time, as Israel's forty years of wandering or the two-and-a-half years of drought announced by Elijah, but these punishments were proclaimed at the first so that the origin of the judgment was understood. Judah was forewarned that she would be in captivity in Babylon for seventy years as a judgment from God (Jeremiah 25:11). The result was discipline instead of mere tragedy, because the people understood that this was by the sovereign will of God rather than the might of the Babylonian army.

Third, in the Bible's specific divine judgments, the relationship between the sin and the destruction that follows is not cause and effect; rather than the natural consequences of their actions, the unexpected occurs. God causes something out of the ordinary to happen as a signature of his divine wrath. The fire and brimstone that rained on Sodom and Gomorrah was not a direct consequence of their behavior, but crashing one's car into a tree could be a direct consequence of drunkenness. Neither was the capture of Canaan by Joshua's army caused directly by Canaan's sin, but a husband's adultery might lead directly to the breakup of his marriage. The unexpectedness of specific divine judgments makes it clear to the spiritually attuned that God is the director of events.

Almost all forms of judgment can be categorized into universal, cause and effect, or specific divine judgment. (The Bible also talks about *final judgment* which involves the permanent division of the lost and saved, but this is after the second coming of Christ.) The following chart summarizes these three types of judgment:

THE JUDGMENTS OF GOD

TYPE	CHARACTERISTICS	EXAMPLES
1. Universal Judgment	All men, women, and children affected; the whole earth affected due to the sin of people.	Certain illnesses, aging and death, toiling in work, pain in childbirth, spiritual death.
2. Cause-and-Effect Judgment		
a. Physical	a. People reaping directly the consequences of their actions.	a. Dying after slipping off a cliff, drinking poison accidentally
b. Moral	b. People reaping directly the consequences of their sins.	b. Drunk driver causing a car wreck, sterility from sexually transmitted disease or abortion, divorce after adultery
3. Specific Divine Judgment	1. Directed toward a) a specific group of people b) at a specific point in time. 2. Announced a) by God or his prophet b) at the beginning of the judgment 3. The judgment is not a direct consequence of the actions or the sins.	The flood, Israel's 40-year wandering, destruction of Korah and his followers, drought of Elijah, destruction of Canaan

AIDS Is Not a Specific Divine Judgment

AIDS is not a specific divine judgment from God directed toward homosexuals because it does not meet the criteria for that form of judgment. Rather, it is a *cause-and-effect judgment* resulting from promiscuous, sinful behavior. The vast majority of those with AIDS contracted it through sexual activity outside of God's boundaries (including both heterosexual and homosexual sin) or by harming their bodies through IV drug abuse.

Some of the victims of the disease, the so-called innocent victims, fall under the category of universal judgment rather than cause-and-effect. Those who contract HIV through no sinful action of their own include transfusion recipients; hemophiliacs; spouses of IV drug users, bisexuals, and adulterers; and babies born to prostitutes. They may live within God's law, at least in most areas of their lives, but have been struck by the disease because of the sinful behavior of another. They are analogous to the family killed by a drunk driver. This judgment on "innocents" is difficult for us to accept from our human perspective; their suffering and death seem senseless and unfair. But God's view is very different. All of us are sinners, and all of us suffer the consequences of living in a corrupt world. One day all will be set right, but until that time creation groans under the weight of mankind's rebellion against God, a rebellion in which we all had a part. Innocence is always a relative condition on this earth.

Even though the majority of the AIDS sufferers are not innocent in the manner in which they became infected, there are several reasons we do not believe AIDS is a specific divine judgment. Basically, the characteristics of the epidemic are unlike all of the characteristics of specific divine judgment.

First, AIDS is not directed only against homosexuals. It is true that in the United States male homosexuals are the group most likely to contract the virus, but transfusion recipients, hemophiliacs, faithful spouses, and babies are also victims. We also cannot say AIDS is directed against homosexuals because the lesbian population almost never contracts it. According to Scripture, female homosexuality is just as sinful as male homosexuality; female homosexuals should be judged just as severely as male homosexuals if this were a specific divine judgment. Moreover, there is virtually no homosexually acquired AIDS in Africa (because there are few homosexuals), while AIDS is spreading rapidly through the heterosexual population.[6] Worldwide, probably more heterosexuals than homosexuals are infected,[7] so God's judgment in this case is not specific. In the U.S. AIDS is now increasing faster among IV drug users, not homosexuals.

Second, no prophet in the biblical sense announced this judgment beforehand. The disease was first recognized in 1981 and existed over twenty years before. Yet only in the last several years have people proclaimed that AIDS is the judgment of God.[8] Specific divine judgment is intended to be instructive for the living. If AIDS were God's specific judgment, we should have seen men and women of God announcing in the early eighties (and before) that the disease was coming.

Third, this disease has not gone against the natural order of things, but rather seems to be a natural consequence of promiscuity[9] and drug abuse.[10] Male homosexuals are experiencing the cause-and-effect results of having multiple sexual partners. Because homosexual males become infected with any sexually transmitted disease at a rate hundreds of times greater than any other group of people,[11] it is natural to expect that they would acquire the sexually transmitted AIDS virus. Further, the most promiscuous homosexual males are the most likely to become infected with the virus. The same is true among heterosexuals: the most promiscuous, including prostitutes, have the highest risk of becoming infected with HIV.[12] IV drug users also have a high rate of various infections related to their sharing of needles. The AIDS virus is just one more added to the list, which includes hepatitis B, other types of hepatitis, pneumonia, and bacterial and fungal infections of the blood, heart, and skin. Clearly, people are getting AIDS as a *natural consequence* of their actions. Fire and brimstone are not raining on the heads of homosexuals, nor is the earth swallowing up IV drug users.

AIDS Is Not a Judgment against the United States

A few Christians suggest that AIDS is a specific judgment against the United States for its moral deterioration.[13] Although the deterioration in our country is lamentable and the response of Christians inadequate, it is hard to equate the AIDS epidemic with judgment on the whole nation for the following reasons.

The AIDS epidemic will peak, as have all epidemics throughout history,[14] after the most susceptible individuals have contracted the illness. Since promiscuity is the risk factor in sexually transmitted diseases such as AIDS, only a small portion of the nation will be infected. It is doubtful that the number of HIV-positive individuals will ever rise above 5 percent of the nation's population. It is true that all of us may pay higher taxes and insurance rates. All of us may have to make decisions about how to interact with AIDS sufferers in the workplace, church, and neighborhood. All of us may be concerned about receiving a transfusion contaminated with HIV. However, these consequences appear to be more of a nuisance than the result of God's anger directed at our nation. The problems we face are markedly different from the utter destruction of Sodom and Gomorrah, the annihilation of many Canaanite cities, and the enslavement of Israel and Judah due to their sins. It is also affecting the U.S. much less severely than the debacle that is occurring in Central Africa. If God were to adequately judge our nation, he would more likely involve us in a nuclear war, an economic collapse, or a series of devastating earthquakes rather than a limited and preventable disease like AIDS.

God Is Not a Machine

We want to be careful not to place limitations on our God. We see no reason why our sovereign Lord could not bring a specific divine judgment on homosexuals or on this country at any time. The swift judgments prophesied in Revelation make that clear. Perhaps the AIDS epidemic is a warning to all of us that God will not be mocked. Western society has wandered far from the Judeo-Christian underpinnings that caused it to be the envy of the remainder of the world. Christians have failed to stem the tide by being salt and light in a compassionate way as we have been commanded to do. We should all get on our knees and pray for mercy over justice and then get about the business of acting as Christ in a dying culture.[15]

WHY THE DIFFERENCE IS CRUCIAL

What difference does it make if we think AIDS is God's specific divine judgment or not? For many people it will make a major difference in how they respond to the epidemic. If this is a specific divine judgment, then many Christians believe we should not try to stop it. In the biblical examples of specific divine judgments, those near the judgment did not fight the hand of God but got out of the way. Lot and his family left Sodom and Gomorrah; Moses and his followers separated from Korah and his followers just before Korah's group was destroyed; Noah did not attempt to dissuade God from bringing on the flood but built an ark to survive it; and not one of Joshua's followers stood in his way as God's army attacked the cities of Canaan. Although King David prayed for God to spare the child born to Bathsheba, he did not go to a physician. In the end, he humbly accepted the judgment of God when it was clear that the sovereign will of God would prevail.

On the other hand, when a universal or cause-and-effect judgment occurred, the men and women of the Bible tried to intervene. People were healed of all sorts of infirmities. Men, women, and children were raised from the dead. The prophets tried to turn the people toward righteous ways which would have restored relationships between spouses, brought children and their fathers together, and resulted in closer relationships with God.

In his novel *The Plague*, agnostic existentialist Albert Camus illustrates this quandary of how to react when calamity strikes. In the novel, a priest comes to the conclusion that the plague is God's (specific divine) judgment and progressively does less and less to fight the illness.[16] When the priest himself becomes ill, he refuses medical treatment. An atheist physician, on the other hand, fights the disease to the point of exhaustion and brings whatever relief he can to suffering people.

Unfortunately, some today are like the priest of Camus, proclaiming or implying that AIDS patients deserve what they have. Though there is some truth in that statement, it fails to acknowledge that those of us with comfortable lives are undeserving of what we have. We are no more deserving of health or plenty than is the dying AIDS patient, except by the graces of God and "the unsearchable riches of Christ." In Luke 13 Jesus warns us against thinking that others are worse sinners just because some misfortune comes upon them. We need to take a careful look at how our Savior acted when cause-and-effect judgment came upon those around him.

THE EXAMPLE OF CHRIST

As followers of Christ, we should model ourselves primarily after his life. Jesus did not see disease as God's judgment but as an opportunity to show God's glory and mercy (John 9:1-3). He consistently touched and ministered to the diseased people, even though he knew they were considered unclean by Jewish law. Jesus consistently ministered to the weak and poor, who, because of their poverty and lack of power, were considered by the self-righteous religious leaders to be under the judgment of God.[17]

Christians are commanded to love; that is to be our most distinguishing characteristic (1 Corinthians 13). Jesus said the two greatest commandments are to love God with all our heart, soul, and mind, and to love our neighbor as ourselves. Everything in Scripture depends on these commandments (Matthew 22:34-40). The apostle John gave perhaps the most penetrating description of God when he said, "God is love" (1 John 4:8). It is true that purity and justice are associated with love, and it can be loving to point out error in another's life. However, Jesus always did this to the downtrodden after tangibly demonstrating his love for them. This was true even in situations involving moral problems. Jesus did not ignore the sin, but he always showed compassion first.

The woman caught in adultery was clearly a sinner (John 8). Moreover, she was reaping a cause-and-effect judgment as a consequence of her actions. She may not have had a sexually transmitted disease, but she carried the social and personal effects of her sin. She was despised by the religious leaders for her transgression and probably suffered from guilt and disgrace. Despite these, the woman was first forgiven by Christ before he told her, "Go and sin no more." The order is crucial and consistent in Jesus' ministry with sinners: first compassion, then a call for change.

The Samaritan woman at the well was morally lax, especially by the standards of the day (John 4). She was reaping the consequences of her immoral life-style, an outcast even among her own people and family. Yet Jesus taught her deep spiritual truths before he said anything about her multiple husbands. It is doubtful that he would have had the opportunity to express those truths to her had he begun the conversation by confronting her with the sinful life she had lived.

Zacchaeus the tax collector was honored to have Christ as a guest before he made restitution to those he had cheated (Luke 19). Zacchaeus had already felt the sting of cause-and-effect judgment for his sin. We know this because of the murmuring against Jesus when he asked to stay at his house. Zacchaeus was a contemptible man in the people's eyes. Yet the Lord saw him as someone who was lost and worthy of seeking and saving.

A most remarkable event in the life of Christ was his anointing by the sinful woman in the house of the Pharisee (Luke 7:36-50). This woman, perhaps a prostitute, was

despised by the Pharisee. She was reaping the natural consequences of cause-and-effect judgment. Yet Jesus showed her
compassion despite the fact that, of all people, he had the
right to be most offended by her life. Jesus then told the
parable of the two men forgiven of debt, one ten times larger
than the other. Who would love the moneylender more,
Jesus asked the Pharisee (and us), the man forgiven little or
the man forgiven much? After the religious leader answered
correctly, Jesus told the woman he had forgiven her sins.
Once her debt was forgiven, she would love him more than
all the Pharisees who thought (wrongly) they owed little.

The religious leaders repeatedly accused Jesus of being
friendly with sinful people, and they were correct. But a doctor must go to the sick to heal, a fact we sometimes forget
today. All of these sinners experienced the cause-and-effect
judgments of being despised by men, alienated from God,
and contemptible in their own eyes. Not once in the Gospels
did Christ treat sinners as despicable unless they were in
positions of religious or political authority and were self-
righteously lording it over the common people. I wonder
what would happen today if Christians would drink or eat
with homosexuals, ask to stay with IV drug abusers, or
allow prostitutes to touch us as Jesus did. Probably many
more of these people would be drawn to Christ from those
actions than from our screaming about their sin, making sarcastic references to their life-style, or caricaturing their man-
nerisms.

It is hard for a spiritually blinded man to see truth in
criticism from a stranger. He will likely become defensive
and belligerent toward his accuser. But let that stranger first
become a comforter, a friend, and let their interaction be characterized by love and forgiveness, then will the blind begin to
see. People came to Jesus because he offered something they
had not experienced before. Here was a pure man, a spiritual
man, who did not take the high place but was willing to
humble himself so that they would begin to see.

There is no question that sin is usually involved in the
acquisition of AIDS. But sinners of every kind deserve to die

according to the law of God. Were it not for the grace of God and the blood of his Son, all of us would be destined for hell. Therefore, let us not be like the priest in *The Plague* who in the end chose to do nothing. Rather, let us model ourselves after Jesus and fight to the point of exhaustion to show God's love and glory to unworthy sinners.

Just as he did for us.

Chapter 13, Notes

1. David Chilton, *Power in the Blood* (Brentwood, Tenn.: Wolgemuth and Hyatt, 1987), 31-46; James McKeever, *The AIDS Plague* (Medford, Ore.: Omega Publications, 1987), 124; and Andrés Tapia, "High Risk Ministry," *Christianity Today,* 7 August 1987, 15.

2. This is the philosophy espoused by *Playboy,* among others.

3. George O'Neill and Nena O'Neill, *Open Marriage: A New Lifestyle for Couples* (New York: M. Evans, 1972). Not surprisingly, this couple later divorced.

4. A. P. Bell and M. S. Weinberg, *Homosexualities: A Study of Diversity among Men and Women* (New York: Simon and Schuster, 1978). The American Psychiatric Association took homosexuality off its list of mental illnesses in 1973.

5. A proposal of the North American Man-Boy Love Association, and from the 1972 Gay Rights Platform adopted by the National Coalition of Gay Organizations, as reported in Enrique Rueda and Michael Schwartz, *Gays, AIDS, and You* (Old Greenwich, Conn.: Devon Adair Co., 1987), 107.

6. Norman Miller and Richard Rockwell, *AIDS in Africa: The Social and Policy Impact* (Lewiston, N. Y.: The Edwin Mellen Press, 1988), 33; C. F. Von Reyn and J. M. Mann, "AIDS—A Global Perspective: Global Epidemiology," *West Journal of Medicine* 147 (1987):694-701; P. Piot et al., "AIDS: An International Perspective," *Science* 239 (1988):573-79; and J. N. Simonsen et al., "Human Immunodeficiency Virus Infection among Men with Sexually Transmitted Diseases: Experience from a Center in Africa," *New England Journal of Medicine* 319 (1988):274-78.

7. The United States had reported a total of seventy thousand cases of AIDS with an estimated 90 percent completeness of reporting as of July 1, 1988, thus accounting for about 70 percent of all *reported* AIDS cases in the world (Centers for Disease Control, "Update: Acquired Immunodeficiency Syndrome [AIDS]—Worldwide," *Morbidity and Mortality Weekly Report* 37 [1988]: 286-88, 293-95. But the reporting of AIDS cases from Africa vastly underestimates the

actual numbers of cases there. Incomplete and delayed reporting of cases in Africa occurs for many reasons: delayed manifestations of disease, limited resources to diagnose the disease, lack of active surveillance systems to identify most cases in both urban and rural areas, apathy and denial of certain governments even to recognize the presence of AIDS in their countries until recently, and lack of access to medical care for many rural residents. Thus, while as of July 1, 1988, the World Health Organization reported 100,410 cases of AIDS from 138 countries, WHO estimates there has been a cumulative total of 250,000 cases of AIDS (J. M. Mann and J. Chin, "AIDS: A Global Perspective," *New England Journal of Medicine* 319 [1988]:302-3). Even if the number of reported cases of AIDS in the United States were 100 percent accurate instead of the estimated 90 percent, and the number of cases of AIDS in the United States was seventy thousand, it still would represent only between 20 to 25 percent of the estimated AIDS cases in the world.

8. David Reagan and Thomas Baker, *What the Bible Says about AIDS* (McKinney, Tex.: Lamb and Lion Ministries, 1988), 7, 13; and Chilton, *Power in the Blood*, chapter 2.

9. H. W. Jaffe et al., "National Case-Control Study of Kaposi's Sarcoma and *Pneumocystis carinii* Pneumonia in Homosexual Men: Part 1, Epidemiologic Results," *Annals of Internal Medicine* 99 (1983):145-51; J. J. Goedert et al., "Determinants of Retrovirus (HTLV-III) Antibody and Immunodeficiency Conditions in Homosexual Men," *Lancet* 2 (1984):711-15; K. H. Mayer et al., "Association of Human T Lymphotropic Virus Type III Antibodies with Sexual and Other Behaviors in a Cohort of Homosexual Men from Boston with and without Generalized Lymphadenopathy," *American Journal of Medicine* 80 (1986):357-63; C. E. Stevens et al., "Human T-Cell Lymphotropic Virus Type III Infection in a Cohort of Homosexual Men in New York City," *Journal of the American Medical Association* 255 (1986):2167-72; W. Winkelstein et al., "Sexual Practices and Risk of Infection by the Human Immunodeficiency Virus: The San Francisco Men's Health Study," *Journal of the American Medical Association* 257 (1988):321-25; and J. McCusker et al., "Behavioral Risk Factors for HIV Infection among Homosexual Men at a Boston Community Health Center," *American Journal of Public Health* 78 (1988):68-71.

10. D.C. Des Jarlais, S.R. Friedman, and R.L. Stoneburner, "HIV Infection and Intravenous Drug Use: Critical Issues in Transmission Dynamics, Infection Outcomes, and Prevention," *Reviews of Infectious Diseases* 10 (1988): 151-58; and E.E. Schoebaum et al., "Risk Factors for Human Immunodeficiency Virus Infection in Intravenous Drug Users," *The New England Journal of Medicine* 321 (1989): 874-79.

11. Randy Shilts, *And the Band Played On: Politics, People, and the AIDS Epidemic* (New York: St. Martin's Press, 1987), 18; and H.

Masur, "Infections in Homosexual Men," in *Principles and Practice of Infectious Disease*, 3d ed., ed. G.L. Mandell, R.G. Douglas, and J.E. Bennett (New York: Churchill Livingstone, 1989), 2280-84.

12. Miller and Rockwell, *AIDS in Africa*, 60, 62, 65.

13. Chilton, *Power in the Blood*, chapter 5; and Reagan and Baker, *What the Bible Says about AIDS*, 40-41.

14. William H. McNeill, *Plagues and People* (Garden City, N.Y.: Doubleday, 1976), 54.

15. We would like to thank two men, Joe Kolb and Ian Rogers, who helped us think through an earlier version of this chapter which was a little mechanistic in tone, as major a problem as the one we were trying to correct. On the other hand, mistakes which remain are ours alone, and these two thinkers are not at fault for them.

16. Albert Camus, *The Plague* (New York: Random House, 1947), 209-10.

17. J. C. Moyer, "Poverty" in *The Zondervan Pictorial Encyclopedia of the Bible*, vol. 4, ed. Merrill C. Tenney (Grand Rapids, Mich.: 1976), 830; and Fred Wright, *Manners and Customs of Bible Lands* (Chicago: Moody Press, 1983), 138.

Even youths grow tired and weary,
  and young men stumble and fall;
but those who hope in the LORD
  will renew their strength.
They will soar on wings like eagles;
  they will run and not grow weary,
  they will walk and not be faint
(Isaiah 40:30-31).

" 'You yourselves have seen what I did to Egypt, and how I carried you on eagles' wings and brought you to myself. . . . Although the whole earth is mine, you will be for me a kingdom of priests and a holy nation' " (Exodus 19:4-6).

But you are a chosen people, a royal priesthood, a holy nation, a people belonging to God, that you may declare the praises of him who called you out of darkness into his wonderful light (1 Peter 2:9).

Chapter Fourteen

A Biblically Based Model for Application

*T*here is an old legend about an eagle's egg that fell out of its nest onto the prairie. An Indian brave found the egg and, being unable to return it to the eagle's roost, deposited it in the nest of a prairie chicken. The mother chicken noticed no difference and so raised the eagle as one of her own. The young eaglet learned to scratch and claw the ground for its food and was never taught to fly for more than a few feet at a time.

One day, when the young eagle had come to full maturity, he saw a bird circling high in the sky on the currents. "How majestic," he thought as he watched the eagle soar on the wind. "Oh, how I wish I could fly like that—with such beauty and grace." A nearby companion overheard the eagle's exclamations of wonder. "You can never be like that magnificent bird, for you are a prairie chicken now, and a prairie chicken you will always be."

And so it was. The eagle who thought he was a prairie chicken grew old and frail. He died having never felt the currents race through his wings or seen the vistas from great heights. He remained a prairie chicken and died not realizing the great position to which God had called him.[1]

* * * * * *

Christians are to soar like eagles, as has our majestic Lord Jesus, yet the old self often grounds us as common sinners. Our forgiveness of others, unceasing joy, and active love for our enemies should make us exceptional. Instead, the church has opted for the political methods of our day to become one more faction promoting its own agenda. Christ never operated in that manner despite living in a time that had similar sins as today. Jesus changed the world spiritually, but also morally and politically, by the renewal of hearts rather than the artificial change of legal coercion. In a moment, we will turn to his life for the model of action. But first we will look at the flawed, secular model that Christians have often followed in the AIDS epidemic.

THE SECULAR MODEL: THE CHOICE OF TWO WRONGS

In disputed areas, most choices are presented erroneously as either-or decisions.[2] This fallacy is prevalent in public issues in the United States, such as with AIDS. Two options are given: Are you liberal or conservative? Are you socialist or capitalist? Do you support recognition of all gay rights or do you want to deny support for homosexuals? Although it may be more convenient to think in such opposites, it also misrepresents reality. Our complex world seldom allows for simple, either-or answers. On the other hand, neither is it automatic that some hybrid between the two extremes is the ideal either.

C.S. Lewis said errors usually come in pairs of opposites; people see one fault and run headlong into the opposite extreme.[3] Charles Colson notes the options of a Christianized or a completely secular government and declares both to be wrong.[4] Herbert Schlossberg characterizes such decisions as the "horns of a dilemma" on which adversaries try to impale their opposition.[5] What typically results, whether in politics, religion, or relationships, is confrontation rather than reconciliation, competition rather than compassion, and strife rather than peace.

Christian alternatives exist that are based on the life and teaching of Christ, and which go against selfish human nature. Jesus faced such choices when tested by the Pharisees, but opted for unique solutions born out of his character. Stone the adulteress or let her go? Jesus gave her forgiveness and told her to sin no more. Pay tax and homage to Caesar or not? Jesus said give that which is unimportant (money) to Caesar, and give that which is important (yourselves in worship) to God. Touch sinners and be unclean or not? Jesus touched the pariahs, but remained pure despite the Law because of his great love for the outcasts.

THE PROBLEMS WITH THE SECULAR APPROACH

If we take an extreme stand for justice in the AIDS epidemic, we will emphasize that homosexuality is an abominable sin, the epidemic is God's judgment, and homosexual men deserve to suffer. Three problems occur in taking this wrong stance. First, we will see homosexual men only as stereotypes, forgetting that there is more to them than their sin; they could be a friend, a relative, or a business associate.

Second, we are altered. We, who are supposed to be active peacemakers, have created tension. We, who are supposed to love all men unselfishly, have become haters of men. We have hurt the outcasts of our society, while also distancing ourselves from God, who will have no part of such "justice." Morality without mercy, void of tears and broken hearts over sinners, is not God's justice.

Third, and not surprisingly, by altering our perceptions of our opponents and by hardening our hearts, we have lost all chance for dialogue with the homosexuals and IV drug users of our culture. If no dialogue exists, then redemption is unlikely. We cannot become fishers of men if we cannot cast our nets into the waters.

THE BIBLICAL WAY OF RELATIONSHIPS

Since secular solutions use reason as the final authority, problems are solved in an abstract way that places proof above people. Commonly, government programs, such as welfare, seem ideal on paper but are disasters in practice because they forget the frailty and grandeur of men. Likewise many thinkers, such as Shelley, Marx, Lenin, Hemingway, and Russell, professed great love for the concept of humanity, while trampling the common people around them.[6] The Pharisees did the same by making the Sabbath and their man-made rules more significant than widows and their own parents. Christians have copied this approach and followed the letter, not the spirit, of the law. Consequently, we remember that sexual immorality is sin deserving of death, while forgetting that the self-righteousness we demonstrate is also a capital sin.

In God's dominion, the important features of life always involve relationships. Jesus said, " 'Love the Lord your God with all your heart. . . .' And . . . 'Love your neighbor as yourself.' *All the Law and the Prophets hang on these two commandments*" (Matthew 22:37-40, emphasis added). This is how it has always been. The Trinity was loving one another before the creation of the world. Then humans were made by God as relational beings. Even before the Fall, God said it was not good for man to be alone. The Hebrews did not discover truth by thought; it was revealed to them by God. Truth is not abstract; it is inextricably bound to the Giver of life. With sin came alienation from God and disruption in our affinity with our fellow men. God's solution was not some rational way out of sin, but a relational way through the Son of God.

The relational aspect of truth was further emphasized when Jesus said, "I am the way and the truth and the life" (John 14:6). He did not say that he had truth or he knew how to find it, but that he is truth. Problem solving must involve relationships or it is not truth. Christians too often copy the world and act by sterile rationalism, using Scripture as proof texts for what is comfortable, rather than accepting the living Word of God as it is (Hebrews 4:12).

TRUTH IN ACTION

Jesus demonstrated his approach to relationships each time he met someone. One of the clearest examples was with the woman at the well in John 4. Few people understand how extraordinary it was that Jesus asked for a drink from an immoral Samaritan woman. His disciples and the woman herself expressed surprise that Jesus spoke with her. Jesus' followers would have been more staggered to learn what he had said during the conversation. To this impure woman, Jesus revealed that he was the Savior, when he was speaking in parables to almost everyone else. The way Jesus spoke with that woman is the model for our behavior with people today.

Similarities

Jesus initiated the conversation with the Samaritan woman by acknowledging their shared humanity. They were both in need of water, and it was this commonality that brought them together. They were also alone and desirous of companionship. He did not sit in silence waiting for her to come to him. He saw their common needs and made himself available. Christ did this especially with the weak and preyed-upon. He treated others as equally important as himself, even though he was far superior to any man.

Sinfulness

Jesus treated the woman with great dignity, despite knowing she was a lowly sinner. He carefully listened to what she had to say, and responded in a natural way as he led her in a conversation about spiritual truths. He did not emphasize that she was the pupil and he was the teacher. Rather he addressed her as a friend before revealing his knowledge of her weaknesses. He spoke to her in the present, momentarily ignoring what had happened in the past. Jesus also looked on her actions in the best possible light, despite her deceptive response to his question about her husband. He said she was correct in saying she had no husband, since she actually had five husbands! He could have rightly called her a liar, but he forgave her of her evil even as he spoke with her. He did not wait until she had shown repentance to treat her as a forgiven sinner.

Service

Jesus served her. He initially asked for something insignificant, a drink of water, then offered her the awesome gift of eternal life. He was not concerned about being seen with her, even when his friends came. He did not alter his actions or the conversation because of what others might think. He was vulnerable and open to the possibility of being rejected. He told her details about himself, while expecting nothing in return. Finally, Jesus gave God the glory for the good that he could give to her. "If you knew the gift of God and who it is that asks you for a drink, you would have asked him and he would have given you living water" (John 4:10). Out of his relationship with his Father, Jesus was able to give to others.

This is our foundational relationship as well. All good human relationships flow from our contact with God. If we have a sustaining relationship above, we will gain the strength, the self-esteem, the purpose, and the openness to love others in the ways that Jesus did. When we meet a prostitute, a drug addict, a practicing homosexual, or a promiscuous heterosexual we should consider that Jesus would treat them just as he treated the Samaritan woman. And because he would, so should we. We ought to look for what is common between us so that we can learn how to serve them. We are to treat them as the lost sheep we once were. We are to look for the best in them, while still realizing their desperate need for our Savior. We should remember that though they are sinners, so are we except by God's grace.

A PARALLEL VIEW

Another description of relating to others is given by the Jewish theologian Martin Buber. His pattern of an ideal relationship emphasizes many of the same characteristics we saw in Jesus' model. Buber said there are two types of relationships, "I-It" and "I-Thou." The former is the ungodly association, and the latter is the godly.

The "I-It" relationship occurs when we treat others as

objects. We (the "I") maintain a certain aloofness and control of the other person ("It") that eliminates many of the aspects of an ideal relationship. First, we tend to think of that person only in the way we have seen him or her in the past, giving the person no chance to change or grow. Second, genuine listening becomes all but impossible since we hear only what we expect to hear based on our preconceived notions. Objects or "Its" do not change on their own. If we cannot listen to them, then we are not totally involved. We have kept back part of ourselves, even as we do not give our all to a piece of furniture, no matter how much we may "love" it. Third, because of this lack of contact, no risk of change in ourselves occurs. The relationship is static. This tends toward exploitation, lack of understanding, and limited fulfillment. The "I-It" relationship has the same fallacies of problem solving as the secular approach given above. If we treat people as "Its," we belittle them, lower ourselves from our high calling as peacemakers, and make dialogue all but impossible.

The "I-Thou" relationship is something altogether different. The prime example of this is God's sacrificial relationship with us. The "I-Thou" relationship is one of giving and receiving. It involves two beings meeting with the best interest of the other in mind. It is a relationship that gives all of oneself, and therefore risks hurt, but also takes a chance on sublime interaction with another. It is a relationship of the present whereby past faults are not held against the "Thou," and the present is seen in the best possible light. Listening and loving can be genuine in this type of relating because the other person is held to be of great value. But the "I-Thou" relationship does not necessarily imply equality, since Buber thinks of God and man in this sort of relationship.[7]

Buber's theology has many mistakes in other areas of thought, but in his conception of authentic relationships, he has captured the true spirit of the Word of God. Taking these ideas from the Old Testament, Buber states the essentials of agape love. God initiates a relationship with us despite the antagonism each of us has shown toward him. The greatest show of love was when God chose to sacrifice his Son to restore the "I-Thou" relationship that had existed in the Garden. Jesus' whole life was one of relating to other people in this way; all were important to him. We can have this fellowship with others if we allow God to give us the strength to soar. We avoid the problems of the secular model by loving our antagonists as God loves us. Then we will seek the best for them regardless of how they treat us. We will not be guilty of degrading them or ourselves, and the possibility of dialogue remains.

THE LIFE OF CHRIST

One of the great strengths of the Bible is that it is more than just a book of wise sayings. The teaching of the character and commands of God are balanced with descriptions of the lives of actual people who show us how to be godly. God's directives come alive as we see men and women live them out.

Although the lives of saints are instructive, Jesus is our ultimate example upon which all our behavior should be modeled. "The Son is the radiance of God's glory and the exact representation of his being" (Hebrews 1:3). One might argue the meaning of his sayings, such as "the meek will inherit the world" or "turn the other cheek," but when the sayings quicken through his life, then the meaning comes alive also. If we are to be true followers of him, we ought to "take up our cross daily" in more than a metaphorical sense. He told us to love our neighbors as ourselves and then described our neighbor as anyone in need (the parable of the good Samaritan). Jesus was the embodiment of a new way that was neither Jewish nor Gentile, but evidence of a new creature. Christ passed the supreme test of love as described by Paul in 1 Corinthians 13:4-7:

> Love is patient, love is kind. It does not envy, it does not boast, it is not proud. It is not rude, it is not self-seeking, it is not easily angered, it keeps no record of wrongs. Love does not

delight in evil but rejoices with the truth. It always protects, always trusts, always hopes, always perseveres.

Jesus was the fulfillment of the Suffering Servant passage from Isaiah 53. And he literally served everyone, from the sinners he had dinner with to the Pharisees he taught, from his own disciples whose feet he washed to all of humanity for whom he gave his life. Servanthood was not a slick public relations maneuver; it was the essential way Jesus acted with people of all positions. This was God come down from heaven to mingle with kings, the powerful, the saintly—NO!; to be around the weak, the unclean, the poor, the dispossessed. Because of that, he was mistreated by the powerful and those who thought themselves righteous. Christ did not pull away when the prostitutes touched him. He did not become indignant when around drunkards. He did not refuse to drink from the hands of a foreign, lascivious woman.

If Christ is our example, dare we pull away from a homosexual with AIDS? We may think of such people as terrible sinners, but as Richard Foster has said, "Once we see the awfulness of sin, we know that regardless of what others have done, we ourselves are the chief of sinners."[8] Ironically, it is only when we deny ourselves that true self-fulfillment comes. We will only soar by becoming servants, as did our Lord.

TAKE THIS CUP FROM ME

Jesus' life was anything but easy. He had no place to lay his head, he was consistently reviled and challenged, people were always demanding something from him. He was tempted by Satan throughout his life. In the end Jesus asked that his ultimate challenge, the cross, be taken from him. Yet because of his great love, his willingness to be submissive to God's will, and his vision of the everlasting while sacrificing the temporal, Christ took up the cross. Why do we think it should be easy for us?

When a young eagle learns to fly, it is not a painless procedure. Mistakes and rough landings occur. It requires a change from the safety of terra firma to that of faith in the invisible wind. For us, that means trusting which way the Wind blows, because the Spirit blows wherever he pleases (John 3:8). But it also involves watching the example of the Father to see how to soar. And the young eagle knows it is never alone, that its Father is always there to cajole, to encourage, and to be that example.

The AIDS epidemic may seem like a blustery storm in the calm of our lives. It may make us feel cold and desire to retreat further into our comfort. But if we withdraw, then we will never reach the position God has called us to ascend. In the next chapter, we will see specific ways within the AIDS epidemic that we might "soar on the wings of eagles."

Chapter 14, Notes

1. Adapted from Charles Swindoll, *Living on the Ragged Edge* (Waco, Tex.: Word Books, 1985), 283.

2. David Fischer, *Historians' Fallacies* (New York: Harper and Row, 1970), 9. Technically this is the fallacy of the false dichotomous questions.

3. George Rekers, *Shaping Your Child's Sexual Identity* (Grand Rapids, Mich.: Baker Book House, 1982), 14.

4. Charles Colson, *Kingdoms in Conflict* (Grand Rapids, Mich.: Zondervan Publishing House, 1987), 46.

5. Herbert Schlossberg, *Idols for Destruction* (Nashville: Thomas Nelson Publishers, 1983), 10.

6. Paul Johnson, *The Intellectuals* (New York: Harper and Row, 1988). There are problems with this book in that Johnson does not give criteria for which intellectuals he chooses to discuss. But he has captured one of the main tendencies among intellectuals in their self-centered egotism which says that they know better than others how to run the world. In the process, they usually forget to order their own household. Schlossberg's *Idols for Destruction* and Johnson's *Modern Times* also confirm this impression. Herbert Schlossberg, *Idols for Destruction* (Nashville: Thomas Nelson Publishers, 1983) and Paul Johnson, *Modern Times* (New York: Harper and Row, 1983).

7. Martin Buber, *I And Thou* (New York: Charles Scribner's Sons, 1958); see *Encyclopedia of Philosophy*, s.v. "Buber, Martin."

8. Richard Foster, *The Celebration of Discipline* (New York: Harper and Row, 1978), 135.

[Jesus said], "Suppose one of you had a servant plowing or looking after the sheep. Would he say to the servant when he comes in from the field, 'Come along now and sit down to eat'? Would he not rather say, 'Prepare my supper, get yourself ready and wait on me while I eat and drink; after that you may eat and drink'? Would he thank the servant because he did what he was told to do? So you also, when you have done everything you were told to do, should say, 'We are unworthy servants; we have only done our duty' " (Luke 17:7-10).

The LORD said to Moses, "Speak to the entire assembly of Israel and say to them: 'Be holy because I, the LORD your God, am holy' " (Leviticus 19:1-2).

[Jesus said], "Be perfect, therefore, as your heavenly Father is perfect" (Matthew 5:48).

We proclaim him, admonishing and teaching everyone with all wisdom, so that we may present everyone perfect in Christ (Colossians 1:28).

Chapter Fifteen

Ministry Arenas

Mark Weaver is a man of action. He heads up the local chapter of the American Family Association, which fights against pornography, bordellos, bookstores, and bathhouses that allow anonymous sex to occur. He is frequently seen as a crusader at city council meetings, a picketer at X-rated theaters, and on the local news reports as a spokesman for the antipornography, antihomosexual citizens. Consequently, he has developed many enemies and has received several death threats. He has been in jail several times for his activities. Sometimes his rhetoric is a little harsh; sometimes his activities seem counterproductive.

Here is another side to Mark Weaver that few people appreciate. He and his wife, Cindy, have hearts of gold for the down-and-out, and they have opened their home over the last few years to several of them. Mark and Cindy became mature believers in an independent Baptist church that considered itself a spiritual hospital, believing that Jesus came to minister to the spiritually sick, not the healthy. That concept has had a lasting influence upon them, as they have compassion for the hurting. Mark and Cindy are about thirty years old and live in a three-bedroom house with three young children. They do not have an abundance of posses-sions, but they believe the Lord has called them to minister to people that the church has traditionally rejected, such as reformed homosexuals, street people, former drug addicts, and ex-convicts. Here are some of the people (with names changed) they have served.

Bill is from a little west Texas town. He has always been small in stature and that tended to isolate him from the other boys. He grew up in a solidly Christian home that was somewhat legalistic. When his parents discovered he had homosexual urges, they prayed for him repeatedly for deliv-erance, but to no avail. Bill married and had a child. Some time later, Bill's wife discovered that he had been a closet bisexual for years, and she left him. Bill was then fired from his job. He was suicidal with nowhere to go. The Weavers took him in for a short time, and by the grace of God and the obedience of two of God's children, he was a changed man. Bill is now strongly involved in Emmanuel Ministries, a reformed homosexual support ministry.

Lyle was a young man who stayed with the Weavers for about a month. He was the son of two demanding pro-fessionals, and was never able to live up to their expecta-tions. He was a small teenager of sixteen when he left home, due to the tension between him and his parents. Lyle later said that all he ever wanted was his father's acceptance, but he had never received it. Because Lyle was small and attrac-tive, he was a set-up for older homosexuals, and he became a male prostitute, both to survive and to gain the approval he had never found. However, he hated having sex with men, and desired to get out of the life-style. When Mark took him in, he had been on the street for two years and was not used to responsibility. But he wanted to please, and he had many positive achievements during his stay with the Weavers. Mark became a father figure to Lyle, because he loved the teenager unconditionally. Lyle is now living in a halfway house in the city and is out of homosexual prostitu-tion.

Harry lived with the Weavers for six months. He had

also grown up in a professed Christian home, which had been dominated by a minister father who lorded over the family. When Harry moved in with the Weavers, he had no money because he had squandered a good income on drugs. His combination of drugs and homosexuality had made him depressed and moody. He was also suicidal despite involvement with the Metropolitan Church, the largest homosexual denomination in America. While living with the Weavers he was a neat houseguest, always helpful around the home, which was especially important at the time, for Cindy was pregnant with her third child. Harry had searched for and found acceptance in the homosexual life-style; unfortunately, he also acquired infection with HIV. Although Harry did not have full-blown AIDS while he lived with the Weavers, pregnant Cindy still had to care for him when he would get routine colds or·stomach viruses. Cleaning up after a nauseated person is one of the less glorious aspects of the Lord's work. Harry eventually escaped from the homosexual life-style and is now involved in a redeemed homosexual support group.

Larry grew up a long way across the tracks from your typical middle-class Christian home. He had accepted the mentality that anything goes, including bisexuality. He had run away from a loveless home at fifteen and had lived on the streets ever since, at least when he was not in jail. He had killed at least two men and had others who were after him. Mark discovered him while picketing a porn shop, and he and Cindy were able to get him off the drugs and alcohol and away from the homosexual environment. The Weavers enjoyed Larry. He was good with their kids and he later told the Weavers that their children's love for him meant more than the love Mark and Cindy had shown him. Mark and Cindy took Larry to church; it was the first time that the forty-year-old man had ever been inside a church building. Larry was with them for seven months, but had to leave because he feared for the Weaver family. With his sordid past, many people were after him, and he feared retribution against his benefactors. Larry has even been afraid to write to them, fearing that would somehow endanger them.

Mark and Cindy Weaver do not see their home as truly theirs; it is God's to do with as he pleases. They say it is wonderfully freeing to give all their possessions to God. Currently they are involved with a group of redeemed lesbians and homosexual men in a weekly support group. Originally, this group met in the Weavers' home and Cindy prepared the dinners. However, the group has outgrown their house and is now meeting in a local church. Too often the reformed criminals, homosexuals, drug abusers, and street people have not been acceptable to God's people. Exceptions exist; we believe God wants these exceptions to be the norm.

Principles from Scripture are always brought to life when they are modeled by godly men and women. Since there is nothing new under the sun, we already possess examples to guide us in our response to AIDS. This is an illness that is analogous in many ways to diseases during biblical times, especially for the manner in which people treated the sufferers. For example, leprosy was thought by many to be terminal, highly contagious, and acquired by sin. What a pitiful group of people were the lepers. No one wanted to be with them. No one, except other lepers, dared touch them. Everyone thought they were condemned by God . . . until the coming of the Son of Man.

The life of Christ is our ideal standard for action. Jesus almost always ministered to people at their point of felt needs, those needs they thought were most pressing. The needs were as serious as the death of a child or a debilitating illness. They were as trivial as lack of sufficient wine at a wedding or hunger pangs of a crowd near the Sea of Galilee. Many of Christ's responses to people in need involved simple acceptance of them as worthy of his time or his touch. If one were to imagine the Son of God in our time, what would he do in this epidemic? He ministered to sexual transgressors and showed love. He approached the untouchable people and placed his hands on them. Those that the conventional religion rejected, Christ accepted with open arms, sins and all. Jesus accepted them as worthy of his love, his touch, and his acceptance—before he spoke of their sin.

SALT AND LIGHT

Jesus demonstrated his love tangibly to the people he met; he taught his followers to do the same. In the Sermon on the Mount, Jesus gave specific instructions concerning godly living: Turn the other cheek during persecution; give someone in need your coat; go twice as far as someone asks; lend money to those in distress; love your enemies; give to the poor in secret. And the consummate command: be perfect even as your Father in heaven is perfect. Not one satisfactory hermeneutical or practical reason exists to allegorize these statements made by Christ. We should not encourage persecution, but when our cheek is struck, are we to retaliate? We are asked—in truth, commanded—to go further, to do more, with no expectations of recompense from the unbeliever. We are to brace ourselves to be cursed, cheated, and slandered. In return we are to love our enemies without conditions. By doing this we concretely show that we are new creatures in Christ, since acting this way runs counter to human nature. So many try to dilute these verses because they are difficult to follow, particularly in a world that demands my due, my choice, my possessions, and my self-centered desires.

One might reasonably ask if perfection is worth attempting, when we know we will certainly fail. Of course it is! If we aim for mediocrity, we will attain no more than that. We will become salt that has lost its saltiness; our light will be hidden under a basket. If we aim for perfection, by the grace of God and with his strength, we might surprise ourselves at how closely we approach it at times.

And Christ does not tell his followers to reach out to others only when it is convenient. If we wait until we are wealthy, until the kids are grown, or until we have our lives well ordered, then we have not followed our Lord's teaching. Life is a process of success and failure, and God uses such challenges to bring us closer to him in relationship, in thought, and in deed. If Mark and Cindy Weaver had waited until their children were older, the men now serving the Lord might be suicide victims. If the Weavers had waited until they had a five-bedroom house, all of these people would have gone through many additional years of misery, and an opportunity may have been lost forever. If the Weavers had waited until it was convenient, they would have waited forever, because there will never be a convenient time for any of us.

SPECIFIC MINISTRY ARENAS

One summer John went fishing with his two young sons. He baited his oldest son's rod with a fly and helped him cast it into the water. For whatever reason, the fish were not interested in the fly, even though they were jumping only a few feet from the shoreline. In the meantime, the younger boy was getting bored with the wait and began throwing rocks toward the leaping fish. John had to stop that boy's antics while trying to determine what was wrong with the lure he was using. Finally he settled on a grasshopper for bait and began catching a number of fish.

Later, as they were leaving the pond, John realized the Lord had shown him a parable. As fishers of men, we require two things: we must use the correct bait, and we must make sure we are not scaring the fish away. For the Christian, the bait is the expression of the love of Christ and the evidence of a transformed life. That bait will draw even the most hardened unbeliever. The second thing required is to keep ourselves and other believers from throwing stones at men by acting in a self-righteous, antagonistic, or mean-spirited manner. A sinner is pushed farther away from the gospel when this occurs. In most ministries these actions seldom transpire, but it happens all too often in ministries to AIDS patients, IV drug users, and homosexual men. With these ideas in mind, we turn to specific groups and methods of ministry.

Ministering to the Christian Community

Leo Tolstoy once said, "Everybody thinks of changing humanity and nobody thinks of changing himself."[1] We are at once the easiest and the hardest to change. We are easiest because no one else requires convincing of the need; hardest because it requires admission of wrongs committed, first to ourselves and then to God. In any case, ministering to the Christian community often begins with ourselves. All of us need to perfect our light to the rest of the world; with most of us, at least in some area of weakness, that light has virtually ceased. Ministering to ourselves in the AIDS epidemic includes education concerning the issues, thought about the needs involved, and consideration given to how our spiritual gifts and available time might be used. Not everyone has the time or leading to be involved directly in AIDS ministry; everyone has the responsibility to avoid throwing rocks in the water, making fishing harder for others.

Next we need to minister to our own children. Evangelical parents have naively assumed that their children would be unaffected by the Playboy philosophy and the attractions of illicit sexuality. The temptations they face are more severe than what we faced, and more severe yet than what their grandparents faced, as we demonstrated in chapter 4. This truth is confirmed repeatedly by surveys that show that born-again Christians, while having dissimilar convictions from the world, have actions that are very similar.[2] We watch the same R-rated movies, laugh at the same television programs that mock our morality, get divorced at a high rate, commit adultery, and become seduced by homosexuality and pornography. Why should we be surprised when our son or daughter sleeps with his or her sweetheart before marriage?

Thankfully, there is evidence that our children want to be chaste until marriage.[3] They have seen the ravages of the sexual revolution and look to us to provide alternatives. As parents we need to set good personal examples by loving our spouses deeply and by refusing to watch movies and television that make a travesty of sound sexuality. Above all else, our children need our time. Abundant, devoted time with them will do more for their self-esteem and fortitude in an antagonistic world than all the material possessions we can give them, all the books on child care we can read, and all the special camps and sports lessons we can pay for. If we do not demonstrate to our children that they are valuable to us by our use of time, why should they value our convictions?

After parents, children are influenced most by their peers and the media. We need to protect our children from undesirable peers by involving them in youth groups that are attractive and instructional. It is still possible to have fun without suggestive jokes, seductively dressed people, or ridicule of others. But in our hypersexualized world, we have often forgotten how. We need to be innovative and encourage enjoyment of God's good gifts such as sports, parks, fellowship, and the support of others.

It is undesirable to shield our children from all worldly influences, since such a philosophical quarantine destroys our credibility with the world while perpetuating the vulnerability of our children when they leave home. The media is everywhere. Sooner or later they will see cable TV or watch rented movies at a friend's house. To tell our children they can't watch TV or movies when all their friends are creates a rift between them and us, and makes movies and television even more enticing. But it is essential that we give them the tools to examine the alluring temptations of modern media. Our children need to understand that no movie, TV program, or song on the radio is merely entertaining; they all carry a message that more often than not is antithetical to Christian morality. Not teaching our children how to critique movies and music is no less dangerous than sending them mountain climbing without ropes or crampons.

Teens should not date before sixteen, and even then they should only date in pairs or in church groups. The earlier that teens date, the more likely they will engage in premarital sex.[4] Even if both the boy and girl have good convictions, in our hypersexualized world the temptations are overwhelming. Some may say this approach is legalistic; in reality it is realistic. It is not being legalistic to keep our four-year-old from playing with fire. Neither is it legalistic to keep our fourteen-year-old from playing with sexual fire. Rather it is proper parental protection.

We ought to instruct one another about the dangers of the sexual revolution. We should be teaching in our Sunday schools methods for critiquing the media. We need to be good examples for our weaker brothers of biblical love and justice toward homosexuals, IV drug abusers, and the sexual immorality. As redeemed homosexuals and HIV-infected people appear in our churches, we ought to roll out the red carpet for them, counter any stands by other Christians to the contrary, and be willing to invite these new members into our homes and fellowship groups.

Ministering to the Redeemed Sinner

The former homosexual man, lesbian, IV drug user, and promiscuous heterosexual have a difficult life as they enter a new world. Not only have they left an addictive life-style, they have also forsaken a whole subculture including friends, personal habits, and various haunts. A new community must be built. If they have a lukewarm reception in the supposedly loving world of Christ, then their life-style change becomes arduous. We need to lead support groups, provide professional counseling, meet for prayer, provide jobs, embrace them when they slip and repent, and open our homes to them so they will feel acceptance. Just as with our own children, new Christians need time, time, and more time with mature, loving brethren. That allows them to learn about our Lord in an intimate fashion and to build a new and attractive world apart from the old, sordid one they came from. Good Bible study and doctrinal teaching are important, but that will be cold and sterile if deep relationships are not involved. Jesus taught with excellence, but his teaching was never divorced from his giving of himself. We are called to do likewise.

Ministering to the AIDS Patient

"AIDS patients die alone." While that may not always be true, too often it is. This should not be; someone needs to be there to show the love of Christ. Myriads of ministers visit those in prison, as well they should. Having AIDS is a type of prison, where the walls are composed of the judgmental looks and attitudes of others, the ostracism of parents, and poverty. AIDS patients are not more deserving of love than other terminally ill patients or prisoners, but thanks be to God, the love of Christ is deep enough to reach all people, regardless of need.

To minister most effectively to AIDS patients, we need to understand the needs they have:

Time. AIDS patients need people willing to spend face-to-face time with them. Giving time does not necessarily mean giving answers. As the dying go through grieving and depression, they simply need someone to go through those experiences with them. It also does not mean presenting the gospel each time you meet. Just being there in a caring way is a more thorough presentation of the gospel than a thousand tracts. Remember, Jesus spoke of giving drinks to the thirsty as an end in itself: "Come, you who are blessed by my Father; take your inheritance, the kingdom prepared for you since the creation of the world. For I was hungry and you gave me something to eat, I was thirsty and you gave me something to drink . . ." (Matthew 25:34-35).

It is a point of tension for evangelicals to recognize how strongly Jesus emphasized works. Salvation clearly comes by grace alone. But somehow in the process of feeding the unlovely, ministering to the dispossessed, and clothing the outcasts, we bring ourselves under the lordship of Christ. Or, as James said, "Faith without deeds is useless" (James 2:20). The Christian who has no good works is like a stillborn child: so much promise of life, yet none to be seen.

Transportation. Many AIDS patients are too weak to drive and cannot afford a taxi (if they could get one to come). They have doctor's appointments, testing to be done, and medicines to pick up. They also need transportation to church, to see friends, and to go to recreational areas.

Meals. Many AIDS patients cannot afford food; many more do not have the strength to prepare food when they can buy it. They cannot simply warm TV dinners, since their chronic diarrhea often requires a special diet.

Support groups. Support groups help the suffering person to see that he is not alone in his disappointment, anger, and grief. Helping a person become involved with a support group allows him to meet others who will also love and accept him.

Financial support. Financial concerns are a major problem for AIDS patients because of the ostracism from family, the inability to work, and the high cost of medical care. Most AIDS patients are young and have limited savings. Although costs for medical care have gone down, some of that reduction has been offset by the mixed blessing of extended life expectancy.

Ministering to the Homosexual and IV Drug-Using Community

Mercy triumphs over judgment (James 2:13), and that should be our order of action, since judgment is the Lord's business, not ours. We ought to be firm in our convictions of the truth of Scripture, which teaches specifically that homosexuality and implicitly that IV drug use are wrong. However, we need not harangue the practitioners of these sins more than those who commit other sins; perhaps a greater measure of compassion is needed because these are such self-destructive sins and because society has rejected those who practice them.

It is entirely possible to have a friendship with a man or woman who practices such sins, while making it clear what you believe. With the aggressive homosexual political activists, it might appear that dialogue is impossible. That has not been our experience. The love of Christ is capable of bridging any barriers. So many of these people are hurting from past experiences of rejection or even physical harassment that meeting a loving challenger is actually a breath of fresh air. Often the activists are aggressive only as a public posture and are open to talk with Christians if true concern is displayed. Also, nothing will gain the attention of the homosexual community faster than when Christians meet the needs of dying AIDS patients. Fishing for men requires love in action, not mere rhetoric of which the modern world abounds.

We can still oppose the agenda of the homosexual community without doing it in a mean-spirited way. Democracies are the best of worlds for Christians because they give us freedom to fish for men, and our bait is far better than anything the world has to offer. So if we lose a few battles within the city councils or in statewide referendums, we do not have to proclaim that the world is coming to an end. We Christians understand the sovereignty of God—until we exit our church buildings. We then act as if each setback is some devastating and irrevocable defeat. By acting that way, we undermine confidence in what we preach. Where is our assurance of the majesty of God? Where is our confidence that the events that happen, happen for a purpose? Christians legitimately can oppose a city ordinance for "gay rights" while remaining friends with an active homosexual. We do not catch fish by throwing rocks at them.

The IV drug-using community is not organized like the homosexual community, nor does it have support from liberal groups in the country. Drug users are divided into two distinct sets. A number of IV drug users are professionals, including doctors, lawyers, and accountants, and some of these are not addicted—they are able to enjoy the high of drugs once in a while without becoming dependent. Most, however, will use drugs more and more frequently and will start having typical addiction problems such as family stress, deteriorating work effectiveness, financial woes, and depression. Christians should befriend these people to help them stay away from drug usage and to be an example of someone who has "peace that passes understanding." Referring them to detoxification hospitals is appropriate; financial support might be necessary through the local churches.

The other group of IV drug users are the destitute poor who support their habit by crime, including selling drugs, stealing, and prostitution. These men, women, and young teens are usually concentrated in urban areas such as the ghettos of New York, Miami, and Los Angeles. Some started in poverty; some were abused in their homes and became runaways. This group is harder to reach and offers significant risk to those ministering to them, which probably should be done under an umbrella organization such as the Covenant House for runaway teenagers. Ministering to the inner city is a foreign mission field, at least in the cultural differences. But Christians should be actively involved in this or supporting those who are.

Ministering to Society

Society, in truth, is an artificial construct in our minds. The main method of ministering to society is to provide light for our local area of the world, loving tangibly those who enter our lives. However, the mass media, the political process, and the educational system must be encouraged to have goals in keeping with God's dictates in Scripture. But—and we emphasize this as strongly as we can—the power of those systems and their antagonism toward the church has been dramatically overestimated by many Christians. For the most part these systems have not conspired intentionally against the church. Rather, the church has hurt herself by failing to live up to the commandments of her Founder. Because of the shrinking world, the national systems appear to have significantly more power than they actually do. The true power of change still descends to the local level, to the congregations providing loving care for their communities, teaching wisdom grounded in God's truth, and giving hope to people with no hope. Having laid that foundation, we will address some of the social issues as if they were separated from the personal ones.

Probably the most important change we could hope for in society is a sex education program in all schools that strongly emphasizes monogamy and gives strong reasons why teenagers should wait until marriage to have intercourse. Young women, who as a group have already paid heavily for the cause of "free love," will be quite responsive if offered confirming evidence that premarital sex is destructive. To be sure, there are interested parties who will want to see the erroneous safe-sex ideas promoted. But if we are united, we will prevail for the simple reason that, in the case of AIDS, science and morality actually teach the same thing.

Christians ought to be involved with the political process, making sure that the American Civil Liberties Union, among others, is not successful in its covert attempt to disenfranchise Christians. (This is one group that does consistently attempt to reduce the freedom of the church.) We need to oppose homosexual legislation firmly but with grace, and we need to continue to write and call our political leaders to let them know where we stand on the various issues that surround AIDS. Given that, we ought to avoid the tendency in the recent past to put all our eggs in the political basket. Although politics is an important area of life, for most Christians political action is one of the least important areas. If we concentrate on making true changes in peoples' hearts, the political actions we desire will fall more easily into place.

We live in a time of mass communication, and we need to be aware of its impact on our lives. One angry Christian screaming epithets at a homosexual with AIDS on national television becomes a very big stone cast in the water. On the other hand, Christians giving money to the dying is also an excellent lure for the fishers of men, as has been demonstrated before.[5] Of course, we do not take up a collection for the dying because it is good publicity, but because it is the right thing to do. Mother Teresa, who won the Nobel Peace Prize a few years ago, in her acceptance speech roundly criticized the secular world for its lack of concern for the weak, including the unborn. She was able to tug at the conscience of the world because of her love for the dying, not because she shouted political slogans.

THE CONSTANCY OF CHRIST

Jesus Christ is unchanging. He would act the same today as he did two thousand years ago. If Christ were in the flesh today, he would still drink with sinners, meet with the lowly, oppose much of what passes for Christianity, and minister to all the needs of people including thirst, hunger, and lack of shelter. By these actions, Jesus was able to attract people to himself; he was using the best bait. He also did not drive people away by his attitude or actions, except the self-righteous religious community which was already running away from him and his teaching.

If we believe that we are to take up our cross daily to follow him, then our actions today are also clear. We are to be servants to the whole world whether they revile us, dismiss our goals, or cast us into prison. Then we can truly follow the words of Jesus when he said, "Come, follow me, and I will make you fishers of men" (Mark 1:17).

Chapter 15, Notes

1. Leo Tolstoy, quoted by Richard Foster in *Celebration of Discipline* (San Francisco: Harper and Row, 1978), 9.
2. A 1984 Gallup poll showed that Christians were similar to non-Christians in many moral areas including sexuality. See Randy Alcorn, *Christians in the Wake of the Sexual Revolution* (Portland, Ore.: Multnomah Press, 1985), 24; John White, *Flirting with the World* (Wheaton, Ill.: Harold Shaw Publishers, 1982), 75; Tim Stafford, *The Sexual Christian* (Wheaton, Ill.: Victor Books, 1989), 12; and Josh McDowell and Dick Day, *Why Wait?* (San Bernardino, Calif.: Here's Life Publishers, 1987), 24.
3. McDowell and Day, *Why Wait?*, 17-19.
4. Ibid., 79. McDowell and Day argue that there exists a direct correlation between age of dating and premarital sex.
5. Tony Campolo, *Twenty Hot Potatoes Christians Are Afraid to Touch* (Waco, Tex.: Word Books, 1989), 14.

PART 4

SOCIETY AND AIDS

Submit to one another out of reverence for Christ (Ephesians 5:21).

You, my brothers, were called to be free. But do not use your freedom to indulge the sinful nature; rather, serve one another in love. The entire law is summed up in a single command: "Love your neighbor as yourself" (Galatians 5:13-14).

To the elders among you, I appeal as a fellow elder . . . Be shepherds of God's flock that is under your care . . . not lording it over those entrusted to you, but being examples to the flock. . . .

Young men, in the same way be submissive to those who are older. All of you, clothe yourselves with humility toward one another, because,

"God opposes the proud
but gives grace to the humble" (1 Peter 5:1-5).

Do nothing out of selfish ambition or vain conceit, but in humility consider others better than yourselves (Philippians 2:3).

Chapter Sixteen

Civil Rights versus Social Responsibility

*I*n a "Focus on the Family" program in the summer of 1988, James Dobson interviewed a mother and daughter with a troubling story. Their identities were hidden by technical means, but their emotions were evident. The mother had been married to the same man for over twenty years and had been absolutely faithful. He was a businessman who left town frequently, but he called her every night he was away. He apparently loved his several children deeply. Although his wife knew their marriage had problems, they were far more serious than she had ever dreamed.

About six months before the interview, the husband was hospitalized with a respiratory ailment. Various tests were done, resulting in the diagnosis of *Pneumocystis* pneumonia. But that was only the secondary diagnosis. The primary diagnosis was infection with HIV. Her husband had AIDS. She was dumbfounded initially and would not believe the diagnosis. But then her husband admitted to being bisexual and having sex with men on virtually all his business trips for the past ten years.

Blood from the wife confirmed that she was infected with HIV as well. By the strength of the Holy Spirit, she had been able to forgive her husband even though he was not repentant. But the children were not so willing to pardon their father. His daughter's voice shook with anger as she described his hypocrisy. She was especially angry about his lack of concern for the death sentence he had given her innocent mother. The father's audacity went further. He was giving speeches to local homosexual groups, claiming persecution at the hands of family and friends.

* * * * * *

Gaetan Dugas will live in infamy for his role in the AIDS epidemic. As we noted in chapter 5, Dugas was identified as Patient Zero, who had been instrumental in the early spread of the disease.[1] Of the first 248 reported cases of homosexual men with AIDS in the U.S., 40 had direct sexual links to Dugas.[2]

Dugas's doctors taught him all the possible ramifications of his illness as it was understood at the time. Despite the probability of AIDS being a sexually transmitted disease, Dugas refused to act on that information. Instead, he continued to have frequent sexual contact with other men, using the typical rationalizations: no one knows for sure if it is contagious; someone gave it to me so it is not my fault if I give it to others; I have to have sex; I cannot stop, so why try. Only the inevitable severe illness and his death stopped him.

Dugas was one of several early cases who spread the disease extensively to other men. He was prolific, not because he was more contagious or less informed, but because he was completely self-centered and addicted to unnatural sexuality. He and others rapidly amplified the infection even while many homosexual men were curbing their habits. He acted within his rights at the time, since no proof existed that AIDS was spread through sexual contact. Others stopped intimacy because of the possibility of spread of this dangerous disease. Dugas, on the other hand, had forgotten his responsibility for his fellow man.

* * * * * *

SECULAR FREEDOM AND PERSONAL RIGHTS

This husband and Gaetan Dugas were men of sin. They were also victims of the age. Their self-centeredness was inflamed by our culture which encourages freedom without boundaries, choices without accountability. Aptly, the cultural observer Tom Wolfe has called this the "Me Generation." *Time* magazine, in its sixty-year anniversary issue of 1983, accurately declared that modern America has deified freedom.[3] Independence and personal choice are so highly valued that little remorse is expressed when others are adversely affected. So society will ignore its duty to the unborn, because women have freedom to choose. A man no longer feels condemned for leaving his family, because he is free to "find himself." And the husband described earlier can speak as a persecuted individual, having spread HIV to his wife, because he is free to act immorally.

Tolerance is the flip side of freedom. It allows one to escape condemnation from others. No guilt feelings from self; no accusations from society. Tolerance demonstrates that no criteria for evaluating right and wrong exist—except perhaps feelings. As Hemingway once said, "What is moral is what you feel good after and what is immoral is what you feel bad after."[4] Obviously, what feels good varies from person to person. So almost anything becomes acceptable as long as messy consequences are avoided such as pregnancy, addiction, or death.

What modern men have forgotten is that our "inalienable rights" must be given from above or they are mere rhetoric. Rights are not intrinsic to the collection of molecules called man or woman. If not endowed by God with transcendent value, then rights will always be at the mercy of the power of the state. And since the modern state has grown enormously in the twentieth century,[5] rights are fragile indeed. Only recently, as the memory of God fades, deprivation of rights has been defined as the right to oppress others through abortion, through claims of First Amendment protection, and through self-indulgent sexuality. The specter of the reign of terror is never too far away.

SOCIAL RESPONSIBILITY FROM CHRIST

The Christian ideal is absolutely different from the secular egoism described above. The biblical accent is on service to others, not personal gain for self. Jesus set the standard not only by his death on the cross, but also by his selfless attitude. He approached the vilest sinners, although the kings of the earth were unworthy to approach him. He washed his followers' feet, although such a job was reserved for the lowliest servants.

Great freedom and personal benefit may occur from being a Christian, but that freedom is always within the boundaries of loving other people before ourselves. Moreover, the love is not dependent upon the merit of the recipient. It requires supernatural strength to love the unlovely, but that is the calling of the church. In a rich spiritual sense Christians no longer have the rights that the secular man is vigorously demanding. Our rights have been deeded to God, because we were bought with a price. Any benefits we have are those he has graciously given, not those we have vigorously fought for.

RIGHTS, RESPONSIBILITIES, AND THE AIDS EPIDEMIC

Elevating the rights of one person beyond what is proper lowers the legitimate rights of others. Especially in the U.S., the tradition of individualism and self-sufficiency comes into conflict with healthy cooperation. Rights breed competition between parties. In contrast, the biblical concept of community is radical in emphasizing service over personal desires. Rights become cooperative. God made us to be interdependent. Christians need to be reminded of this because the tendency toward self-centered individualism is bred into us by our culture.

In the AIDS epidemic, three groups interact: the HIV-infected individuals and their supporters; the health care workers, including physicians, nurses, and lab technicians; and the rest of society. Each of these groups has duties toward and proper expectations from the other two (see diagram). If these are not balanced then some members of society suffer and injustice is done. Let's look at the responsibilities of each.

PATIENTS

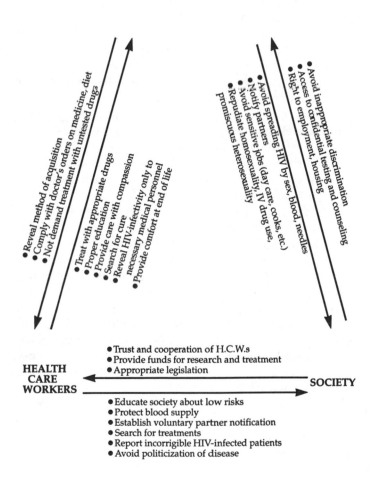

HEALTH CARE WORKERS

SOCIETY

- Trust and cooperation of H.C.W.s
- Provide funds for research and treatment
- Appropriate legislation

- Educate society about low risks
- Protect blood supply
- Establish voluntary partner notification
- Search for treatments
- Report incorrigible HIV-infected patients
- Avoid politicization of disease

Text within the figure:

Left arrow (Patients → Health Care Workers):
- Reveal method of acquisition
- Comply with doctor's orders on medicine, diet
- Not demand treatment with untested drugs

Left arrow (Health Care Workers → Patients):
- Treat with appropriate drugs
- Proper education
- Provide care with compassion
- Search for cure
- Reveal HIV-infectivity only to necessary medical personnel
- Provide comfort at end of life

Right arrow (Patients → Society):
- Avoid spreading HIV by sex, blood, needles
- Notify partners
- Avoid sensitive jobs (day care, cooks, etc.)
- Avoid homosexuality, IV drug use,
- Repudiate promiscuous heterosexuality

Right arrow (Society → Patients):
- Avoid inappropriate discrimination
- Access to confidential testing and counseling
- Right to employment, housing

Health Care Workers

In the past, doctors and nurses treated many patients with contagious, incurable diseases. Doctors often acquired plague through the cough of dying patients. Nurses contracted cholera while cleaning up sufferers after bouts of diarrhea. Many died helping others with these and other illnesses. A professional risk was incurred that was recognized by all. But due to vaccines and antibiotics, those trained in the late forties and early fifties were the first generation that did not worry about risks. Physicians had to readjust in the eighties to the reality that an accidental needle-stick could be life-threatening. Consequently, many refused to treat patients with AIDS, although such prejudice is considered unethical.

Moreover, until modern times, medicine was primarily seen in the West as a calling from God to serve others, not as a means of attaining social status and wealth. The reality of calling and the riskiness of medicine have vanished over the last fifty years with the secularization of medicine and the discovery of antibiotics and vaccines.

Health care workers owe services to people infected with HIV. Physicians and nurses are to provide good, compassionate medical care prolonging life, alleviating suffering, and providing counseling and education. Part of that time should be spent teaching patients how to avoid spreading the disease to others. Medical professionals should cooperate in clinical studies to help discover future treatments. All health professionals should hold to strict confidentiality, letting only assistants within the practice and necessary consultants know the diagnosis. Confidentiality should be adhered to for any disease, but especially with HIV infection, since so many people fear AIDS and treat its victims poorly.

Health care workers owe society proper education to minimize the risk of acquiring HIV disease. Physicians should protect the blood supply through proper screening of donors and testing the donated blood. Ongoing research should be conducted to search for treatments and to further lower the risk from transfusions. Physicians have the responsibility to protect the uninfected by notifying partners whenever possible, such as the wife of a bisexual man. Since such notification is usually impossible without cooperation, strong encouragement must be given to the patient to notify partners. The physician should remind his patient that he has a moral obligation to inform sexual and IV-sharing partners and that HIV is now a treatable, although incurable, illness. AZT and other therapies prolong life, so the earlier someone is informed of possible infection with HIV, the better. Patients who refuse to curb their dangerous activities should be reported to public health authorities. It is also incumbent upon physicians and public health departments to evaluate data as objectively as possible to avoid politicization of the disease. For example, if "safe sex" is the misnomer we have suggested, then we should avoid using this deceptive terminology.

The HIV-infected Patient

The patient should be responsible to the health care team to provide as much information about possible ways that he caught the virus. He is responsible to take good care of himself and follow the advice of his doctors in taking medication, changing his diet, keeping routine appointments, and avoiding high-risk behavior that might spread HIV to others. If he is having trouble following this advice, he needs to explain why so that the therapy can be altered or support groups can be suggested to maximize his own care and avoid spread to others.

The patient does not need to announce to others that he is infected with the virus (as he would if it were a casually contagious disease). The person infected with HIV needs to tell others with whom he has shared needles or had intimate contact that he is infected. He owes it to the uninfected members of society to avoid high-risk behavior even if they want to have sex or share needles. He ought to be understanding that people are fearful of the unknown and that some will not want to be around him even if it is safe. He should avoid donating blood, semen, or organs, and if possible bypass sensitive occupations that might alarm the public, such as being a cook or day-care worker. If he has acquired

HIV through personal choices such as IV drug use or promiscuous sexuality, he should admit his error and renounce such activity.

Society

The public's primary responsibility is to treat HIV-infected patients as people, not pariahs. The public should provide funds to pay for the necessary care, just as it does for indigent patients with other self-caused illnesses. The public should provide opportunities for HIV-infected individuals to have jobs insofar as they are able, to have proper housing, and to have friendships with non-infected people. Society should be willing to help as they would for any ill person. Individuals should keep confidential any knowledge of the infection with HIV or how the patient got the disease.

The public needs to have reasonable expectations for cures, take appropriate public health measures, and avoid sexual contact or needle-sharing with HIV-infected people. Legislation needs to be enacted that carries penalties for lapses of confidentiality and discrimination directed at HIV-infected individuals. It also should include penalties for repeated, purposeful spread of the virus by the infected. No support for quarantine should be entertained, since it is unnecessary except under extreme cases involving the most recalcitrant infected person. Even then, the goal should not be punitive but restorative through education and counseling. Society should be able to inquire about different aspects of the disease but needs to trust to a reasonable degree the information on AIDS coming from the medical profession.

If all three groups will act appropriately, then the epidemic will more quickly come under control, a level of trust will develop that encourages cooperation, and better treatment will occur for the patients.

TO TEST OR NOT TO TEST, THAT IS THE QUESTION

Controversy has raged ever since 1985 when the HIV antibody test became available. Current testing for HIV utilizes two tests, the screening ELISA and the confirming Western Blot, a reliable combination. The main issues revolve around confidentiality, mandatory testing, partner notification, and the stigma and symbolism of the test.

Confidentiality is the main issue from the homosexual viewpoint. In communities such as San Francisco, where half the homosexual population is infected with HIV, the test could be misused to stigmatize homosexuals. Even with the new openness in the homosexual community, most prefer to remain "in the closet" and are fearful of their positive test results being made public.

Confidentiality usually should not be an issue since doctor-patient interaction is private. If someone in the church has a drinking problem and is getting counseling, he would be understandably upset if the pastor announces that fact in the Sunday morning service. The doctor-patient relationship has been likened legally to the same circumstance.

But exceptions do exist. Evidence of child abuse within the family must be reported to authorities. If a man admits to his psychiatrist that he is planning to kill someone, the psychiatrist is duty-bound to report the situation to the police. Diagnosis of a severe, casually transmitted disease such as pulmonary plague negates confidentiality and requires temporary quarantine to protect others. In our own community, a restaurant's water supply was contaminated with salmonella, causing a number of people to be hospitalized. Because of the bad publicity, the restaurant quickly closed even when the source of contamination was eliminated. Were the owner's civil rights violated by reporting the contamination? Not in this case, since public welfare transcended the right of this man to have a successful business. The key issue in all these cases is that a duty to report exists because other victims' rights and health must be considered.

As we discussed in the chapter on the prevention of HIV disease (chapter 8), the only testing that seems to reduce the spread of the disease is voluntary, confidential testing. Mandated testing would be inordinately expensive, be easy to avoid in most cases, test people who are at low risk, and actually increase spread because potential HIV carriers would likely avoid testing while continuing their high-risk behavior. Partner notification usually can be done only with cooperation since most patients are homosexuals or IV drug users who have many sexual or drug-sharing partners known only to themselves. Mandated testing would be appropriate in cases of rape or incest.

LAWSUITS AND AIDS

The only risk a known carrier presents to the public is to have intercourse or share needles without informing his partner of his infectious state or to repeatedly attempt to donate blood. Although those who engage in immoral sexual activity bear some personal responsibility for the consequences of their behavior, our legal system has already addressed some grievances from partners who received a venereal disease through sexual intercourse.[6] Most of these have been private lawsuits where the plaintiff sues for negligence, battery, or fraudulent misrepresentation. In some states, statutes have been enacted making transmission of venereal diseases a crime, although not all of these states have added HIV disease to their list of sexually transmitted diseases.[7] Rock Hudson's male lover was able to sue and win a large settlement from his estate for Hudson's misrepresentation of his HIV status. A few cases of at least temporary confinement have occurred due to charges of attempted murder when a known HIV-infected person attempted to bite or spit on another individual or when a prostitute continued to ply her trade despite knowledge of her infection.[8]

The problem with most lawsuits that involve consensual sexual activity is proving who is the source and who is the recipient of the illness. If two promiscuous homosexuals or heterosexuals are involved, it is difficult to prove who transmitted the infection. Both have engaged in high-risk activity and each could have acquired HIV from another source. It would be different if one person were monogamous (as was the wife in the story at the beginning of this chapter) or one person had received medical treatment for HIV infection without informing a new sexual partner.

Lawsuits involving transfusion transmission of AIDS are likely to be far more successful. Indeed some major lawsuits have already been settled for large sums of money, and many more are being processed now. One San Francisco blood bank had at least seven lawsuits in process in 1989. Liability premiums have increased dramatically in the last few years for the blood-banking industry.[9] The plaintiffs have the advantage of being totally innocent in their acquisition of the disease, being able to establish that the transfusion caused the HIV infection (since donors can be traced), and suing hospitals or blood banks which have "deeper pockets" than an individual with HIV disease.

SUGGESTED ACTIONS

The biblical perspective of personal responsibility for actions, instead of the secular position emphasizing the rights of individuals, allows for a more reasonable balancing of individual and social obligations. Although partner notification in general is impossible without cooperation from the patient, the patient has a strong moral duty to notify as many partners as can be found. Moreover, those individuals who have engaged in high-risk behavior in the past ought to know their HIV status before potentially exposing others to AIDS. Not knowing is a lame excuse for a promiscuous homosexual or IV drug user. A rapist should have to undergo immediate testing and repeat testing in three and six months to determine his HIV status for the victim's sake. Any patient should be obligated to test for HIV infection if a nurse is pricked with the needle used to draw blood from him. Confidentiality and counseling should occur in all such cases based on the results of the test.

From a Christian viewpoint, it is good to recall that we are all sinners and that we are all sinned against. Balancing compassion and justice becomes a more realistic objective if we remember that many of the homosexuals and IV drug users had abusive homes and that society has encouraged immoral sexuality for some time.

THE RIGHT TO WORK

It should be illegal to fire someone for being infected with HIV, as long as he is able to do the job, since HIV is not a danger to fellow workers. Potentially, an HIV-infected person could cause irreparable harm to a business if the infection were generally known and he worked in a sensitive area such as meal preparation or child care. Although not medically warranted, it would be reasonable to ask such an employee to voluntarily move to a less sensitive area within the company or to find the employee an equally satisfying job elsewhere. As long as this option is not abused, all parties involved (the employer, the employee, and the public) are treated compassionately (see chapter 17 on economics).

HOMOSEXUAL RIGHTS?

Homosexuals should have no special rights outside of those guaranteed to all members of our society. The homosexual life-style is sinful and should not be given tacit approval by repealing laws that make sodomy a crime. To give approval to homosexual sex is analogous to giving approval to adultery, drunkenness, or prostitution. On the other hand, Christians should protect the basic needs homosexuals have for jobs, housing, and medical care.

One of the common misconceptions about law is that "you cannot legislate morality." That is patently false. Almost all legislation has some moral dimension. It is difficult to enforce laws that regulate private and consensual acts, but the laws should remain nonetheless. In a post-Christian culture such as ours, anything that is legal will soon attain respectability, as has occurred with pornography. We should not make incest or drug abuse legal simply because they are difficult to enforce. If all such laws were withdrawn in our self-centered society, immoral behavior would increase.

Christians should not become vindictive toward gay rights activists. Christ provided the proper method of action. He clearly condemned immorality, yet did not harangue sinners. He made it clear that their sin was wrong. Then, by the integrity of his character and the truth of his message, he convinced them that his was the right way. If our light shines brightly by showing love and providing care for those who hate us, making sacrifices of time and money for sinners, then the darkness will be great and people will be drawn to God's light like a moth to a light in the blackest night.

DRUG USER RIGHTS?

IV drug users have no more rights than other citizens, but because of their precarious state they are more likely to be despised, used, and neglected. Many are trying to dull the ache of poverty, pain, and pessimism. Only one in seven are in a drug treatment program, and even then the results are not impressive. Treatment centers are unsuccessful because they do not remove the social problems that caused the person to start drugs originally. Without committed relationships, little hope for change exists. Here is a desperate group of people ready for the gospel—if they can see the reality of it in God's people.

A large problem in reaching this group is that many within the church who have the time and resources to help are white while most of the drug users are Hispanic and black. Although they may be distant from many of us culturally, they are not as culturally removed from our brethren in the minority churches. It is time that we get together to solve these problems with black, brown, and white churches working together to form the only rainbow coalition that truly exists.

THE RIGHTS OF SCHOOL CHILDREN

A few years ago Ryan White, a hemophiliac teenager with AIDS, was chased from his hometown because he wanted to go to school. Fortunately, the town where he moved accepted him. Open meetings with physicians and parents there helped avert another panic. Part of the irony is that Ryan was discriminated against because he had the complete syndrome, even while many asymptomatic children with HIV disease are in schools all over the country. No child should be treated as Ryan was.

Why do parents of such children want them to go to school where they will be exposed to many illnesses? External infections are usually not the problem for AIDS patients, but reactivation of infections they have already had. Particularly in older children, who have already been exposed to many ailments before infection with HIV, the dangers of going to school are small. The danger they pose to other children is nonexistent.

Many parents think the educational advantages of a classroom setting outweigh the advantages of private tutors. Children with other serious illnesses profit greatly from being with their peers and being treated as much as possible as regular kids. Their morale is better, they can accept the necessary therapy more readily, and they are happier. Children tend not to live any longer than adults once complete AIDS develops. However, with the extension of life by AZT and soon other drugs, the odds are that AIDS will become a long-term chronic illness such as cystic fibrosis, muscular dystrophy, and diabetes. To keep such children out of school, to make them feel like outcasts, is to lack compassion.

THE RIGHTS OF PROSTITUTES

Surprisingly, many people are concerned about the rights of prostitutes. Prostitutes have been unfairly vilified as spreaders of HIV. They are actually responsible for few cases in the U.S. (Africa is a different story). Also, an unfair double standard exists when their patrons do not receive a similar condemnation. Some have suggested that prostitutes be licensed and routinely examined to ensure that they are HIV-free, since it is unrealistic to stop the world's oldest profession.[10] Christians should condemn the patrons as strongly as the prostitutes, but to accept prostitution as inevitable and make it legal is not responsible, since it will increase the exploitation of women and give tacit approval to sin. All sins will occur, but are we to make drug use, adultery, prostitution, and murder legal because they are inevitable?

PRISONER RIGHTS

Prisoners are treated differently from the rest of society, but still have certain legal protections. Courts have stated that all prisoners have rights to reasonable living standards, to visit with loved ones, to practice religion, to exercise, to protest conditions, to have access to the courts, to have adequate protection from prison violence, and to have fairness of the rules for each prisoner.[11] With the current crisis in overcrowding few prisons adequately meet these criteria, which has resulted in court orders to improve circumstances.

A number of states practice mandatory HIV testing of all prisoners.[12] A prisoner's chances of being infected are much higher than those of the average person for several reasons. First, a large number of drug users are incarcerated for various crimes. Most HIV-infected inmates became infected from IV drug use before imprisonment (92 percent in one study of New York prisons) rather than through homosexual activity. Second, in some prisons drugs are smuggled in, allowing for further spread of HIV disease among prisoners if precautions are not taken. Third, an enormous amount of homosexual rape occurs for sexual gratification and as a method to humiliate other prisoners.[13] Consequently, the spread of AIDS within prisons is a real possibility.

Wardens have had difficulty addressing these problems due to lack of funds, hysteria among guards and cellmates of infected inmates, overcrowding, and the cost of necessary reforms to stop rape and drug use within prisons. Here are the true outcasts of our society whom few people want to be bothered with. This is also a place ripe for the gospel because of the despair and hopelessness. HIV-infected prisoners should receive proper medical care, which has not usually occurred in the past. If the HIV-infected prisoner is not known to be sexually violent, then it is unfair to lock him in solitary confinement as has been done.[14] Prison ministries should be encouraged to address the physical, psychological, and spiritual needs of these special prisoners. The gospel has been given to set the captive free, including those behind bars.

THE RIGHT TO THE GOSPEL

Some of the most difficult issues in this epidemic concern the rights and responsibilities of those involved. Christians have a difficult task because we must stand up for the integrity of Scripture, which means condemning sin, while showing service to a dying world. The way of Christ is the way of the servant. He reached out to all, even those whose spirits were marred by the sin in their lives. Never did Jesus deny someone the right to follow him. We should maximize the rights of others to commit to him by being ambassadors with no rights of our own. This means ministering to people the world calls pariahs: homosexuals, drug users, prostitutes, and prisoners. But the captives will be set free as we point to the One who is the Way, the Truth, and the Life.

Chapter 16, Notes

1. Randy Shilts, *And the Band Played On: Politics, People, and the AIDS Epidemic* (New York: St. Martin's Press, 1987), 130.

2. The first cluster of AIDS cases was reported initially by the Centers for Disease Control. ("A Cluster of Kaposi's sarcoma and *Pneumocystis carinii* Pneumonia among Homosexual Male Residents of Los Angeles and Orange Counties, California," *Morbidity and Mortality Weekly Report* 31 [1982]:305-7), then more extensively and formally in *The American Journal of Medicine* in 1984 (D. M. Auerbach et al., "Cluster of Cases on the Acquired Immune Deficiency Syndrome: Patients Linked by Sexual Contact," *The*

American Journal of Medicine 76 [1984]:487-92). Shilt's Patient Zero (Dugas) was linked to these original scientific articles in a review article in 1989 (S. C. Holmberg et al., "Biologic Factors in the Sexual Transmission of Human Immunodeficiency Virus," *The Journal of Infectious Disease* 160 [1989]:117).

3. Roger Rosenblatt, "What Really Mattered," *Time* , 5 October 1983, 24-27.

4. Hemingway quoted in Randy Alcorn, *Christians in the Wake of the Sexual Revolution* (Portland, Ore: Multnomah Press, 1985), 74.

5. Rosenblatt, discussing views of Paul Johnson, in "What Really Mattered," 24-27. See also Paul Johnson, *Modern Times* (New York: Harper and Row, 1983), which chronicles the rise of the modern state.

6. Donald H. J. Hermann, "Torts: Private Lawsuits about AIDS" in *AIDS and the Law*, ed. Dalton and Burris (New Haven, Conn.: Yale University Press, 1987), 158-66.

7. Ibid., 166.

8. John F. Decker, "Prostitution as a Public Health Issue," in *AIDS and the Law*, 88.

9. Joshua Hammer, "AIDS, Blood, and Money," *Newsweek*, 23 January 1989, 43.

10. Decker, "Prostitution as a Public Health Issue" in *AIDS and the Law*, 89.

11. Urvashi Vaid, "Prisons" in *AIDS and the Law*, 236.

12. Ibid., 235.

13. Ibid., 237-38.

14. Ibid., 241.

"No one can serve two masters. Either he will hate the one and love the other, or he will be devoted to the one and despise the other. You cannot serve both God and Money" (Matthew 6:24).

At the end of every three years, bring all the tithes of that year's produce and store it in your towns, so that the [priests] . . . and the aliens, the fatherless and the widows who live in your towns may come and eat and be satisfied, and so that the LORD your God may bless you in all the work of your hands (Deuteronomy 14:28-29).

The LORD will guide you always;
    he will satisfy your needs in a sun-scorched land
    and will strengthen your frame.
You will be like a well-watered garden,
    like a spring whose waters never fail
(Isaiah 58:11).

"Do not store up for yourselves treasures on earth, where moth and rust destroy, and where thieves break in and steal. But store up for yourselves treasures in heaven, where moth and rust do not destroy, and where thieves do not break in and steal. For where your treasure is, there your heart will be also" (Matthew 6:19-21).

Chapter Seventeen

Economics and AIDS

I f what Christ says is true—where our treasure is, there resides our heart—as the children of this age are wont to be intent upon
getting things that make for delight in the present
life, so believers ought to see to it that, after they
have learned that life will soon vanish like a
dream, they transfer the things they want truly to
enjoy to a place where they will have life unceasing.

We ought, then, to imitate what people do
who determine to migrate to another place, where
they have chosen a lasting abode. They send
before them all their resources and do not grieve
over lacking them for a time, for they deem themselves happier the more goods they have where
they will be for a long time. But if we believe
heaven is our country, it is better to transmit our
possessions thither than to keep them here where
upon our sudden migration they would be lost to
us. But how shall we transmit them? Surely, by
providing for the needs of the poor; whatever is
paid out to them, the Lord reckons as given to

himself (Matthew 25:40). From this comes that notable promise: "He who is kind to the poor lends to the LORD" (Proverbs 19:17). Likewise, "He who sows bountifully shall also reap bountifully" (2 Corinthians 9:6). For what is devoted to our brothers out of the duty of love is deposited in the Lord's hand. He, as he is faithful custodian, will one day repay it with plentiful interest. Are our duties, then, of such importance in God's sight that they are like riches hidden for us in his hand? And who would shrink from saying this, when Scripture so often and openly attests it?[1]

John Calvin

* * * * * *

THE FOUNDATIONS OF BIBLICAL ECONOMICS

The Bible has much to say about money and its approach is vastly different from the secular one. The contrast includes:

God owns everything. The Lord God has said, "The world is mine, and all that is in it" (Psalm 50:12). We do not own possessions; we are merely caretakers of them.

God entrusts people with possessions for a time. God loans possessions to people in variable amounts to test our stewardship. In his grace, God may cause us to prosper. "Wealth and honor come from you" (1 Chronicles 29:12).

Money directly competes with God for our attention. Jesus made the contrast stark. Serve God or serve money; you cannot do both. This makes money a tool to use in the world and not an end in itself.

God will provide all our basic needs. "So do not worry, saying, 'What shall we eat?' or 'What shall we drink?' or 'What shall we wear?'. . . But seek first his kingdom and his righteousness, and all these things will be given to you as well" (Matthew 6:31,33).

Since we have received freely, we are to give. "Freely you have received, freely give" (Matthew 10:8). By giving to people, who bear the mark of God's image, we are investing in what is vital.

In chapter 12 we concluded that America has deified sex; it has become the ultimate in many people's lives. Money is also a god; the difference is money has been sacred for so long that most Christians have forgotten when it was not so. When capitalism diverged from God in the eighteenth century, the importance of "being" (who we are) was replaced with "having."

God and Money are competing deities and their kingdoms function in opposite ways. God's kingdom is one of giving; Money's is one of taking. God's kingdom is relational; Money's is transactional, so people are exploited for gain. Modern psychology, with its focus on personal benefit (self-actualization) over family or society, enhances the world of Money. The ethic of eros also operates like Money in that it is a self-centered, grasping desire, rather than the giving love of agape.

Money always controls the person, never the reverse. In this sense the church has been seduced by the lord of this world. Christians try to raise enormous sums of money for ministries to evangelize, when the limitation on evangelism is never tied to money. After all, why does God need *our* money when he owns everything? Money is extremely important, not for what it can buy but for what it does to the heart. As Jacques Ellul said,

> We are therefore called to use our wealth so that our actions announce to the watching world that election is free, that grace is abundant, that a new creation is promised and that God owns all things. The important thing is never again the wealth itself or the social forces or economic power it represents, but only the spiritual reality to which it points.[2]

We as a church have failed to do this, and so the world which acts consistently according to its god, Money, can rightly criticize us for not being consistent with our God, Yahweh. "Honor the LORD with your wealth, with the first-fruits of all your crops" (Proverbs 3:9). If we do not give him the best, then we have placed the lord Money above the Lord God.

THE AIDS EPIDEMIC

As the number of people who develop AIDS increases, money issues will become more significant. Many have worried that AIDS patients will cause financial instability for insurance companies, certain cities, and the country as a whole. However, projections into the next few years indicate that the amount spent for each HIV-infected patient will be forty to eighty thousand dollars from the time of diagnosis to death. This is not out of line with other serious illnesses such as cancer, renal disease, or heart disease. Some cities, such as San Francisco or New York, will be more severely affected because of their higher numbers of AIDS patients. Yet even in these cities the increased costs are not prohibitive even without additional national assistance.[3]

How the Christian community responds economically in the following areas will affect our overall witness to the homosexual community and to society at large. Our most valuable witness with money will be when it is given along with our time, friendship, and prayers. The love we demonstrate and the hope of Christ we offer will have lasting importance beyond the financial assistance, but the funds are the tool needed to open the door.

The Individual

We often talk about the AIDS epidemic as an abstract problem, but we need to be reminded that the statistics are the sum of individual sufferers. Each of these souls has his own trials, fears, and struggles to relate. One of the main struggles involves economics.

Many have asked, "Why should we give money to people with AIDS since they have reaped what they have sown?" No attitude is more against the spirit of Christ. Jesus gave his life, a far more significant commodity than money, to individual sinners in the same situation as those with AIDS today. Such questions are equivalent to making money more significant than people. We should not dole out funds contingent on the perceived worthiness of the recipient. We are to be discerning in our choices, but such discernment comes through walking by faith. Too often, such reticence to help others is disguised materialism rather than spiritual wisdom.

The type of economic help AIDS patients need varies. Some churches will have in their body many HIV-infected individuals who need assistance. Others will not have any (particularly in churches with older members), but will be located in a large urban area where many people with AIDS reside. In some churches a member will have a relative with AIDS who can be helped. Others might have a fund-raiser for an area organization that ministers to AIDS patients. Most of the needs of AIDS patients can be provided with small amounts of money but large amounts of time. Shopping for groceries, cooking meals, or providing transportation are all ways of helping meet those needs. As one observer noted, "AIDS is a virulent one-way ticket to poverty."[4]

AIDS in the Workplace

In most cases, the asymptomatic person infected with HIV has every ability to continue to work, some for as long as ten years. (That time will likely become longer as AZT and other drugs prolong the symptom-free period.) Consequently, a person with HIV can maintain a productive, self-sustaining life for some time, which will help keep down the overall costs to society.

The hysteria surrounding AIDS causes employers and fellow employees to discriminate against HIV-infected workers. An Ohio restaurant owner fired a man with twenty-two years experience when his infection was anonymously disclosed.[5] A popular pediatrician in Dallas had to close his business when a reporter decided to go public with his knowledge of the doctor's infection with HIV. Over the last decade, many people lost their jobs when their HIV status became known. Recent polls suggest many employers would fire HIV-infected individuals despite the Centers for Disease Control's affirmation that no danger exists to other workers or the public even in restaurants, doctors' offices, or day-care centers. Loss of job should not be one of the burdens these men and women have to bear.

Christians should not oppose a sinner's working, only his homosexual or drug involvements. It is still illegal in many states to practice homosexuality (and in all states to use IV drugs), and he can be opposed on those and scriptural grounds. But it is never morally wrong to work except in an immoral profession such as prostitution. Therefore, on one day we can vigorously support a man's right to work regardless of what other co-workers think of him. On the following day, we can just as vigorously oppose the same man's justification of his homosexuality or IV drug usage, again regardless of what others think of him. This was the way of Christ.

An adult with full-blown AIDS may be unable to work at all or may work inadequately, but the evaluation of his ability to work should be based on his job performance, not his HIV status. Mitigating factors such as longevity and contributions to the growth of the business should also be considered, just as with a worker who is impaired by alcohol, cancer, or marital problems. It might seem unfeeling for businesses to lay off laborers who can no longer work well, but unproductive employees can be the difference between a business's survival and failure. Compassion comes at another level, not here.

The responsibility of a Christian employer will vary depending on the circumstances, but Jesus' teaching gives us general guidelines: We are to go the second mile, treat our employees as we would want to be treated, and always show them respect as befitting those who bear the image of God. Christian-owned companies should give special benefits to all their employees (not just AIDS patients) that guarantee a stipend and insurance for a time if the company has to release them. Christians ought also to help people find another, less demanding job if they are weakened by AIDS. God will honor our faith in his provision when we go this extra mile for others.

Housing

Housing is a special economic need of AIDS patients because they are often evicted due to the fears of others. The extent of this fear was demonstrated when the home of a family in Florida that had two children with HIV disease was destroyed by an arsonist. Rock Hudson's home in California was difficult to sell after his death even though it was advertised for less than half its market value. Discrimination against someone due to illness should be opposed by everyone. Although homosexuality and IV drug use should have no special protection, all people need shelter. The Christian community should guarantee that AIDS patients have a place to stay even if it is in our own homes.

However, homosexuality or IV drug use should not be allowed to be promoted on one's property, just as one should not allow any other illegal activity. If a homosexual man lives in a rental home that I own and advertises a party that includes sadomasochism, I have the right to ask him to leave. (It would be appropriate to ask him to stop the promotion of his homosexuality, and if he agreed, to allow him to stay.) This might seem harsh to the world, but it is not if Christian morality is consistently applied to other sins. In other words, it would be reasonable to ask the homosexual man to leave my property if I also am ready to ask any heterosexual to leave who advertises wife-swapping.

The key question is, What will we allow to be presented as the norm for our society? Most homosexuals until recently were satisfied to keep their activities quiet, and were left alone. The homosexual culture began challenging this in the forties and fifties as the number of homosexual bars increased. The "out of the closet" mentality became a battle cry with the 1969 Stonewall Inn riot. All state antisodomy laws are properly written to punish homosexual acts, not homosexual tendencies, but the American Civil Liberties Union and others disparage such laws, suggesting that police are camping in people's bedrooms. That is mere inflammatory rhetoric. Although homosexual acts were illegal in all fifty states before 1960, the laws were not applied oppressively against homosexuals unless public indecency or molestation occurred. Mutually consenting adults could engage in homosexual acts without fear as long as they did it in their homes and did not try to promote the normalcy of those acts.

The Old Testament has similar laws against homosexual acts, which state that a man who committed sodomy (or adultery or bestiality) would be stoned. But how many people does Scripture say were stoned for sexual sins? Absolutely none. Since two witnesses were required, the law was almost unenforceable. If any were caught and stoned, it was not recorded and must have been a rare event. Any person who practiced homosexuality in ancient Israel did so cautiously. The person did not admit his or her form of sexual intimacy, nor proclaim that homosexuality was an "alternate life-style," because he or she would be executed. (The one near-stoning, the woman caught in adultery, was probably a set-up by the religious leaders to test Jesus. If so, it was quite hypocritical because only the woman was going to be stoned, the man perhaps being in cahoots with these so-called righteous men.) The importance of the laws lay not in catching illicit sexuality but in standing as a testimony to society that homosexuality, adultery, and bestiality are not acceptable.

In some states, it may be within the letter of the law to refuse to lease a home to a known homosexual. However, it is more in keeping with the example of Christ to assist such a person. Jesus was around drunkards. He took one of the wicked tax-gatherers into his inner circle. He allowed immoral women to touch him. Jesus came into direct contact with sinners much more than the isolated middle-class church does today. How much more likely is a man to consider the claims of Christ if we provide for his needs than if we deny him access to basic housing? This is a complex area, but such are the results of a fallen world.

The one legitimate reason to evict anyone is nonpayment of rent. No discrimination exists if an AIDS patient is asked to leave for failure to pay rent because that obligation is required of all alike. The property owner should not be expected to subsidize an AIDS patient's living expenses. If a patient is asked to leave by a Christian landlord, he should be cared for as fully as possible. Alternate places to live, including the landlord's own home, should be available. Sanctuaries for the dying within loving homes will do more to draw these and others to Christ than almost anything else we could do. Christ taught us to give to those in need and no condition of spiritual perfection was required.

Health Insurance

Serious conflict occurs with insurance and AIDS. The main disputes involving individual policies have been over the legality of requiring pretesting with the antibody test and the possible discrimination against practicing homosexuals as higher-risk individuals. The insurance companies argue that the HIV test is vital to determine an individual's risks. Their opponents argue that to be HIV-positive is not to have the disease. However, as we noted earlier, it is more appropriate to think of HIV infection as a disease with a long asymptomatic period, so it is fair to use the test for some rate decisions since HIV does increase the companies' costs. But the test should be uniformly applied. If a company tested someone for HIV, it should test all in that age group. In the past, some men who were judged effeminate were forced to take an HIV test while other men were not.

The other problem has been the difficultly in estimating the costs for an HIV-infected individual. As the epidemic ages, these costs will be easier to project and higher rates could be set for those infected. The answers to these dilemmas vary for each company and from state to state, and the situation remains in flux.

Controversy will grow in group policies also because

some areas of the country are "higher risk." Is it fair for a resident of California to pay higher rates on medical insurance than someone living in Maine, simply because more people per capita have AIDS in California? It probably is for two reasons. First, the people in California (among other areas) have passed laws and city ordinances that have encouraged homosexual activity, fostering an environment that enabled HIV to spread widely. Therefore, a certain guilt exists for the state as a whole. Second, supply and demand make certain areas of the country more expensive to live in. Increased insurance premiums might simply be one more cost of living in a high-risk AIDS area, whether that be California, Florida, or New York. In a fallen world, it is impossible to make everything perfectly equitable.

Some suggest that we outlaw the HIV test for pre-insurance physical exams so that the costs for treating AIDS patients are spread to all companies equally. Another option is to have the government assume the care of all AIDS patients. State and local governments are already caring for AIDS patients to a large degree, since the patients often lose their jobs, exhaust their savings, and end up in county hospitals, which are tax-supported. Citizens will pay for the care somehow because we do not let people die in the streets. Though we may balk at paying for illnesses that are the direct result of sin, AIDS patients are not the only ones who receive such care. We continue to care for the alcoholic with liver disease, the obese with heart disease, and the smoker with lung disease. We should be no less compassionate toward AIDS patients.

Christians should be as compassionate as possible, helping AIDS patients make payments for insurance premiums, doctors' visits, and medication. If we are willing to show a skeptical world that a dying homosexual man is more vital to us than our money, then we demonstrate that our treasure lies with eternal things such as the souls of other men, rather than with worldly possessions.

Life Insurance
Life insurance is a separate issue from health insurance for several reasons. First, while it is obvious that people need

medical care, no one can argue that life insurance is necessary. There is no true need, since no direct benefit to the individual exists. Second, the vast majority of life insurance policies are individual rather than group policies so the insurance companies assume a greater risk. If someone knew he had less than six months to live and he could hide that fact from the insurance company, then he would likely take out as large a policy as possible. Prior to the widespread knowledge of AIDS, many homosexual men did exactly that. Consequently, the amount paid out to the beneficiaries of patients who died from AIDS-related complications was five times as high as other death policies ($250,000 versus $50,000).[6] Third, the amount of the payout is determined at the time of the agreement in life insurance and is often much higher than with medical insurance. A person who develops AIDS might die quickly from pneumonia, making the insurer pay a few thousand dollars for medical care. But the life insurance company pays the full amount of the policy, often in the hundreds of thousands of dollars.

It might seem compassionate to allow HIV-infected people to take out large life insurance policies, but it is hardly realistic. It is like gambling with marked cards—the one in the know wins easily at the expense of the other players. If life insurance can be obtained without HIV testing, then the amount paid out will either bankrupt the insurance companies or force everyone else to pay much higher rates. It is reasonable to allow insurance agents to request HIV testing from everyone or from those with symptoms of HIV disease. The person applying for insurance may refuse to be tested, but then he or she gets no insurance. Some companies have developed programs whereby the person with HIV can get life insurance but at considerably higher premiums. As with medical insurance, the regulations vary from state to state.

Christians should go further where families are involved. The main benefit for the one covered by a life insurance policy is the knowledge that his family will have sufficient money to care for their needs when he dies. Christians should not provide hundreds of thousands of dollars to a surviving family, since that goes far beyond basic needs, but we should take seriously James's charge to care for widows and orphans by opening our homes and our pocketbooks (James 1). A church's reassurance that they will care for the survivors of an AIDS patient will offer great comfort to him and clearly demonstrate the compassion of Christ.

Research Money

Homosexual activists and some scientists alleged that insufficient money was provided initially for research on AIDS. They accused the government agencies that decide the outlay of funds of being unconcerned about a disease that primarily affected homosexual men. Some underfunding probably occurred because scientists are attracted to research they enjoy; investigating the behavior of homosexual men is not attractive to most. That reluctance is understandable, but if it was based on the view that homosexual men are of less value than others, then the decisions made were immoral. However, many other legitimate reasons existed for delayed funding, and current research may be overfunded given the number of infected individuals and the qualified scientists available to do research.[7]

A homosexual writer compared the number of deaths from AIDS with the numbers from toxic shock syndrome and Legionnaire's disease and said that much more was spent per death in these tragedies than on the AIDS epidemic.[8] But it is illegitimate to compare the funding for AIDS research to these other diseases that burst quickly on the scene, acquiring a notoriety that made research money more readily available. Both toxic shock and Legionnaire's disease appeared in a straight-forward manner and required less medical sophistication, making their investigation much easier. AIDS is much more complicated than either toxic shock or Legionnaire's disease (which were simple bacterial illnesses) and so requires complex research techniques most laboratories are unable to perform.

Research is developed over time. Scientists have to cultivate ideas, write proposals, get approval from boards and ethics committees, and acquire expensive equipment. When AIDS was discovered, few retrovirologists existed in the country. Research money depends on the recipient being capable of using the money efficiently. It would have been foolish to give large sums of money to 99 percent of the doctors in this country, who did not know what a retrovirus was, much less what to do with one in a research setting. Since no new epidemic of any magnitude had happened in recent memory, it was natural to think that the few men with *Pneumocystis* pneumonia and Kaposi's sarcoma were only isolated cases rather than the harbinger of thousands of deaths. The few scientists who realized the significance of the epidemic were young and lacked the renown that might have hastened the acquisition of grants. AIDS is akin to cancer because of its slow onset, its variety of manifestations, and the complicated treatment and therapy it requires that often lasts for years. Truthfully, patients suffering from almost any disease could also claim that too little has been done for them.

Ironically, physicians were providing the advice necessary to avoid AIDS even before the illness was discovered. For years doctors had counseled homosexual men to decrease the number of their sexual partners to avoid other venereal diseases. Physicians and social workers had advised IV drug users to stop sharing needles because of the spread of other blood-borne infections. But this advice was ignored by both groups. It is doubtful that more research money early on would have made any major difference, since no cure is likely even in the near future despite years of research and the expenditure of millions of dollars.

More money might have made a difference in one area, however. More research might have identified the cause sooner, allowing quicker protection of the blood supply. Even if this had been done, only a few thousand lives would have been saved, virtually all of them outside of the homosexual and IV drug-using communities.

Determining the flow of research funds is a complicated process. The amount of money spent is limited and is often not directly related to results. Millions can be spent wastefully if the researchers are unqualified. Some might argue that the disease that causes the most deaths should get the most money, but this approach belies the complexity of the decisions. Should chronic illnesses that seldom cause death, such as asthma, allergies, premenstrual syndrome, or dermatitis, receive no research money? Should deaths of the aged, as in heart disease and most cancers, be counted equally with deaths of younger people, as in drug abuse and alcoholism? Should an illness that is on the upswing in numbers, such as AIDS, receive more support than stable illnesses such as hypertension and kidney disease? Should illnesses that are often self-caused, such as lung cancer, cirrhosis, and AIDS, receive fewer dollars than those that are not, such as brain tumors, rheumatoid arthritis, or leukemia? Should illnesses that seem more likely to have breakthroughs in the near future be given special consideration? How much money should be spent on basic research that has no immediate application but may be extremely significant for future therapies? How do we guarantee that diseases of minorities, such as sickle-cell anemia, obtain proper financial assistance? Should we spend more money for Third World diseases, such as malaria and gastroenteritis, that kill far more than most Western illnesses?

The way most research grants are determined is probably the best approach generally. A scientist becomes interested in a certain disease that he is qualified to study. He then writes a proposal for the goal of his work, including the need for the research, the cost of new equipment and salaries for lab assistants, and the length of time for the project. All of this is submitted to experts in the field who determine the project's validity. Certain biases, personality conflicts, and different philosophies for research make this an imperfect process, but it is better than responding to every wail from special interest groups.

THE INDIVIDUAL AND MONEY

Homosexuals have accused institutions of failure in this epidemic.[9] Certainly, the medical community, government, research institutions, media, and others could have worked better in some areas. But the primary failure still must be placed on the individual for his own actions. It is individuals who act, not groups, and almost all people involved with the AIDS epidemic have acted sinfully. We Christians too have fallen short of our role as care-givers to the needy. We also should repent and bring our actions more in line with the actions of Christ. No deeds are more immediately convincing to the secular world than when Christians give their homes and money to those they disagree with morally. If Christ could give his life for sinners of all types, shouldn't we be able to give our possessions?

CHRIST AND MONEY

No man was personally less interested in money than Jesus Christ. He was supported by followers, but only with the bare necessities of life. Imagine! The Lord of all the universe with barely the clothes on his back and no pillow for his head. It is a sad irony that the Lord, who owns all yet possessed none of it while on earth, is consistently offered Mammon by his followers. What Christ truly desires is the same thing that he gave: life and dedication. Only by giving our lives to him do we show that he is truly Lord.

Christ was not personally concerned about wealth, but he was concerned with how it affects the heart. The widow who gave two cents so excited him that he called his disciples over to tell of her deed. It was not the two cents that mattered but her heart for God. Christ asked the rich young man to give up all that he had. When he did not, Jesus did not fret that some charity was poorer than it could have been. The money was not important; the condition of his heart was what mattered. When the woman poured perfume on Jesus' head, she was criticized for wasting what could have been sold and the money used to feed many people. But what mattered was not the value of the perfume but the condition of her heart and of the hearts of those who criticized her. Christ is watching the condition of our hearts in the AIDS epidemic. Will we choose the Master or Mammon?

Perhaps the greatest example of Mammon versus God occurred not in Jesus' teaching but in his life. For the True God, who would give his life freely, was bought for a mere thirty pieces of silver. He could have stopped the transaction with a legion of angels, but he did not. He knew the spiritual work he was about to accomplish was far more important than the money. Since we live in a world that considers money sacred, we need to be careful that we do not make the material realm more important than the spiritual. When we do, we exchange a few coins for the majesty and infinite worth of the Lord Jesus Christ.

Chapter 17, Notes

1. John Calvin, *The Institutes of the Christian Religion*, vol. 1, ed. John T. McNeill (Philadelphia: Westminister Press, 1960), 827.

2. Jacques Ellul, *Money and Power* (Downers Grove, Ill.: InterVarsity Press, 1984), 68.

3. D. E. Bloom and G. Carliner, "The Economic Impact of AIDS in the United States," *Science* 239 (1988):604-610.

4. D. E. Rogers, "Federal Spending on AIDS: How Much Is Enough?" *The New England Journal of Medicine* 320 (1989):1623.

5. Mark Rothstein, "Screening Workers for AIDS" in *AIDS and the Law*, ed. Dalton and Burris (New Haven, Conn.: Yale University Press, 1987), 140.

6. Mark Scherzer, "Insurance" in *AIDS and the Law*, 191.

7. W. Winkenwerder, A. R. Kessler, and R. M. Stolec, "Federal Spending for Illness Caused by the Human Immunodeficiency Virus," *The New England Journal of Medicine* 320 (1989):1598-1603.

8. Randy Shilts, *And the Band Played On: Politics, People, and the AIDS Epidemic* (New York: St. Martin's Press, 1987), 110.

9. Ibid., xii-xiii.

Not many of you should presume to be teachers, my brothers, because you know that we who teach will be judged more strictly (James 3:1).

You must teach what is in accord with sound doctrine (Titus 2:1).

Jesus said to his disciples: "Things that cause people to sin are bound to come, but woe to that person through whom they come. It would be better for him to be thrown into the sea with a millstone tied around his neck than for him to cause one of these little ones to sin. So watch yourselves" (Luke 17:1-3).

Therefore, as God's chosen people, holy and dearly loved, clothe yourselves with compassion, kindness, humility, gentleness and patience (Colossians 3:12).

Chapter Eighteen

Education and AIDS

I attended a conference on AIDS in which a portion was dedicated to the means of educating various groups, including teenagers, minorities, and the general population. One of the speakers was an ethicist, who identified himself as a Baptist minister. His presentation troubled me, so I went up after the lecture to question him.

This ethicist had asserted that sex education was vitally necessary from the middle schools on up. He also said that sex education was not a moral issue but a health issue. So I asked him what his goals were for sex education, knowing it can be used to instill biblical morals or to manipulate children into accepting any form of sexuality.

He was evasive, but I kept pressing him to find out what he truly wanted. This Baptist minister finally admitted that he thought homosexuality was a legitimate expression of sexual love. He did not accept the scriptural passages that condemned it, nor the accuracy of what Jesus reportedly taught about sexuality. In short, he had a low view of Scripture and merely chose what he thought was "true." His form of sex education would reflect these views.

I left that conference angry at this man for two reasons. First, he claimed to be a Baptist minister, which was true on paper but deceptive in spirit, since few Baptists condone what this man accepts. Second, he did not reveal what he meant by sex education. If this were a health issue instead of a moral issue, as he claimed, then the sex education he should teach is the one taught in Scripture: absolute monogamy within heterosexual marriage. That alone will reduce the spread of HIV disease. But that was clearly what he was *not* going to teach.

Either this man lacks integrity, because he would not say what he truly believed, or he thought he was being honest in his presentation but had become foolish in his thinking. I do not know which it was. It is easy to assume the former since this is a well-educated man with a doctorate and seminary training. However, remember what Malcolm Muggeridge said:

> Education—the great mumbo jumbo and fraud of the ages—purports to equip us to live and is prescribed as a universal remedy for everything from juvenile delinquency to premature senility.
>
> For the most part it serves to enlarge stupidity, inflate conceit, enhance credulity, and put those subject to it at the mercy of the brainwashers with printing presses, radio, and television at their disposal.[1]

Maybe this man foolishly believed that he was teaching truth honestly.

* * * * * *

Sometimes the assault on traditional values is straightforward and intense. At other times it comes disguised, a wolf in sheep's clothing, as with this Baptist minister. In either case it is vital for all believers to weigh instruction carefully regardless of the source.

Is Education the Way to Stop the AIDS Epidemic?

Many have said that public education is the most effective way of stopping the AIDS epidemic.[2] Those who make this claim are naive about education's potential. Their optimism assumes that people will act responsibly if taught, refusing to spread HIV by selfish behavior. But that is exactly what happened early in the epidemic[3] and continues to happen today. Education involves moral instruction that gives direction to the data collected. Even with proper teaching, people will still sin and spread HIV. Historically, education has had a limited effect in stopping other venereal diseases.[4]

Education imparts knowledge from the moral point of view of the teacher. If I teach safe sex to teenagers, implicit in that instruction is the idea that teenagers will not abstain from sexual activity. If I teach an IV drug user how to get free, sterile needles, then implicit is the idea that supplying sterile needles will save lives. Those assumptions may or may not be true. Both the overt instruction and its moral assumptions must be evaluated to avoid adopting anti-Christian ideas. Like fish in water, we often breathe in our culture and its values without questioning what we have taken in.

Many types of education exist. Parents are the most important instructors, but are becoming less so because often both parents are working. Under these circumstances children do not stop learning, they merely learn from different sources, including friends, day-care teachers, and television. Secularization has become so complete in public schools that in recent years, U.S. history texts have been rewritten to virtually exclude our religious heritage.[5] In quantity of time, no teacher at home or in school matches television. The average American watches two hundred times as much television as he spends reading books.[6] And children watch more than adults. Music, films, other people, and the church are also educators.

AIDS EDUCATION

Those who believe that education is the primary way to stop the AIDS epidemic believe that several forms of instruction are needed. Each of these has its own characteristics.

The Mass Media

Homosexual activists have accused the mass media of doing a poor job of education in the AIDS epidemic. Originally, reporters and news anchors were understandably nervous reporting on AIDS since it was primarily a disease of homosexual men.[7] Full discussion would reveal distasteful homosexual bedroom practices. Moreover, HIV disease is not easy to understand with its esoteric discussion of T-helper cells and opportunistic infections. Also, no one in the media knew how big this epidemic would become. In light of the limited behavior change of high-risk groups and the skewed portrayal by the media of so-called "safe sex," it is unlikely that more publicity in the early days of the epidemic would have made much difference.

The media started with preconceived notions that hamstrung it as a force for education. A 1980 poll of leading television and newspaper journalists revealed a strong liberal bias: 86 percent of those polled seldom or never attended church, 75 percent thought homosexuality was normal, over 50 percent thought adultery was acceptable, and 90 percent thought abortion was a woman's right. In all categories Americans see these issues quite differently. Another poll of television writers and producers showed similar results.[8] No wonder opinion polls show the press has only a 16 percent approval rating.[9]

The national media has limited ability to stem the AIDS epidemic for several reasons. First, only a portion of the population closely reads the newspaper and the weekly newsmagazines. Many of the people who need to be reached, such as IV drug users, people on the street, and teenagers, are the ones least likely to read such sources.

Second, early reports were often sensational to increase

interest. Skewed reporting has occurred in several ways. Casual contagiousness or mosquito transmission of HIV has been implied even in prestigious newspapers, since this affects the general reader more than stories on IV drug use or homosexual practices. New findings have been written so as to suggest that a cure was imminent. Eye-catching headlines have altered the content of stories, transforming an incremental scientific advance into a possible cure. Research on vaccines, the studies on drugs, and many other stories were given an optimistic tilt where optimism was unwarranted. Such reporting instilled false hopes in AIDS patients, while limiting behavioral change in high-risk groups who thought a cure would soon be available.

Third, media leaders wrongly accept the idea that better-educated people are more moral. Since the media-makers have more schooling than most Americans, they have assumed a patronizing attitude toward the public, offering deceptive stories that make their views appear more reasonable than they are.[10] A similar stance was taken by the ethicist described at the beginning of this chapter who altered his speech to make it more palatable for others. As the polls indicate, the ethical positions of the media elite are suspect despite their educational achievements.

Fourth, the national media believe overwhelmingly in individual free choice. If a man and a woman want to commit adultery or use drugs, it is acceptable since supposedly no one is hurt. A child can be aborted because a woman's freedom is more important than "fetal tissue." If homosexual men want to have fifty or more "lovers" a year and have anonymous sex with four men in an evening, the media will not criticize them because they do not want to restrict freedom. The national media start with a different set of values than most people and are blind to their own biases. The media moguls simply cannot fathom how someone can come to a conclusion different than theirs.

Finally, the media accept sexuality as an activity that no one could realistically refrain from for even a brief time. Gandhi held such a fascination for Western intellectuals in part because by choice he was able to abstain from sex and material possessions. The West, having little self-control, considered him saintly. With these foundational beliefs, education on AIDS by the national media will suit homosexual activists. The media portray homosexual men sympathetically, conveniently leaving out the distasteful tendencies of extreme promiscuity, drug use, and recurrent venereal diseases. Anyone who suggests homosexuality is sinful is a bigoted homophobe. Condom use is presented favorably, ineffective though it may be, since the promiscuous want it promoted.

General Education

In the spring of 1988 the largest single mailing of information on AIDS was sent to every household in America. This distribution was arranged by C. Everett Koop, then the U.S. Surgeon General. It told in detail the cause of HIV disease, its method of spread, the risk groups involved, and how to stop it. Koop became a controversial figure among evangelical Christians for discussing the use of condoms for AIDS prevention, after briefly promoting abstinence and monogamy in the pamphlet.

In 1987 some magazines and newspapers began accepting advertisements for condoms. Problems exist with simple condom commercials void of instructions. Condoms are not absolutely safe, as we noted in chapter 8, although they are promoted as the answer to stopping the epidemic. Also, the goal of condom ads is to sell a product, not educate people. They are not likely to describe the difficulty of proper usage, the chances of a tear, or correct disposal techniques. Most sexually active people are well aware of the availability of condoms; the question is whether they will use them properly.

Abstinence from immoral sexuality and drug abuse is the only completely effective way to prevent AIDS. The Surgeon General's report and other educational pamphlets mention abstinence, but usually only in passing. Far more emphasis needs to be placed on the fulfillment of a monogamous relationship as well as the need for family stability and for the emotional well-being of children. To merely mention chastity and monogamy before going on to a much longer explanation of condom usage is to leave the impression that condoms are the only way to prevent AIDS. And in emotional and sensitive issues like this one, impressions may mean everything.

CHRISTIANS, CHASTITY, AND CONDOMS

Should the Christian community only emphasize chastity in marriage as the way of stopping AIDS? Should Christian doctors never mention condoms or methods for sterilizing needles for fear of contaminating ourselves with the immoral activities of others? Those who suggest this course of action are naive. Most of the evangelical community is sheltered from the harsh realities of the world. Jesus understood the reality when teaching about the model of lifetime commitment between a man and a woman in marriage. He admitted that exceptions to the rule exist if one partner commits adultery. Moreover, he argued that Moses gave a writ of divorcement because of the hardness of the Jews' hearts. If God's chosen people, who had seen his miracles in Egypt, experienced his presence daily in the cloud above the Tabernacle, and had Moses as their leader, could have hardened hearts, how much more a lost person in our day?

In the 1980s, over 80 percent of unmarried males and over 60 percent of unmarried females engaged in sex before they turned twenty.[11] Do we want the church to appear to sacrifice these kids by trying to block any attempts to reduce their risk of AIDS? Monogamy and abstinence must be presented in a very favorable light, but we underestimate the power of sexual addictions to cause teenagers to stumble. We underestimate despair in an addict who thinks no alternative to his problems exists except the high of drugs. We underestimate the pervasiveness of our sexualized society to cause even the redeemed to fall. Is a person who is accustomed to having sex with fifty or a hundred people a year going to stop easily? Without emotional support from the church, is a lonely, single mom going to refuse the men who come into her life? We live in a sordid world where many of these people have been emotionally and physically abused. A large portion of the promiscuous homosexuals and straights, male and female, are convinced that the only way they can achieve a relationship, emotional fulfillment, and feelings of self-worth is to be sexually active.

Our opposition to government and private attempts to teach an immoral sexual ethic will never be effective if we do not offer realistic alternatives. We will simply be dismissed as a fringe group offering other-worldly answers to very real problems. The way is prepared for change among millions of people who are watching the Christian community's response to AIDS. We need to produce educational pamphlets that present in a positive light the Christian position on sexuality, not simply denounce what everyone else says. We need to be active examples of caring to show concretely the meaning of Christianity. And we need to realize that before someone can be saved, he must be kept alive to see the love of Christ in his people. That is the educational alternative to the "just say no" or "just use condoms or clean needles" positions.

How do we justify discussing condoms and clean needles? The lost have no power to change their lives, and too few Christians are in a position to minister to these people. It takes time to establish relationships, set up programs, and penetrate a hardened heart. While we are feverishly promoting such ministries, anything that prevents infections, prolongs life, or treats complications, while not as good as a change in heart, is better than the alternative of death. Yet we know that ultimately our goal for sinners is salvation, not just stopping immoral activity. Once they come to Christ, he can empower them to sanctify their lives.

EDUCATION TO HIGH-RISK GROUPS

Many funds have been spent on educational materials that will never be seen by the public for they are targeted at specific subcultures such as homosexual men, IV drug users, or minorities within ghettos or barrios. Consequently, the posters and pamphlets use street language, jargon, and sometimes graphic sexual drawings to be effective.[12] These are often supported by federal grants and because of their crudeness have caused some controversy.

Ideally, governmental expenditures should not promote immoral activities, and these pamphlets promote "safe sex" and clean-needle use rather than abstinence. However, given the current climate within the targeted groups, little else could be expected. If Christians merely oppose these groups at the point of values, minor headway will be made and the world will think we care more about our moral dictates than about the people acquiring HIV. Rather Christians ought to oppose these materials on scientific grounds, showing the ineffectiveness of the recommended actions. Christian physicians could point out the unacceptably high rate of HIV spread even when condoms are used. We could show that funds used to teach addicts how to clean needles could be used more effectively in drug treatment clinics to get people off drugs. Christians might apply for funds for church-run drug programs, which have proven more effective than agency programs because the church-run programs offer relational and spiritual help. If we approach this problem in these ways, then the world will see that we are primarily concerned about the individuals affected.

Another form of pseudo-education is particularly nefarious because it exploits the ill. This is the underground literature that promotes unproven and illogical therapies. Most of these therapies, which include vitamin treatments, psychic surgery, meditation, ozone therapy, and untested drugs (such as a protein from a Chinese root and a blood thinner promoted in Japan), are costly and give unwarranted hope for cures. They often represent the schemes of unscrupulous people taking advantage of the AIDS sufferer's desperation. However, some of these hazardous therapies are promoted by an organized group of people with AIDS, who hope against hope that some of these will be the miracle cure they are searching for.[13] Whole books have been written describing the positive results of Eastern philosophy. Some patients have gone to France, the Philippines, and Mexico for various therapies. Others have been able to get pirated tablets of AZT prior to its release in this country.

No one wants to die at the relatively young age of most AIDS patients. The desire for any hope will spur men and women to seek improbable cures. As Christians, we should be concerned about two dangers. First, effective therapies may be delayed or unnecessary side-effects may be caused by the pseudo-therapies. Second, patients may become entwined in false spirituality, since so many of these hopes are given a New Age slant. Because many AIDS patients believe they have been abandoned by the church, a lot of the desperation they experience is born from a spiritual vacuum. It would be a great tragedy for this epidemic to open many to spiritual needs only to have them look to the East for answers because Christians have shown love inconsistently. Our education to them should include compassionate and sensitive explanations of the dangers of these so-called therapies. If Thoreau was correct that most men lead lives of quiet desperation, how much more so these people?

SEX EDUCATION

Compulsory sex education is the most controversial form of general education. It has been routinely maligned by most conservative Christians at the same time that agencies such as Planned Parenthood have hailed it as a panacea for all our problems. The AIDS epidemic has further heightened the tension in this dialogue since death is now added to the issues of sexuality, pregnancy, and population control. This has become an important debate, made more so since the evangelical C. Everett Koop has been a proponent of public sex education even into lower grade levels.

Some Christians who are adamantly against sex education argue that any form increases promiscuity.[14] So-called value-free sex education presents various forms of extramarital sexuality as equivalent to sex within marriage. For the value-free educators the goal is to prevent pregnancy and sexually transmitted diseases rather than premarital sexual activity. To their embarrassment, both teenage pregnancy and sexually transmitted diseases have increased despite their sex education classes. In a Harris poll commissioned by Planned Parenthood in 1986, teens who had sex education courses were 50 percent more likely to engage in promiscuous sexual activity than those who had not.[15] This occurs because the teaching itself encourages teen sexuality, outweighing the "benefits" of instruction about contraceptives. Some quotes from materials being used will show the disturbing teaching our teens are receiving:

> Everyone must develop his own set of principles to govern his own sexual behavior (High school psychology).

> The place, the opportunity, and their bodies all say "Go!" How far this couple goes must be their own decision (Grades 7-12 sex education).

> Adolescent petting is an important opportunity to learn about sexual responses and to gratify sexual and emotional desires without a more serious emotional commitment (Grades 9-10 health).

> Contrary to past belief, masturbation is completely harmless and in fact can be quite useful in training oneself to respond sexually (Grades 9-10 health).

> A person with variant sexual interests is not necessarily bad, sick, or mentally ill. . . . Rarely is any physical harm done to the child by child molesters and exhibitionists (Grades 6-12 homemaking).[16]

Not only is this type of sex education anathema to most evangelical Christians, it would also be upsetting to most non-Christians. Well-known psychiatrists such as

Elkind and Bettelheim do not like value-free sex education any more than we do.[17] This sort of indoctrination by secular-minded educators has the hidden agenda of making their personal ethics everyone's morality. There is nothing "value free" about it.

SEX EDUCATION OR NO, IS THAT THE QUESTION?

Those Christians who reject sex education altogether have rightly rejected the type of sex education we have just looked at, but their implication that we have thereby eliminated sex education outside the home is naive. Many teenage girls watch afternoon soap operas, which average 1.5 incidents of extramarital sex per hour. Each year, about two-thirds of those between the ages of fourteen and sixteen see the top five R-rated films, with immoral sex implied or enacted an average of eight times per film.[18] In the mid-seventies magazines for teenage girls were giving advice such as: "There is no right or wrong about sex, except, of course, the moral rights or wrongs such as using a reliable contraceptive," and "There is no reason why a girl shouldn't carry a sheath around with her all the time, so that if the situation arises when she wants to sleep with a boy, she can ensure he wears one to make intercourse safe."[19] About 70 percent of all pornography, including the hard-core variety, ends up in the hands of boys under eighteen.[20] Teenage boys observing this fantasy world of compliant, available girls naturally try to mimic such activities in real life.

Some Christians might smugly think that such is not the case for their child who does not go to R-rated movies or look at pornography. But Planned Parenthood admitted that illicit sex occurred twenty thousand times on television in one year, most of it during prime time.[21] As one author keenly questioned, "How many . . . seductions did your grandparents see as children? Probably a grand total of none. . . . How many . . . have your children seen? Hundreds—most of them thousands. . . . Through the media, [they've] been taught daily since childhood that sex outside of marriage is not only okay, but fun, exciting, perfectly normal, and generally free of consequences."[22] If you don't own a television your child will likely see sexual acts watching TV at a friend's house. Moreover, peers will mindlessly speak the same propaganda since they know of nothing better. No age is more prone to peer pressure than the teenage years. Teens do not usually see premarital sex as immoral but rather as a route to acceptance and closeness.[23]

Sex education in the public schools is coming whether we want it or not. Sex education is already taught to some degree in 93 percent of high schools.[24] In a public poll conducted in 1986, 86 percent of the parents said sex education should be taught in the schools.[25] That poll was conducted when only ten thousand deaths from AIDS had occurred. How high will that percentage be when the death toll is above a hundred thousand . . . or one million? Parents no longer feel adequate to teach about sex or sexually transmitted diseases. Studies show that less than one-fourth of all parents have *ever* talked to their teens about sexual intercourse.[26] Parents are scared about AIDS and feel inadequate to discuss sex.

The secular world will not sit idly while thousands of teenagers acquire HIV infection because of lack of information. Within all schools we need sex education that is founded on Christian principles. It is absolutely incontrovertible that AIDS has been fanned by nonbiblical sexual morality. If responsible Christian leaders will become involved in the debate on sex education, a real opportunity exists to establish moral teaching. If we avoid the issue, Planned Parenthood, moral relativists, and homosexual leaders will provide the curriculum, and destructive sexuality will be perpetuated.

Others agree with the Christian position on sexuality. The White House Domestic Policy Council has called for "education based on fidelity, commitment, and maturity, placing sexuality within the context of marriage."[27] Parents traditionally have more influence upon the local school boards than upon Hollywood or upon New York publishers.

Christians can stonewall and say their child will never participate in sex education, but how does that provide light in the darkness? Christians today need to marshal their influence to push for sex education that is healthy for the whole of society.

CHRIST AND EDUCATION

Jesus Christ is the greatest educator of all time. His was not a sterile, intellectual teaching, but one that was vibrant with truth and the expectancy of changed hearts. His teaching was always placed within the framework of relationships with others and with himself, for nothing else is eternally important. His instruction reverberated with love. Moreover, he taught us to do the same, although we have largely given up the task:

> "You are the light of the world. A city on a hill cannot be hidden. Neither do people light a lamp and put it under a bowl. Instead they put it on its stand, and it gives light to everyone in the house. In the same way, let your light shine before men, that they may see your good deeds and praise your Father in heaven" (Matthew 5:14-16).

It is time to remove the bowl and let the light of the Son shine forth from us.

Chapter 18, Notes

1. Malcolm Muggeridge, quoted in Charles R. Swindoll, *Living on the Ragged Edge* (Waco, Tex.: Word Books, 1985), 23.

2. Jane Harris Aiken, "Education as Prevention" in *AIDS and the Law*, ed. Dalton and Burris (New Haven, Conn.: Yale University Press, 1987), 90.

3. See Randy Shilts, *And the Band Played On: Politics, People, and the AIDS Epidemic* (New York: St. Martin's Press, 1987).

4. Allan M. Brandt, "AIDS in Historical Perspective: Four Lessons from the History of Sexually Transmitted Diseases," *The American Journal of Public Health* 78 (1988):367-71.

5. Paul Vitz, discussed in Marvin Olasky, *The Prodigal Press* (Westchester, Ill.: Crossway Books, 1988), 17. Also an Associated Press report in the *Austin American-Statesman*, 26 May 1986, said that even the liberal group People for the American Way had demonstrated the paucity of religion in public school textbooks.

6. Peggy Charren, "Children's Television: A Conflict of Interests," *Pediatric Annals* 14 (December 1985):789; and Neil Postman interview, "TV's 'Disastrous' Impact on Children," *U.S. News and World Report*, 19 January 1981. Adults watch fifteen hundred hours or more of television a year while reading only an average of two books a year. Children spend 20 percent more time in front of the television than in school each year.

7. Shilts, *Band Played On*, 172, 510.

8. Quoted in Olasky, *Prodigal Press*, 116.

9. Ibid.

10. Ibid., 67-68.

11. Josh McDowell and Dick Day, *Why Wait?* (San Bernardino, Calif.: Here's Life Publishers, 1987), 21.

12. See Douglas Crimp, ed., *AIDS: Cultural Analysis, Cultural Activism* (Cambridge, Mass.: MIT Press, 1987), 232, 260-63.

13. Joshua Hammer, "The AIDS Underground," *Newsweek*, 7 August 1989, 50. See also Shilts, *Band Played On*, 489, 492, 537.

14. David Chilton, *Power in the Blood* (Brentwood, Tenn.: Wolgemuth and Hyatt, 1987), 49-50.

15. Ibid. See also Jeff Nesbit, "Teen Pregnancy Found to Rise Despite Sex Education, Prevention Efforts," Knight-Ridder News Service, *Austin American-Statesman*, 10 February 1986.

16. John Vertefeuille, *Sexual Chaos* (Westchester, Ill.: Crossway Books, 1988), 163-64.

17. Elkind says the "new programs sometimes seem to be condoning, if not advocating, teenage sexuality" (David Elkind, *The Hurried Child* [Reading, Mass.: Addison-Wesley, 1981], 57); Bettelheim adds, "I think such [sex education] classes are a danger and that they are implicated in the increase in teenage sex and teenage pregnancies" (quoted in Elkind, *Hurried Child*, 60).

18. Clif Cartland, *You Can Protect Yourself and Your Family from AIDS* (Old Tappan, N. J.: Fleming H. Revell Co., 1987), 58.

19. Margaret White, *AIDS and the Positive Alternatives* (Basingstoke, U.K.: Marshall Pickering, 1987), 7.

20. Kenneth Kantzer, "The Real Sex Ed Battle," *Christianity Today*, 17 April 1987, 16.

21. John D'Emilio and Estelle B. Freedman, *Intimate Matters* (New York: Harper and Row, 1987), 274.

22. Randy Alcorn, *Christians in the Wake of the Sexual Revolution* (Portland, Ore.: Multnomah Press, 1985), 103.

23. Cartland, *You Can Protect Yourself*, 128.

24. George Howe Colt, "Teen Sexuality: Making Choices in Treacherous Times," *Life*, July 1989, 26.

25. Cartland, *You Can Protect Yourself*, 14.

26. Vertefeuille, *Sexual Chaos*, 169; and McDowell and Day, *Why Wait?*, 379.

27. Cartland, *You Can Protect Yourself*, 159.

On this mountain the LORD Almighty will prepare
    a feast of rich food for all peoples,
a banquet of aged wine—
    the best of meats and the finest of wines.
On this mountain he will destroy
    the [death] shroud that enfolds all peoples,
the sheet that covers all nations;
    he will swallow up death forever.
The Sovereign LORD will wipe away the tears
    from all faces;
he will remove the disgrace of his people
    from all the earth.
        The LORD has spoken
(Isaiah 25:6-8).

"I will ransom them from the power of the grave;
    I will redeem them from death.
Where, O death, are your plagues?
    Where, O grave, is your destruction?"
(Hosea 13:14).

Since the children have flesh and blood, [Jesus] too
shared in their humanity so that by his death he might
destroy him who holds the power of death—that is, the
devil—and free those who all their lives were held in
slavery by their fear of death (Hebrews 2:14-15).

When the perishable has been clothed with the imper-
ishable, and the mortal with immortality, then the saying that is written will come true: "Death has been
swallowed up in victory" (1 Corinthians 15:54).

Chapter Nineteen

AIDS, Plagues, and Death

*T*he boy was taken to the auxiliary hospital and put in a ward of ten beds which had formerly been a classroom. . . . The infection was steadily spreading, and the boy's body putting up no resistance. . . .

[Later] the child had come out of his extreme prostration and was tossing about convulsively on the bed. From four in the morning Dr. Castel and Tarrou had been keeping watch and noting, stage by stage, the progress and remissions of the malady. . . .

The doctor's hands were gripping the rail of the bed, his eyes fixed on the small tortured body. Suddenly it stiffened, and seemed to give a little at the waist, as slowly the arms and legs spread out X-wise. From the body, naked under the army blanket, rose the smell of damp wool and stale sweat. The boy had gritted his teeth again. Then very gradually he relaxed, bringing his arms and legs back toward the center of the bed, still without speaking or opening his eyes, and his breathing seemed to quicken. Rieux looked at Tarrou, who hastily lowered his eyes.

They had already seen children die—for many months now death had shown no favoritism—but they had never yet watched a child's agony minute by minute, as they had been doing since daybreak. . . .

And just then the boy had a sudden spasm, as if something had bitten him in the stomach, and uttered a long, shrill wail. For moments that seemed endless he stayed in a queer, contorted position, his body racked by convulsive tremors; it was as if his frail frame were bending before the fierce breath of the plague, breaking under the reiterated gusts of the fever. Then the storm-wind passed, there came a lull, and he relaxed a little; the fever seemed to recede, leaving him gasping for breath on a dank, pestilential shore, lost in a languor that already looked like death. When for the third time the fiery wave broke on him, lifting him a little, the child curled himself up and shrank away to the edge of the bed, as if in terror of the flames advancing on him, licking his limbs. A moment later, after tossing his head wildly to and fro, he flung off the blanket. From between the inflamed eyelids big tears welled up and trickled down the sunken, leaden-hued cheeks. When the spasm had passed, utterly exhausted, tensing his thin legs and arms, on which, within forty-eight hours, the flesh had wasted to the bone, the child lay flat, racked on the tumbled bed, in a grotesque parody of the crucifixion. . . .

The occupants of the other nine beds were tossing about and groaning, but in tones that seemed deliberately subdued. . . . Only the child went on fighting with all his little might. Now and then Dr. Rieux took his pulse—less because this served any purpose than as an escape from his utter helplessness—and when he closed his eyes, he seemed to feel its tumult mingling with the fever of his own blood. . . .

The child, his eyes still closed, seemed to grow a little calmer. His clawlike fingers were feebly plucking at the sides of the bed. Then they rose, scratched at the blanket over his knees, and suddenly he doubled up his limbs, bringing his thighs above his stomach, and remained quite still. For the first time he opened his eyes and gazed at Dr. Rieux, who was standing immediately in front of him. In the small face, rigid as a mask of grayish clay, slowly the lips parted and from them rose a long, incessant scream, hardly varying with his respiration, and filling the ward with a fierce, indignant protest, so little childish that it seemed like a collective voice issuing from all the sufferers there. Rieux clenched his jaws, Tarrou looked away. . . . Father Paneloux gazed down at the small *mouth, fouled with the sores of the plague and pouring out the angry death-cry that has sounded throughout the ages of mankind. He sank on his knees, and all present found it natural to hear him say in a voice hoarse but clearly audible across the nameless, never ending wail: "My God, spare this child!"*

But the wail continued without cease and other sufferers began to grow restless. The patient at the far end of the ward, whose little broken cries had gone on without break, now quickened their tempo so that they flowed together in one unbroken cry, while the others' groans grew louder. A gust of sobs swept through the room, drowning Paneloux's prayers, and Doctor Rieux, who was still tightly gripping the rail of the bed, shut his eyes, dazed with exhaustion and disgust.

When he opened them again, Tarrou was at his side.

"I must go," Rieux said. "I can't bear to hear them any longer."

But then suddenly, the other sufferers fell silent. And now the doctor grew aware that the child's wail, after weakening more and more, had fluttered out into silence. Around him the groans began again, but more faintly, like a far echo of a fight that now was over. For it was over. Castel had moved round to the other side of the bed and said the end had come. His mouth still gaping, but silent now, the child was lying among tumbled blankets, a small, shrunken form, with tears still wet on his cheeks.

Albert Camus, *The Plague*[1]

* * * * * *

We have quoted at length from Camus's portrait of a dying child to remind us of the repulsiveness of death. Death is not supposed to be attractive, for it is the evidence of the victory of the enemy. In most Western societies such scenes are hidden from the public, being too distasteful for our viewing. Our cinematic versions of death are tame by comparison, even though plenty of blood and guts are shown. These scenes are mild because it is not the death of the body that is difficult to watch, but the fading of the soul within that body. Our society's repression of suffering and death allows us to exist with a sense of immortality that belies the ticking of the clock that brings death closer. We need to feel that pain a little to help remind us of the important things in life and to increase our compassion for the person suffering. We are strongly moved by Camus's description of the death of a child; we should be as strongly moved by the death of young men and women in the AIDS epidemic.

Jesus was. The death of a young man moved him to weep at the victory of death, even though he knew Lazarus's life would soon be restored. It is an incredible portrait of the One who would conquer death, distraught that he had temporarily lost to the adversary. Perhaps at that moment, Christ was weeping not only for Lazarus, his friend, but also for the millions of deaths that had already occurred and would yet occur. Christ knew his victory over death would soon be seen in his friend's case, and eventually for all time when death is cast into the lake of fire (Revelation 20:10-15). Yet he allowed himself to feel the pain of the current crisis. So should we.

DEATH: THE WORST PROBLEM?

Death is a severe problem. But if one is a Christian, it is not the worst problem. For the Christian, selfishness, materialism, personal peace without concern for others are worse challenges than death. Death realistically can be called sleep for the Christian, because it has indeed lost its sting; it has lost its victory. Not that we are always peaceful with death, even if we have complete assurance of salvation. The pain often associated with death is genuine, as are the disappointments in separation from family, missed opportunities, and sins committed, even though forgiven. But there is joy mixed with the bitter taste of death. The relationships lost here will be regained in eternity. The mistakes of this life change into the consistency of the next. The seeing through a glass darkly becomes the clear vision of our heavenly Father.

No such consolation exists for the non-Christian. Death is the inevitable victor. Life ceases and the whole exercise seems pointless. That is why man without God struggles against death so vigorously. At one time the secular world believed that to eliminate the Christian views of death and afterlife would result in a more casual approach to extinction. But the opposite has happened because those who bear the image of God believe they are more than mere dust.[2] Freud thought that religion was created in part because people were too immature to face mortality. In his maturity he thought he could face death without God, but as he aged, he became increasingly less self-assured. Besides, Freud thought he would attain immortality in his writings. When he saw his disciples fall away and modify his theories, he realized his books would not endure as he had thought and he felt fear.[3]

By staying healthy, by enjoying life fully, the non-Christian mitigates the thoughts that in the end, life is futile. How can the secular man die peacefully? It would seem that he merely stops struggling, having no energy left to fight his adversary. In the Western world, one can enjoy the pleasures of life, numbing the soul with food, sex, wine, drugs, education, or work before the final day of reckoning occurs. AIDS is a cruel disease, taking those small comforts away. It is a sudden dose of reality for people who have been living life in the fast lane. Like a man in a warm, fur coat falling into an icy pond, the artificial warmth is snatched away.

Our time celebrates youth and beauty much as the ancient Greeks, in part to create an illusion of vitality. Suffering must be hidden. So most people die in the hospital, instead of at home as they did in the nineteenth century. Our senior citizens are placed in nursing homes and our borderline mentally ill are institutionalized. Children with special problems such as deafness or blindness are bussed to separate schools. With amniocentesis we search for abnormal babies so we can destroy them before we see them face to face. In television, movies, and advertisements, we see the youngest and most attractive men, women, and children, despite the graying of our society.

Physical death is not the worst problem for secular

man, although he thinks it is. The worst problem is not that the world may die in a nuclear holocaust or that the greenhouse effect will warm the globe and change our climate. His worst problem is sin which separates him from his Creator. But his pain is significant, and we who know the security Christ brings must never underestimate the distress he feels or tries to deaden in various ways.

ALONENESS

The iciness of death is a shock that restores some perspective concerning what is truly important in life. Even such a hardened atheist as Jean Paul Sartre admitted a belief in an afterlife shortly before his death (to the dismay of his close friends).[4] Therefore, the proximity of death is an opportunity for the gospel. The time is made even more opportune by the virtual certainty that one will be alone as the end approaches. Many AIDS patients die utterly apart from family and friends. Parents have often rejected their homosexual or drug-using child. Non-Christian friends do not want to be reminded of their own mortality, so they slowly drift away. In the end only pain, hunger, nausea, and absence of dignity remain. And after death has come, most AIDS patients expect only cold emptiness.

No man, woman, or child should die so utterly alone and without hope because Christ, by dying bereft of friends and family, provided a new people, a new family to reach out to all of mankind. No person is so decadent, no life so wasted, no sins so grievous that the Son of God cannot overcome. These people still contain within them the glorious image of God no matter how much filth they have allowed to tarnish that image.

THE DEATH WISH AND AIDS

It is amazing that so many homosexual men continue to risk death from AIDS. It is true that the risky behavior has been curtailed through fewer sexual partners and the use of condoms. However, homosexuals may be drifting back to their previous habits of promiscuity and no condoms.[5] More IV drug abusers are using sterile needles and avoiding sharing needles with other users, compared with the habits of the past. However, in most communities over half the addicts continue high-risk use of needles, at least part of the time.

This seeming death wish is not so unreasonable if seen from their perspective. Virtually all homosexual males and IV drug abusers are hurting people. Many of the homosexuals have had distant or absent fathers, have been seduced into the life-style by prostitution or experienced homosexual men, or had their guard lowered by the use of drugs. The IV drug users often come from impoverished or abusive homes. Many of the drug users started when they were kids on the street after being kicked out of their homes. The only thing some of the younger ones have to sell is their bodies. In an America that makes freedom of choice the ultimate good, it is easy for some men to justify sleeping with young teenage boys or girls. We should not be surprised when these children turn to the rush of alcohol and drugs to escape the pain of their memories, self-hatred, and guilt over their actions.

The drugs and sex become addictive and so it is simplistic to expect the drug user and the homosexual to "just say no." If they say no, the pain is still there. The pleasure of addiction is real, and to them it is worth risking death to avoid the unanesthetized pain. They will be able to change more easily if an alternate life without drugs and sex can compete with the misery. Such an alternate life must be relational. Lasting joy and true significance only occur in relationships with other people and with God. Drug treatment centers and psychologists who counsel homosexuals to change have a low success rate because their treatments do not include developing caring relationships with other people. So what may appear to us, in the comfort of our middle-class existence, as a death wish, is the opposite. The addict wants to live, but without the agony he experiences while off the ambrosia.

In some ways promiscuous sexuality is more difficult to escape than drug use. Our society largely refuses to condemn promiscuity as wrong (unlike drug use), because most people are confused about their own values. Moreover, this hypersexuality is attractive because it is a counterfeit of what most young people are looking for: intimate, personal relationships. That is why the sexuality becomes more frequent, more intense, more perverse, and completely empty. The "rush" of the orgasm gives a sense of something real, of a deep affinity with another person. But the promise fades away and the person continues to search for a better technique, a more pleasing partner, or a better combination of sex with drugs or alcohol. The risk of death through sex is understandable if emptiness reigns apart from it.

For Christians to berate IV drug users or homosexuals for the sin involved is to miss the point. They are often tortured by their own self-condemnation. Some patients are even relieved when they find out they actually have full-blown AIDS instead of being merely HIV-positive.[6] That is partly related to the difficulty of waiting for the disease to declare itself; it also may be related to feelings of guilt and a desire to be punished for their sins.

SUICIDE AND ABORTION

Many men with AIDS consider suicide to avoid the pain and suffering at the end. Many women consider abortion to avoid having a child who is likely to die from AIDS. Should these be viable options?

Suicide is always available to people who truly want life to cease. They cannot be locked up in suicide prevention wards forever. The pain is controllable with drugs; the true needs of people are not. That is where the love and acceptance of others comes in. Hospices run by Christians should be one method of making compassion available. Churches should be at the forefront in establishing and financially supporting such efforts to love the unlovely. Christian doctors could provide medical care without charge and could teach neighbors that the hospice presents no danger to their neighborhood.

Probably all of us have had fleeting thoughts of suicide when life has been difficult. But to be with someone who consistently entertains such thoughts can be unnerving. Most of these people simply need a friend to be with them. They need a person who will sit and listen as they describe their pain. They need to be touched by another human being who truly wants to be there. And they need hope—hope that there is something better beyond death, hope that they can be forgiven for the mistakes they have made, hope that their life has not been wasted. The Christian can provide all of these. Moreover, the type of hope we offer is very different from what the world offers. The world's hope is usually baseless, a sentimental wish for something better. Our hope is substantive, and it is not baseless because it rests on the finished work of Jesus Christ. No one should die alone without being offered that hope.

Christians can provide a difference as well in the issue of abortion for an HIV-positive pregnant woman. It is currently estimated that only 30 percent of infants born to women infected with HIV will come down with AIDS. To automatically abort all babies of women with HIV infection, as some have suggested, hardly makes sense. It is inconsistent to sacrifice the unborn and then extend mercy to the adult AIDS patient. For society to be selective in its compassion is the ultimate in discrimination.

After these infants are born, Christians should be available to provide the compassion they need, whether they are infected with the virus or not. To help care for the infected infants requires time, fortitude, and conviction to show God's love during their shortened life. The uninfected infants need the same, since many of them soon become orphans. "Religion that God our Father accepts as pure and faultless is this: to look after orphans and widows in their distress. . ." (James 1:27).

THE STAGES OF DEATH

The fear of death strips most people of the facades they have spent a lifetime erecting. Consequently, most people go through similar stages when confronted with death, whether they are powerful politicians or impotent street people. It is helpful to discern these stages so as to be proper ministers to the dying.

Most people initially deny the possibility of death when they discover they have a terminal illness. Then anger often ensues against God, against all those who have wronged them, against the impotence of the physicians, and against themselves for perceived failures. Anger is too intense an emotion to last for long, especially if one is fighting a debilitating illness. Then a bargaining phase ensues involving God or family members or the doctors. "I will be good for the rest of my life if you get me past this illness, God." "I will give all my money to this hospital if you cure me, doctor." "I will never commit infidelity again if you stay with me through this struggle." As the bargaining proves unsuccessful, depression begins and can last for various lengths of time. Eventually, the patient gives in and accepts the death to come.[7] These stages are interchangeable and important to understand when dealing with a dying patient. They are expected reactions. The dying person may not necessarily want others to respond to each stage, but he needs a group of friends there to help him go through the process.

What the dying person needs most from others is heartfelt compassion and willingness to listen to the hurts. In those circumstances, the caregiver may be pressed to say something profound or to establish meaning where there is no apparent meaning. The ministering friend may desire to fill the quiet time with empty talk when silence may be far more healing. A caring relationship is worth far more to the dying patient than gifts or wisdom. A time will come after the quiet when sharing the truths of God will be appropriate. But that will come after the minister has shown the terminally ill person that he has significance even in the midst of his suffering and helplessness. Christ demonstrated such compassion to the sinners around him. He gave little time to the rich and powerful, but all the time in the world to the weak. "Let the little children come to me," he said, not because they were profound but because, as some of God's creatures, they were important.

AIDS: The Twentieth-Century Plague?

Some people have compared AIDS to the bubonic plague that struck Europe in several epidemics in the last millennium. At one point AIDS was called the "gay plague" when it was thought to attack only homosexual men. Others have said it is a plague sent from heaven to punish a group of rebellious people. Still others have claimed that it will strike as many people as the Black Death (the most virulent assault of bubonic plague) that attacked Europe in the mid-1300s, killing up to a third of the population. Is the metaphor of AIDS as plague a good description or a deception? Two questions are involved. First, will AIDS kill as many people as the plague? Second, will AIDS cause equivalent changes in society as the bubonic plague did?

Medically, AIDS is unlike the plague. Throughout history, the illnesses that exacted the greatest numbers of lives were all casually contagious (smallpox, cholera, influenza) or spread through insect vectors (bubonic plague, malaria, typhus). AIDS will never approach the high number of deaths of the plague because it is neither. Syphilis is the sexually transmitted disease that has caused the most havoc in history, yet it has caused far fewer deaths than bubonic plague.

The casualties of AIDS have increased rapidly because of the long incubation period. Most of the people who died of AIDS in the eighties contracted the disease before it was medically known. A similar effect would occur if a well were contaminated with a slow but irreversible poison that took about ten years to kill. People would continue to use the well for a number of years and so many people would be poisoned. Like syphilis prior to antibiotics, AIDS will become a chronic cause of death in that some people continue to drink from the poisoned well in spite of the known danger. The numbers will slow as more people have the experience of watching a friend or acquaintance die of AIDS.

AIDS is like the plague in social effects. Until recently, historians underestimated the impact of new diseases on society.[8] When a malady causes large loss of life, enormous cultural and social changes result. The bubonic plague strongly affected religion and was thought to have brought an end to the domination of the Catholic church. The bubonic plague showed the church's impotence in the face of the pestilence. Unfortunately, the disease also revealed the cowardice of many church officials as they fled before its path. Many economic changes occurred because of the shortage of laborers, and many historians think this sounded the death knell for feudalism. If that is true, then the plague ushered in the modern states with all their benefits and curses.[9]

AIDS has already had a major impact on our society, far beyond what the numbers of ill would warrant. Modern communications has magnified the importance of AIDS and made it a celebrity,[10] leading to many of the changes. Image, not reality, is most important in our age of visual communication, and AIDS has an impressive image; one only has to look at the daily paper to see its notoriety. It is this infamy that has led to the disproportional social effects of AIDS.

Newborn tetanus kills over one million children every year according to the World Health Organization. This disease usually occurs due to unsanitary deliveries in undeveloped areas of the world. One million deaths each year means that this illness annually kills twenty times the total number who have died during the AIDS epidemic in the U.S. Many reasons come to mind as to why AIDS is more famous than neonatal tetanus or most other diseases. Some are reasonable and some are not. All of them energize the social changes of the AIDS epidemic.

> 1. AIDS is a new illness and so is fascinating to watch as it unfolds; other diseases that kill many more people have existed since the beginning of modern medicine.

> 2. AIDS is a stigmatized disease because of its association with homosexuality and IV drug use.

Not many people openly admit they have AIDS if given a choice.

3. AIDS kills mostly men and women in the prime of their lives. Newborn tetanus or heart disease kills mainly the very young and the very old, people who are less valued by our production-oriented society.

4. AIDS is a lethal First World disease. Multiple illnesses in the Third World kill many more people than AIDS, but these are devalued. People in the developed world naturally worry about threats that affect them personally, but some of this devaluation of Third World diseases is related to latent racism and cultural discrimination. Does a mother in Africa feel any less pain for the death of her baby than does a woman in America?

5. AIDS is feared like cancer in that it often causes a slow, disfiguring, painful end.[11] Fear of AIDS has been recently classified as an obsessive-compulsive disorder related to its notoriety.[12]

6. AIDS challenges some of the basic beliefs of our society and so has had a major impact on the West similar to the impact from the plague.

THE SOCIAL EFFECTS OF AIDS

Effects on Ideas

Some of society's most cherished myths have been challenged by the AIDS epidemic. First, AIDS challenges the idea that medical advances have eliminated the danger of severe epidemics. As recently as 1983 a noted historian of disease suggested that we are beyond major infectious epidemics in the West.[13] AIDS is the first pandemic since the dawn of antibiotics.

Second, AIDS challenges the idea that man and his technology can do anything if he sets his mind to it. This is one virus that is unlikely to be cured in the near future, and most of society knows it.

Third, AIDS challenges the idea that sex is risk free. That has been a fallacious idea for a long time. Nonetheless, it took AIDS to finally bring the point home.

Fourth, AIDS attacks the idea that personal pleasure or self-fulfillment is always good. Personal pleasure in the form of promiscuous behavior can be deadly.

Fifth, AIDS is challenging the idea that male homosexuality is a normal, healthy life-style. Despite the outward signs of solidarity and belligerence, many male homosexuals are questioning their behavior as they see their friends die.

Sixth, AIDS is challenging the American concept of individualism. People are not islands completely separate from others. The biblical concept of connectedness and community is a much more realistic way of ordering society.[14]

Finally, AIDS is forcing the church to look at the myth of sexual purity among Christians. The body of Christ is going to see more and more of its members admitting past homosexual liaisons, heterosexual adultery, and unwed pregnancies leading to abortion. Hopefully, the church will rise from her slumbers to address realistically this crisis too long kept quiet.

Effects on Behavior

Some positive modifications in behavior have come from the epidemic, and they should not be ignored. Many have changed their sexual and drug using behavior, and the numbers will increase as the general population begins to see people dying of AIDS. More homosexuals are renouncing their sexual addiction, many turning cautiously to Christ. If other homosexuals are ministered to in a Christ-like manner, then many more will turn from their destructive habits. The AIDS epidemic has caused many to turn toward God because it has shaken up man's smug confidence in his own capabilities. Perhaps man is not the one in control of a supposedly mechanistic world.

Some Negative Effects

A large number of lawsuits are beginning and more are on the horizon in our already litigious society. Many are legitimate (such as suits by infected transfusion recipients in 1982-1985); others are questionable as people seek to redirect blame for their irresponsible choices (such as the suit by Rock Hudson's lover). Research dollars will be less available for other worthy efforts. Taxes and the costs for medical insurance are likely to rise as the few thousand cases turn into hundreds of thousands each year. The epidemic has created a new group of pariahs: the future ill, those who are HIV-infected yet not sick. Already a new form of discrimination based on fear has resulted. People are once more turning to the state as our secular savior, despite government's proven inefficiency. AIDS has contributed to a dramatic drop in medical school applications, conceivably diluting the quality of future practitioners. Blood banks, which have always had difficulty getting sufficient donations, are having severe shortages, since people are afraid that somehow they might get AIDS by giving blood. Openness in discussing sexual matters has led to changes in television and advertising, and threatens the innocence of children exposed to sexual issues long before they need be. AIDS further encourages what Susan Sontag calls the Apocalypse From-Now-On phenomenon, the tendency for many futurists to constantly point to various problems as unsolvable, which results in social panic out of proportion to the difficulties at hand.[15] The AIDS epidemic is a major challenge, but it will not lead to the Apocalypse.

As more HIV disease enters the heterosexual population, we could see homosexual men progressively becoming scapegoats subject to increased gay bashing. In the Black Death in the fourteenth century, Jews were murdered for poisoning the wells that supposedly caused the plague. Although homosexuals have more responsibility in this plague than Jews did in theirs, it is still wrong to claim that they are the cause. All of society is guilty for laying the foundation for the sexual revolution with its promiscuity; homosexual men merely happened to be the most promiscuous.

As with plagues in the past, AIDS is having a large impact on our society, but the number of actual sick is much smaller. So AIDS is plague-like in social ramifications, but not in numbers of deaths.

THE CHRISTIAN RESPONSE TO SOCIAL UPHEAVALS

The modern world has essentially eliminated the concept of sin and replaced it with the concept of disease (of alcoholism, insanity, substance abuse, and so on). People become machines that are not responsible for the state of their lives. The secular man cannot adequately explain the whys and wherefores of the AIDS epidemic. He tries to dismiss it as simply another virus, but it is far more than that, as we have seen.

One advantage the Christian worldview has over others is its ability to explain tragedy, such as plagues, wars, and other disasters. However, Christians have explained these problems too narrowly by placing all the blame on the individual offenders. In doing that we have adopted the modern American ideal of individualism, that we are responsible only for ourselves, which goes against biblical teaching. Although individuals face God for their own sin, Judeo-Christian culture has always emphasized community and the often corporate nature of sin. The whole Canaanite culture was destroyed for the terrible evil of those involved in religious prostitution and child sacrifice. When Achan sinned, the whole nation of Israel suffered a reverse in battle. When the people had fallen into sin even the righteous, such as Daniel and Jeremiah, were displaced with the unrighteous.

The Christian nation within the West has had the responsibility to leaven the whole lot with good leaven. In that responsibility we have failed for several decades and cannot wash our hands clean of the whole matter. Just like Pilate, we delude ourselves if we think we are completely free of responsibility for the death around us. In the many ways that we have left our first love, we are responsible. In the manner in which we have adopted the errors of the culture around us—its materialism, racism, pursuit of personal comfort, and greater concern for the score of the ball game than for dying homosexuals—then we have sinned.

There is no golden age of Christianity, but at least in the past the church was more responsive to suffering in the world. Christians set up the leper colonies, hospitals, and orphanages, not secular philosophers. Christians gave large funds to support medical missionaries, to relieve famine in the world, and to provide for the dying. Christians started the Salvation Army and other local organizations in every city ghetto in America to provide for the homeless, the drunkards, and the poorly clothed. But recently we have allowed the government to take over our responsibilities, and the government is a poor replacement. At the most it can supply assistance without relationship, which fosters dependence and degradation. Assistance without true relationship provides only survival; Christians have the opportunity to provide life, and that more abundantly.

Recent events provide some basis for hope that things may be changing. We see more and more people taking up the plight of the unborn. We are seeing a new evangelical outreach to the homeless, the runaways, and the hungry. We see that the biblical teaching of the evangelical church can be merged with the "social gospel" and still retain its force for change. We are beginning to understand Christ's teaching that when we feed or clothe the poor, we also do the same for him.

THE DAY DEATH DIED

This is a chapter full of woe. Woe for the suffering of a child. Woe for the suffering of many people with disease. Woe for our failures to provide light in a dying culture. But by God's grace, no chapter of life need end in woe.

Two millennia ago a remarkable event occurred when the God-man gave his life on the cross. The last great enemy Death exacted one more lifeless body, seemingly his greatest triumph. But when that body rose from the tomb, Death suffered his greatest defeat.

Thank God that Jesus preferred to die than to live without us.[16] And because of that, no one ever need die without hope again.

Chapter 19, Notes

1. Albert Camus, *The Plague* (New York: Random House, 1948), 190-95.

2. Os Guinness, *The Dust of Death* (Downers Grove, Ill.: InterVarsity Press, 1973), 33.

3. Anthony Campolo, *Partly Right* (Waco, Tex.: Word Books, 1985), 141.

4. Norman Geisler, "The Collapse of Modern Atheism," in *The Intellectuals Speak Out about God*, ed. Roy Abraham Varghese (Chicago: Regnery Gateway, 1984), 136.

5. H.V. Fineburg, "Education to Prevent AIDS: Prospects and Obstacles," *Science* 239 (1988): 592-96; M.H. Becker and J.G. Joesph, "AIDS and Behavioral Change to Reduce Risk: A Review," *American Journal of Public Health* 78 (1988): 394-410; and L.H. Calabrese et al., *AIDS Research* 2 (1986): 357.

6. Earl Shelp and Ronald Sunderland, *AIDS and the Church* (Philadelphia: The Westminister Press, 1987), 45.

7. See Elisabeth Kübler-Ross, *On Death and Dying* (New York: Macmillan Publishing Co., 1969).

8. See William H. McNeill, *Plagues and People* (Garden City, N.Y.: Doubleday and Co., 1976).

9. See Philip Ziegler, *The Black Death* (New York: Harper Torchbooks, 1969); and Robert Gottfried, *The Black Death* (New York: Macmillan Publishing Co., 1983).

10. Susan Sontag, *AIDS and Its Metaphors* (New York: Farrar, Strauss & Giroux, 1988), 83.

11. Ibid., 38, 41.

12. Judith Rapoport, *The Man Who Mistook His Wife for a Hat* (New York: E.P. Dutton, 1989), 146-49.

13. William McNeill quoted in Sontag, *AIDS and Its Metaphors*, 57.

14. Robert Bellah et al., *Habits of the Heart* (New York: Harper and Row, 1985), 282.

15. Sontag, *AIDS and Its Metaphors*, 88.

16. See the moving song by Michael Card, "Could It Be," from the "Present Reality" album, Sparrow Records, 1988.

"Then the King will say to those on his right, 'Come, you who are blessed by my Father; take your inheritance, the kingdom prepared for you since the creation of the world. For I was hungry and you gave me something to eat, I was thirsty and you gave me something to drink, I was a stranger and you invited me in, I needed clothes and you clothed me, I was sick and you looked after me, I was in prison and you came to visit me.'

"Then the righteous will answer him, 'Lord, when did we see you hungry and feed you, or thirsty and give you something to drink? When did we see you a stranger and invite you in, or needing clothes and clothe you? When did we see you sick or in prison and go to visit you?'

"The King will reply, 'I tell you the truth, whatever you did for one of the least of these brothers of mine, you did for me' " (Matthew 25:34-40).

If your enemy is hungry, give him food to eat;
    if he is thirsty, give him water to drink
(Proverbs 25:21).

The Spirit and the bride say, "Come!" And let him who hears say, "Come!" Whoever is thirsty, let him come; and whoever wishes, let him take the free gift of the water of life (Revelation 22:17).

"*No eye has seen,*
    no ear has heard,
no mind has conceived
    what God has prepared for those who love him"
(1 Corinthians 2:9).

Chapter Twenty

Warnings and Opportunities

M y name is Tom. Three years ago I became a Christian after being in the homosexual life-style for about ten years. My life as a practicing homosexual was a miserable existence. However it was an improvement over what I had before.

I grew up in a small Texas town where football was king, and I was the biggest kid in my class. I remember being harassed as early as grade school because I enjoyed books, art, and music rather than sports. One of my uncles was an All-American football player, and I knew there was no possibility of me coming close to his accomplishments in sports. So I never tried. My heart was not in it. I grew up being called "queer" and "faggot" by many of the kids and even some of my family members.

My father was distant and did not support me when I needed it. I realize now that he treated me just like he was treated by his dad, but for a long time I hated him. I remember when I graduated salutatorian that his only comment was, "Leave it to him to finish second." Neither was my mother as supportive as she could have been.

My family went to a traditional church. Many of the schoolmates who had mistreated me also went to the same church. Their mistreatment I could understand since kids frequently display a mean streak. However, when I was an older teenager, I found out that some of the parents, including adults that I had looked up to in the church, were also accusing me behind my back of being homosexual. That was the beginning that carried me away from the church.

I went to college still thinking I was heterosexual, but ceased going to church. My junior year I met a coed whom I cared for deeply. She became pregnant, and we planned to get married since we thought we were in love. Two days before the wedding, I found out she had aborted my baby. I had always wanted to have children and I could not believe she would do that without talking to me first. I flew into a rage and immediately drove back to college. I was angry at the whole world: my father and my family, my home-town, the church and God, and now women.

When I ran back to college I did not decide to get involved in the homosexual scene, it was just something I drifted into. I met one guy who introduced me into the life-style; he loved me deeply. After we were together for a few months, I remember going to a gay bar. It was the first time I remember being totally accepted by a group of people. No one could call me sissy or queer here, since some men were adorned in dresses and many were more effeminate than I was. After a lifetime of emotional deprivation and harass-ment, this seemed to be wonderful. I would soon find out it wasn't.

I began getting into drugs, especially speed. Thankfully, I am deathly afraid of needles so I never got into IV drugs. I also began a quest for my emotionally absent father. I was attracted to older men who were emotionally supportive. I never went to the gay baths, but I had a series of relationships with older men that were never fulfilling. I did not see women anymore and totally dedicated my life to the homosexual community. After some years I was having more and more sex with men and was using drugs frequently. I was on a slow death spiral like a moth coming closer and closer to the flames. Then the Lord started working a miracle in my life.

A friend and lover of mine became a Christian and started sharing the gospel with me. We ceased being intimate, but that just made me more angry at the God I had rejected. But my friend continued to love me and spend time with me. And he shared the love of Christ with me. I had heard all the verses before about the sinfulness of homosexuality, but now I saw them in a new light, because of the compassion of my friend. He accepted me despite my sin and that was something I had not seen from church people before. He also shared verses about Jesus' compassion for sinners even before they gave up their sin. I especially like the story of the prodigal son from Luke 15. That son was as low as a man could get and yet his father accepted him. I had never been accepted by my father, and I didn't feel accepted by my heavenly Father either. Yet here was Jesus, whom so many called the Savior, saying that his Father was ready to accept a son who had wasted his inheritance on riotous living and was eating with the pigs like an animal. After several months and much time with my Christian friend, I realized he had something I wanted. I craved to know the acceptance of my Father and the cleansing of my Savior.

I was still heavily into speed at the time and so the Lord had to bring me to himself in the midst of the rushing highs and the crashing lows of the drug. By his grace and preserving miracles, he did. But it was not an easy road out; it never seems to be for any man in the homosexual life-style. My escape has been typical. I think five major barriers have to be crossed before escaping that type of life. Other sinful addictions have two or three of these barriers, but few sinners have more obstacles to pass than the homosexual male before coming completely to Christ.

The first barrier is that I, like virtually all homosexual males, had deep scars in my life. I had been hurt by many people including family members and people who called themselves Christians. Change involves admission of wrongness and willingness to face hurts from the past that had been numbed by the sex, drugs, and alcohol.

The second barrier to overcome is the need to separate from the culture that one identifies with. The homosexual life-style involves a whole counterculture to the straight world. Therefore, one must not only cease having sex with other men, but one must also stop the drugs, parties, vacations, and cruising that are integral parts of being gay. These habits often have been practiced for years. For ten years of my life I had been engaged in activities that made it easy to meet other homosexual men. All of that had to stop.

I have never seen anyone who could continue in the parties and drugs while stopping the sex.

The third major barrier is that one must give up one's strongly established identity within the homosexual community. One so strongly identifies with homosexual activities and the homosexual mentality that it requires a 180-degree reversal in thinking to become a Christian. The homosexual propaganda says "Gay is beautiful" and "I am gay," not "I choose to do gay activities." To deny all the creeds of the homosexual community that one has accepted for years is not easy.

The fourth major barrier is that a homosexual man must leave a safe, cohesive group where he is comfortable and accepted, even if miserable, to go back to the hurtful world of the straight community. That is the main reason an alternate world of love and acceptance must be seen to draw the homosexual out of the life-style. It was especially difficult for me to leave the emotional attachments of men I deeply cared for. I was betraying them in a sense and going over to the world that had persecuted these same friends. Coupled with that is the fact that few heterosexuals can identify with the life you have left. Most feel uncomfortable around you and are not sure how to establish a relationship. Redeemed homosexuals are caught between two worlds.

A final barrier to overcome is that the Christian world tries to convert homosexuals with rational arguments that not only destroy one's identity but also attack one's friends. Quoting Scripture without demonstrating love is only one other form of gay bashing, as homosexuals see it. A homosexual man does not have to be told that homosexuality is wrong according to the Bible. We have heard those verses so many times we can probably quote them from memory. I think most homosexuals know deep down that something is wrong; I certainly did, as did many of my friends who have escaped and come to Christ. I have never seen a homosexual man come to Christ by Scripture-quoting. They [homosexuals] only come to him by Christian loving. The Christian community will reach homosexual men when it undertakes the same sacrificial love that Jesus did when he chose to go to the cross.

The church I attend now is a haven for hurting people. In the building, there is a conspicuous sign that says: YOU ARE SAFE

HERE. My prayer is that churches across the country will adopt that motto for themselves. Then a real hope will exist for the homosexual men dying of AIDS and the others who are dying spiritually, dying in homosexuality.

* * * * * *

In his convicting testimony Tom shows us that it is a formidable undertaking for a man to escape from homosexuality on his own. Only with sincere love and complete acceptance from Christians is that likely to occur. But the same could be said for almost any addiction. It is natural for Christians to feel uneasy when first confronted with sinful lives so dissimilar to our own, whether it involves homosexuality, IV drug abuse, or promiscuous heterosexuality. But we should recall that we experience most of life in common with such people. We are created in the image of God, as are they. We have jobs to work, bills to pay, and food to cook, as do they. We are continually in need of God's grace in our lives, as are they.

We do not want to minimize the thoroughness of the sin in their lives, but they do not practice sin continuously. To call them homosexual men or IV drug users is a misnomer; those labels identify their behavior during only a small portion of their day. We forget that we can minister to such a person in numerous ways throughout the day without being sullied by the sin he or she may commit later. Jesus was our model for such activities. He met with the sexually immoral, he spoke with the social outcasts, he touched those others were afraid to be around.

SEARCHING FOR A HEART OF GOLD

Many differences exist between Christianity and the world, but one stands out in our mind as an important closing reminder. God judges a man not only by his actions but also by his thoughts. "Man looks at the outward appearance, but the LORD looks at the heart" (1 Samuel 16:7). Jesus went further, saying that sin, even grievous sin such as adultery and murder, begins in the mind (Matthew 5). We Christians cannot force someone to change his life. We cannot force the IV drug user to quit, the playboy to stop sleeping around, or the homosexual to stop sleeping with other men. We cannot even change the attitudes and actions of other Christians. Only one person can be directly affected and changed by my thinking, and I am that person. It may be easier to see the sin in others. It may be easier to require change in others. But God looks at our hearts as well as theirs.

Francis Schaeffer wrote a book called *True Spirituality* that he reread every year to remind himself of the ways he was to think and act. In the final chapter of the book, he answered this pivotal question: Can spiritual living or faith ever be taught? Schaeffer's answer: "Yes, faith can be taught, but only by exhibition."[1] Jesus said, "Follow me, and I will make you fishers of men." He meant far more than just walking after him. We are to walk his walk, to live life the way he did. It is not enough for us to give lip service to what we believe. Our faith without works is dead.

WARNINGS

In the case of the AIDS epidemic the church has not been walking the walk of our Lord. Too often we have approached homosexuals like Tom, not with the truth of Scripture, but with the haughtiness of self-righteousness. We have failed, by our example, to teach the IV drug user about the personal sacrifice of Christ. We have been too quick to condemn the promiscuity of the prostitute while excusing too readily our own lusts. We have looked on the dying AIDS patient from afar and gloated that he received his just deserts, forgetting that our sins are just as deserving of death were it not for Christ's sacrifice for us.

THE GOOD SAMARITAN REVISITED

The story of the Good Samaritan is so familiar to us that we forget its power and intent. Jesus told this parable to answer the question, "Who is my neighbor?" In other words, "Who am I to love?" Here is a modern retelling of that story:

An inner-city youth was kicked out of her home as a young teenager because not enough food was on the table. She begged and stole for a few months, but had to start turning tricks to survive. The psychological pain she endured became unbearable, so another prostitute helped her to minimize the pain with the high of cocaine that she sniffed daily. Eventually sniffing wasn't enough, and she began injecting the drug into her veins. After a year of this, she became sick with fever and passed out near the place where she solicited customers. She looked awful because she was very thin, sick with fever, and had vomited all over her clothes.

A pastor on his way to an inner-city revival meeting saw her and quickly crossed the street to avoid her since he was running late. She is beyond saving, he thought to himself. I must minister to the living.

A little later, a youth leader at the evangelical church came walking down the street hoping to witness to the neighborhood. He saw the teenage girl and turned away, thinking she probably brought all of this on herself. What's more, he had too many other duties to worry about one more down-and-out teenage hooker.

Fortunately, another prostitute named Tammy, who had just accepted the Lord as her Savior a month before, came by and saw the girl. Tammy was by no means perfect, having trouble escaping from the drugs that had also taken hold of her life. She had even turned three tricks a week before to get a few more drugs. But she had repented of this sin and genuinely had the love of God in her heart. She was getting counseling from a local Christian group and would stop the drugs and prostitution, she was sure.

Tammy carried the young teenager to her own apartment, cleaned her up, put some of her own clothes on her, and gave her something to eat. The teenager still looked quite ill, so Tammy called a taxi and took her to the hospital, spending the last ten dollars she had on the fare. The girl was hospitalized in serious condition, and Tammy stayed with her even though she didn't know the girl's name. After two weeks the girl was well enough to be discharged, and Tammy took her home and cared for her despite already difficult circumstances.

Jesus asked, "Which of these three do you think was a neighbor . . . ?" The expert in the law replied, "The one who had mercy. . . ." Jesus told him, "Go and do likewise" (Luke 10:36-37). The excuse might be given that it is appropriate for ex-hookers to love hookers and for former homosexuals to love homosexuals. But Jesus never allows that exemption for us. Our neighbor is every man or woman we have contact with, regardless of our natural attraction to their person and character. We will deserve the title "fishers of men" when we realize that our neighbor is the prostitute soliciting on the street, the IV drug user overdosing in an alley, the homosexual frequenting a gay bar . . . or the businessman mugged on his way to work.

Jesus never said the Christian life would be effortless; he said in Matthew 5 that it would involve persecution, turning the other cheek, and giving up our possessions. At the Last Judgment every circumstance of our lives will be examined, our actions as well as the motivations of our hearts. Perhaps the harlots and drug users will get into heaven more readily than many who are considered leaders in the church. God's warning to all of us is the same one John the Baptist gave to the Pharisees whose heart-change he doubted, "Who warned you to flee from the coming wrath? Produce fruit in keeping with repentance" (Matthew 3:7-8).

Nothing is more startling about the moral teaching of Scripture than the many verses that say we are to love our enemies. And that love is to be love in action, not the pseudo-love of saying, "Be warm and be filled," as we walk on the other side of the street from a dying teenager. No man or woman has sunk so low in sin, disease, and decadence that we should not reach out to him or her. This is not easy to accept, but it should remind us of our frailty as we attempt to live our lives for our Savior. We need to willingly admit our weakness and ask God for the strength to do the right thing.

THE TRANSITION

Warnings and opportunities in God's kingdom are two sides of the same coin. What he sends is a curse for one and a blessing for another, depending on how it is received. We think the same can be said for the AIDS epidemic. How can suffering and death, even if self-caused, be an opportunity for blessing? Perhaps the following true story will illustrate what we mean.

John loves to hike in the mountains. One day he went hiking with his sister, and they came to a snow-topped ledge. It was only two feet wide and about thirty to forty feet across to the other side. An icy slope dropped away from the ledge and at the bottom of the slope was a lake. One slip and the victim would fall down the slope and into the icy lake with virtually no hope of escape. But John foolishly wanted to go across the ledge, and he set out first. About half way across, some of the rock gave way, and he began to slide down the perilous slope. He accelerated faster and faster with no way to stop himself. By God's grace, a boulder was jutting out from the slope. As John continued to slide, his legs buckled under him, and he crashed into the rock. Had he been two feet to his left or right he would have missed this rock formation and plunged to his death.

This now-wiser man slowly recovered his senses and painstakingly crawled back up the slope along the path he had slid down; precariously he inched his way back to the arms of his relieved sister. He then had to hike down the mountain, assisted by his sister, with a broken kneecap, a bruised body, and an embarrassed ego. All the way down, despite his many pains, he was thanking his God who had graciously preserved him.

For the sexually immoral and for the society that has tolerated such destructive behavior, the AIDS epidemic can be read as a morality play. The signs of danger, such as increasing divorce, illegitimate children, and sexually trans-mitted diseases, have been ignored just as John ignored the danger before him on the snowy ledge. Society set out on an even more dangerous course. Finally, the ledge has given way and there is no way to stop the slide except by the grace of God. Our culture and the church need to throw themselves at the feet of our sovereign God and ask for mercy. As Os Guinness said of the West in 1973, "A culture rivaling Rome for inhumanity, ahead of Assyria in the catalogues of cruelty, surpassing Sodom and Gomorrah for its perversions, dare not plead for justice. That would mean only the silence of God, the judgment of being left to the consequences of our settled choice"[2] And our sins far surpass what was occurring in the early seventies.

But pain may be incurred even in God's grace, just as John was injured as he was saved from falling to his death. For some it might mean watching a friend with AIDS die, while being personally preserved. Others might have to go through the agony of withdrawal as they try to give up heroin. Another may have his life under a cloud because he is infected with the AIDS virus and awaits the destruction of his immune system. Another may have already reached that point as his immune status is poor and he awaits the coming of the opportunistic infections and death.

Is it grace to have one's life telescoped down so that only a few years or months remain? Yes it is, if in the process a prodigal son may return to his Father's loving embrace. God speaks to us in our pleasures, but shouts to us in our pain, C.S. Lewis once said.[3] This life is fleeting compared to the world to come, and if God must use pain and suffering to gain our attention, then so be it. The warnings existed long before the coming of the AIDS epidemic; AIDS is merely a step-up in intensity.

Lack of love for others is probably the sin that makes us Christians least like our Savior. But other sins should not be forgotten. Too many in the church have slipped down other icy slopes of materialism, self-righteousness, personal comfort in a dying world, and lack of forgiveness (even though so much has been forgiven them). Many bemoan the fact that Christians have little influence in our secularized world. They tell us our influence is undermined by the plots of secular humanists, conspiracies in the New Age movement, political actions by liberals, bias by the left-wing media, or conspiracies in the educational system. Christians have had little input into the modern world, but it is not for those reasons, which are only convenient scapegoats.

Christians have little influence in our society because we are not walking in the footsteps of our Master. If each of us would take up our cross each day and consider seriously what that means, then we would have great influence in the world. When we begin to show the compassion of the Lord Jesus—when we begin to tangibly reach out to a suffering world, when we begin to care for our enemies as much as for ourselves, when we are willing to die for our persecutors—then we will have taken hold of our heritage and reestablished tremendous influence on all areas of society. Just like the Lord Jesus.

The warning signs God has given to the unbelieving world in the AIDS epidemic are also given to Christians. The AIDS epidemic, borne of a decadent society, points out our own worldliness and consequent failure to win over our culture.

THE OPPORTUNITY

We are not responsible for the sin in the world, but we share in it when we have done less than our best to act as light. If there is limited light in the world, why should we be surprised when the non-Christian world acts as if it is in darkness? It is time to remove our light from under the basket. It is time to let our light shine boldly on the mountaintop.

The first event that occurs before a change in direction is a disavowal of the original path; in this case that might mean repentance for many Christians. An admission of wrongdoing is a difficult experience, but of all people, Christians should be most capable of admitting failure for three reasons.

First, because we have gone from darkness into light, we have the wisdom and power of the Holy Spirit available to us. If we ask for truth in our own lives, he will be faithful to reveal it to us. We delude ourselves if we do not acknowledge our need, for heartfelt change requires an intense spiritual battle.

Second, at some point prior to our regeneration, we admitted our guilt before God. Christianity is the only major worldview predicated on man's fallenness and need for change from above. To admit partial mistakes at various points in our life should be much easier.

Third, unlike the secular world, we do not depend on our rightness in deeds for our self-worth, but upon our rightness in being sons of the living God. To admit that our deeds have been ill-conceived does not destroy our worth. To become different by becoming more dependent on God is an act that separates us completely from the non-Christian world. It is at that point that we become truly available for God's service.

Charles Colson, in his book on politics titled *Kingdoms in Conflict*, recognized that change that makes a difference is change that begins at the grass-roots level.[4] He had been at the very pinnacle of power in the Nixon administration, yet came to realize that political power is in many ways impotent. He gives many examples of "little platoons" of godly people who are making a difference because they are loving people with their whole heart. Such love can come only from above. When we see more Christians acting in selfless love, we will be worthy of becoming fishers of men.

Look at the fields! They are white for harvest! The opportunities are boundless! What group of people is more open for the good news of Jesus Christ than those who are dying through consequences of their own actions? Look at all the homosexual men who would see the love of our Lord as we minister to their dying friends. What great numbers of IV drug users could come clean through the power of God's love, perhaps the only strength greater than a chemical addiction. How many doctors and nurses could be impressed with the compassion of the church as we carry AIDS patients to their clinics, give food and financial assistance, and invite those patients into our homes? How many family members could be affected as we offer to be peacemakers between estranged parents and their sons?

It is time for Christians en masse to lose our lives so as to gain them, to love others before ourselves, to take the servant's position and wash others' feet, and to be willing to take up our cross for a dying world. Then the influence of the intellectual children of Bertrand Russell, Margaret Mead, John Dewey, and Alfred Kinsey will fade away because they do not have the truth of God. Only we who know the Creator can provide lasting solutions for a dying world. That is the command we have been given and that is the cross we must take up. For his glory.

Chapter 20, Notes

1. Francis Schaeffer, *True Spirituality* (Wheaton, Ill.: Tyndale House Publishers, 1981), 169.

2. Os Guinness, *The Dust of Death* (Downers Grove, Ill.: InterVarsity Press, 1973), 367.

3. C. S. Lewis, *The Problem of Pain* (New York: Macmillan Publishing Co., 1962), 93.

4. Charles Colson, *Kingdoms in Conflict* (Grand Rapids, Mich.: Zondervan Publishing House, 1987), 253-64.

Glossary*

ABSTINENCE. Voluntary self-restraint from an activity, such as sexual intercourse.

ACQUIRED IMMUNODEFICIENCY SYNDROME (AIDS). The end-stage of infection from persistent HUMAN IMMUNODEFICIENCY VIRUS, characterized by a constellation of infections and cancers known to occur only when the IMMUNE SYSTEM has been weakened or destroyed.

AIDS BLOOD TEST. See ELISA and WESTERN BLOT.

AIDS-RELATED COMPLEX (ARC). A group of symptoms, signs, and infections that suggest progressive immune destruction from HUMAN IMMUNODEFICIENCY VIRUS, but not to the degree necessary to be called AIDS. This term is used less often now, as HIV infection is now seen as a continuum of steadily deteriorating immunity.

AIDS VIRUS. See HUMAN IMMUNODEFICIENCY VIRUS.

ANTIBIOTIC. A chemical or substance, either found in nature or formulated in the laboratory, that inhibits the growth of or kills microorganisms and can be taken either orally, by injection, or intravenously to treat infections.

ANTIBODY. A protein produced by cells of the IMMUNE SYSTEM to neutralize or eliminate material recognized as foreign to the body (such as bacteria, toxins, and VIRUSES). The presence of an ANTIBODY directed against a specific ANTIGEN (as measured in the laboratory) is evidence of previous infection by that ANTIGEN.

ANTIGEN. A substance which is not part of the body (i.e., foreign to the body) and which induces an ANTIBODY response by the IMMUNE SYSTEM.

AZT. The first approved medication for the treatment of HIV infection. AZT inhibits an enzyme (REVERSE TRANSCRIPTASE) necessary for HIV's replication in the T-HELPER CELL.

BIOPSY. A medical procedure whereby a piece of tissue is removed surgically for study in the laboratory under a microscope.

BISEXUAL. One who has sexual intercourse with both sexes.

CASUAL CONTAGIOUSNESS. Refers to the ease of spread of an infectious disease that would occur during normal day-to-day activities between individuals. Examples include microorganisms spread by respiratory droplet encountered by talking, coughing, or sneezing (e.g., measles, tuberculosis, and influenza) or spread by hand contact (e.g., colds, skin infections, and certain viral diarrheas). Excluded from this type of transmission is sexual contact (sexual intercourse) or sharing of needles and syringes between intravenous drug users.

CENTERS FOR DISEASE CONTROL (CDC). This branch of the
federal government, based in Atlanta, Georgia, is
responsible for investigations of outbreaks of illnesses
(new or old), tracking SEXUALLY TRANSMITTED DISEASES,
and recommending infection control policies for
hospitals, among other duties.

CHEMOTHERAPY. Treatment of cancers and malignancies with
drugs.

DNA. Deoxyribonucleic acid, a double-stranded building
block of genetic material found in genes and chromo-
somes in the nucleus of bacteria, VIRUSES, fungi, animal,
and plant cells.

ELISA, or ENZYME-LINKED IMMUNOSORBENT ASSAY. ELISA is a
laboratory method of determining the presence of
antibodies produced by the IMMUNE SYSTEM. In regards
to HIV it is very sensitive to detect all individuals with
HIV antibodies. But by being so sensitive, it will also
occasionally produce a positive test result (called a
false-positive), even when the individual being tested
has not been infected with HIV and made antibodies to
HIV. For an HIV ANTIBODY test to be a "true positive" or
"confirmed positive," an ELISA blood test is done
twice and if positive both times, a second test (*see*
WESTERN BLOT) is performed. Then if the WESTERN BLOT
is positive, one is said to have HIV ANTIBODY.

EPIDEMIC. A sudden appearance of a disease in a population
involving many persons at one time and which is
continuously present.

FACTOR VIII. The congenitally missing protein in HEMOPHILIA
needed for normal blood clotting. FACTOR VIII is
commercially available, being extracted from
thousands of units of plasma (obtained from blood
donors), then given intravenously to hemophiliacs,
causing their blood to clot properly.

HEMOPHILIA. An inherited defect in the blood clotting mechanism. HEMOPHILIA is manifested almost exclusively in males and is characterized by easy bleeding, both internally and externally. Supplementation of FACTOR VIII is required to prevent hemorrhages.

HETEROSEXUAL. One who is attracted to or has sexual intercourse exclusively with persons of the opposite sex.

HUMAN IMMUNODEFICIENCY VIRUS (HIV). The official name for the VIRUS that causes AIDS, but also called the AIDS VIRUS. Older names included HTLV-III or LAV (for human T-cell lymphotropic virus #3 and LYMPHADENOPATHY virus, respectively).

HIV ANTIBODY. A protein produced by the IMMUNE SYSTEM in response to infection with HIV. Presence of HIV ANTIBODY in one's blood stream is currently determined by two methods used in conjunction with one another, the ELISA and WESTERN BLOT blood tests. If these tests show that HIV is present, that is evidence of exposure to and infection with HIV.

HOMOSEXUAL. One who is attracted to or has sexual intercourse exclusively with persons of the same sex.

IMMUNE SYSTEM. The organ system of the body responsible for protecting and defending the body against damage from foreign substances and microorganisms. It is a delicately coordinated interaction between many different types of white blood cells, including lymphocytes, leukocytes, and the MACROPHAGE/MONOCYTE.

IMMUNODEFICIENCY. A state characterized by suppressed function or destruction of cellular elements of the IMMUNE SYSTEM. The result is to leave the person

susceptible to various microorganisms normally
contained, killed, or eliminated from the body. HIV is
Acquired and by its destruction of T-HELPER CELLS
causes Immunodeficiency, which in turn results in a
Syndrome of many OPPORTUNISTIC INFECTIONS and
cancers (thus the acronym "AIDS").

INCUBATION PERIOD. The period of time from actual entry of a
microorganism causing an infection to the time of first
symptoms and signs of the infection.

INTRAVENOUS DRUG USAGE (IVDU). The injection of drugs into
one's veins by needle and syringe.

KAPOSI'S SARCOMA (KS). A cancer or uncontrolled growth of
cells surrounding blood vessels. Prior to AIDS, KS was
only rarely seen as a slow-growing tumor in older men
or an unusually malignant variety in Africa.

LYMPHADENOPATHY. Abnormal swelling and enlargement of
lymph nodes, which are part of the IMMUNE SYSTEM.
Diffuse lymphadenopathy refers to this condition in
many lymph nodes in several parts of the body
simultaneously.

MACROPHAGE/MONOCYTE. A specialized white blood cell of
the IMMUNE SYSTEM that normally ingests and destroys
microorganisms. Unfortunately in the case of HIV
infection, HIV actually survives in the
MACROPHAGE/MONOCYTE, rather than being destroyed
by the cell's chemicals. Serving as a haven, the
MACROPHAGE/MONOCYTE is believed responsible for
actually taking HIV into the brain tissues, a sort of
"Trojan horse" event.

MONOGAMY. Marriage and/or sexual intercourse with only
one partner.

OPPORTUNISTIC INFECTIONS (OI). Infections that occur only when the body's IMMUNE SYSTEM is not working properly or portions of the IMMUNE SYSTEM have been destroyed. Usually in the case of AIDS these infections are relapses of previously dormant infections and are "opportunists" once IMMUNODEFICIENCY develops.

PNEUMOCYSTIS CARINII PNEUMONIA (PCP). The most common opportunistic infection in AIDS patients. *Pneumocystis carinii* is a ubiquitous microorganism previously thought to be a protozoan, but recent findings suggest genetic characteristics of a fungus. The most common manifestation is pneumonia, characterized by fever, breathlessness, and nonproductive cough.

RETROVIRUS. A family of VIRUSES characterized by a unique enzyme, REVERSE TRANSCRIPTASE. Within one of the subfamilies of retroviruses called lentiviruses are several animal VIRUSES and two human VIRUSES (HIV-1 and HIV-2). These lentiviruses persist despite action by the IMMUNE SYSTEM, probably by passing cell to cell.

REVERSE TRANSCRIPTASE. An enzyme, produced by HIV and needed for the incorporation of HIV's genetic material into the host cell's genetic material for eventual replication.

RNA. Ribonucleic acid, a single-strand of genetic material found in the nuclei of some VIRUSES, but also in the cytoplasm of VIRUSES, bacteria, fungi, animal, and plant cells.

SEXUALLY TRANSMITTED DISEASES (STDs). Infections that are spread via the physical contact from sexual activity between two individuals.

SPERMICIDE. A chemical placed in the vagina that kills sperm. Nonoxynol-9 is a commercially available SPERMICIDE also shown in the laboratory to be lethal for HIV.

T-HELPER CELLS. A part of the IMMUNE SYSTEM that directs and augments the immune response against foreign material and microorganisms. It is this very specialized immune cell that HIV preferentially invades, replicates in, and then destroys. Since the T-HELPER CELLS function like a conductor of an orchestra or a quarterback of a football team, their destruction by HIV infection results in an "acquired immunodeficient" state, rendering one helpless against various infections and cancers.

VACCINE. A substance that when given to a person results in the IMMUNE SYSTEM producing an ANTIBODY that provides protection to the individual against a particular disease.

VIRUS/VIRUSES. The smallest of all microorganisms, containing genetic material (in the form of the RNA or DNA) and proteins, but unable to reproduce outside living cells.

WESTERN BLOT. A very specialized and technically difficult laboratory method for determining the presence of HIV antibodies. This technique is used on blood that has been tested positive twice for the presence of HIV antibodies using the ELISA test. If the WESTERN BLOT test is interpreted as positive (demonstrates presence of HIV ANTIBODY), one is said to have a "true" positive result or a "confirmed" positive ANTIBODY test.

*Taken in part from *AIDS: A Guide for Survival* (Harris County Medical Society and Houston Academy of Medicine, 1987); *Stedman's Medical Dictionary* 22d ed. (Baltimore: The Williams & Wilkins Co., 1972); and with the assistance of Steven W. Parker, M.D.

Select Bibliography

Alcorn, Randy. *Christians in the Wake of the Sexual Revolution.* Portland, Ore.: Multnomah Press, 1985.

Alcorn covers comprehensively the many aspects of the sexual revolution, including causes and effects and methods to turn the process around. Although this is an excellent book, Alcorn does not put enough emphasis on basic social changes in America that have been the driving force behind the revolution and that will make reversal, even in the age of AIDS, that much more difficult.

Bellah, Robert et al. *Habits of the Heart.* New York: Harper and Row, 1985.

This book, written by several sociologists, discusses the important issues facing individuals in the 1980s. The authors explore the tendency of society to think in psychological terms while showing the importance of commitment, family, and religion to give the full life.

Colson, Charles. *Kingdoms in Conflict*. Grand Rapids, Mich.: Zondervan Publishing House, 1987.

> Colson shows clearly the difficulties involved in trying to make a government Christian and shows why that should probably not be our main goal anyway. He has a strong emphasis on the power and compassion of grassroots Christianity to effect positive changes in our culture.

Crabb, Lawrence. *Understanding People*. Grand Rapids, Mich.: Zondervan Publishing House, 1987.

> Probably the best work Crabb has done since it lays a firm foundation for "Christian" psychology. He asks the basic questions most Christian psychologists have overlooked.

D'Emilio, John and Estelle Freedman. *Intimate Matters: A History of Sexuality in America*. New York: Harper and Row, 1988.

> This book deals with the history of sexuality in America from an academic point of view. It is well written for a scholarly book, but tends to be descriptive and accepting of all forms of sexuality, which is not surprising since D'Emilio is a homosexual. It therefore has major blind spots such as an uncritical acceptance of the Kinsey Report data despite its many errors and refusal to see the great damage the "free love" movement has caused.

Elkind, David. *The Hurried Child*. Reading, Mass.: Addison-Wesley, 1981.

> Psychologist Elkind shows how the modern world has tended to force children into adult roles with resulting promiscuous sexuality, revolt against parents, and childhood anxiety.

Ellul, Jacques. *Money and Power*. Downers Grove, Ill.:
InterVarsity Press, 1984.

Ellul talks about what money is; most Christian
authors talk about what money does. He thereby
points to the intrinsic dangers of money, although he
goes too far by claiming money is evil in itself. The first
half of the book is still highly recommended.

Guinness, Os. *The Gravedigger File*. Downers Grove, Ill.:
InterVarsity Press, 1983.

Guinness provides the needed balance for the "ideas
make history" of *Idols for Destruction*. As a sociologist,
he sees how our society and culture effect changes in
the way people think. The book is written similarly to
C.S. Lewis's *The Screwtape Letters* in that each chapter is
a letter from an enemy agent to a subordinate showing
how social changes brought on by the church have dug
a grave for Christianity.

Johnson, Paul. *Modern Times*. New York: Harper and Row,
1983.

Roger Rosenblatt, senior editor of *Time* magazine, has
said that Johnson has a conservative axe to grind.
Maybe so, but he does it exceedingly well, documenting
his interpretation of the twentieth century better than
most liberals do. He traces the fall of absolutes and why
that directly caused the carnage of our century. The
only disappointment is that the book ends abruptly, not
calling for the need to return to the absolutes that the
whole book would seem to point to.

_____. *Intellectuals*. New York: Harper and Row, 1988.

A somewhat disappointing book after *Modern Times*
(although still worth reading) which claims that most

intellectuals of the left are self-centered and far more interested in the abstract idea "humanity" than the real life humans around them. Although that is probably a true tendency, Johnson never explains why he chose to talk about the particular men and women he did and so dilutes his theme.

Keysor, Charles, ed. *What You Should Know about Homosexuality*. Grand Rapids, Mich.: Zondervan Publishing House, 1981.

This excellent book discusses thought on homosexuality in the Old Testament, in the New Testament, from the point of view of the patriarchs, and in psychology. It is particularly good at laying to rest the liberal theologians' attempt at making homosexuality acceptable from a scriptural perspective.

Kilpatrick, William. *Psychological Seduction*. Nashville: Thomas Nelson Publishers, 1983.

This psychologist does an admirable job of criticizing the aims of the "humanistic" psychologists such as Carl Rogers, Rollo May, Virginia Satir, and many more. In this fallen world, "self-actualizing" psychologies have tended to translate into selfishness and have encouraged bad choices such as divorce, abortion, and personal aggrandizement.

Kübler-Ross, Elisabeth. *On Death and Dying*. New York: Macmillan Publishing Co., 1969.

This classic book describes the stages a dying person goes through including denial, anger, bargaining, and acceptance, and is a good book to read for those who might minister to HIV-positive individuals. Her most recent books, including one on AIDS, are badly marred by New Age thinking. However those do not detract from the quality of *On Death and Dying.*

McDowell, Josh and Dick Day. *Why Wait?* San Bernardino, Calif.: Here's Life Publishers, 1987.

This book discusses the teen sexuality crisis; it shows why teens have sex and gives a number of good reasons to wait. The authors allow teens to speak for themselves which is a strength since teens will be more affected by the words of their peers than by abstract ideas from adults.

Olasky, Marvin. *Prodigal Press.* Westchester, Ill.: Crossway Books, 1988.

Olasky teaches journalism at the University of Texas. In this book he shows how the media that was once Christian in emphasis and morality has fallen away. Moreover, he develops the different methods that "truth" is presented in the media and what is necessary to return this wayward child home.

Packer, J. I., ed. *The Best in Theology.* 4 vols. Carol Stream, Ill.: Christianity Today, Inc.

This recent yearly series of books brings together the best articles in various areas of theology written by evangelical scholars. Although many of the articles may be too esoteric for the tastes of the lay reader, for the most part they are well written and accessible to those with limited theological backgrounds.

Postman, Neil. *Amusing Ourselves to Death.* New York: Viking Penguin, 1985.

This is the most important book I have read outside of Scripture. Postman shows how our conversion to a visual culture (television, movies) from a print culture has caused fundamental changes for the worse in our society. Television has not merely detrimentally affected our society; it has altered it so that relationships, church services, and effectively all areas of our society now rely on superficial entertainment to be successful. Postman, a communications professor, has managed to convey the problem in clear-cut fashion in a short book.

Richards, Larry and Paul Johnson, M.D. *Death and the Caring Community.* Portland, Ore.: Multnomah Press, 1980.

This book has the strength of dealing with dying from an abstract, scriptural, and personal point of view since Johnson was dying of cancer at the time it was written. It demystifies dying, taking the fear away from those who might be called to minister to the terminally ill.

Schlossberg, Herbert. *Idols for Destruction.* Nashville: Thomas Nelson Publishers, 1983.

Schlossberg deals lucidly with the various ideas men have used to replace God. These "idols" take a number of forms which he develops in depth. He seems to think too highly of free markets, perhaps forgetting that capitalism too can be an idol.

Shilts, Randy. *And the Band Played On: Politics, People and the AIDS Epidemic.* New York: St. Martin's Press, 1987.

Shilts is a homosexual journalist who has followed the AIDS epidemic for a San Francisco newspaper since 1982. Considering his biases, he gives an accurate chronology of the epidemic while being even-handed in his criticism of various institutions for their failures at different times. His biggest weakness is that he does not emphasize the failure (sins) of individuals and that even if those criticized institutions had operated in the manner that Shilts wanted, it would have made little difference.

Stafford, Tim. *The Sexual Christian*. Wheaton, Ill.: Victor Books, 1989.

Stafford deals thoroughly with the challenges Christians face in the area of sexuality and how even committed Christians are vulnerable to sexual sin. He explains how our society's thinking on sexuality has changed from that of commitment to a crisis in true intimacy. (*See also* John White. *Eros Defiled*. Downers Grove, Ill.: InterVarsity Press, 1977.)

Swindoll, Charles R. *Living on the Ragged Edge*. Waco, Tex.: Word Books, 1985.

Swindoll does an admirable job of taking the Book of Ecclesiastes and applying it to today, showing that life "under the sun" is tedious, disappointing, and hopeless. However, life with God can transcend these problems, albeit not without difficulty and trials.

Ziegler, Philip. *The Black Death*. New York: Harper Torchbooks, 1969.

This readable academic book discusses the various aspects of the terrible series of bubonic epidemics of the 1300s that caused one-fourth of Europe to perish. Of special interest is the social changes that resulted from the carnage, some of which have parallels to the AIDS epidemic of today.

Scripture Index

Genesis
2:18 258
2:25 . . . . 250, 259
3 269
6:5 272
15:16 272
18 272

Exodus
19:4-6 286
20:17 162

Leviticus
5:3 184
13:45-46 184
18:21 272
18:22-23 . . . . 228, 234
19:1-2 298
20:1-5 272

Numbers
12:10 128
14 272
14:18-19 22
16 272

Deuteronomy
14:28-29 334
22:22 228
28 270

1 Samuel
16:7 395

2 Samuel
12 272

2 Kings
23:10 272

1 Chronicles
29:12 336

Psalms
50:12 336
145:9 14

Proverbs
3:9 338
4:18 210
19:17 336

Ecclesiastes
2:11 233

Isaiah
25:6-8 370
40:30-31 286
53 295
55:7 136
58:11 334
64:6 136

Jeremiah
25:11 273
32:17 184

Ezekiel
1:9 82
5:1 82
16:49-50 . . . . 237, 243
18:21-22 34
18:23 14

Hosea
8:7 112
13:14 370

Amos
4:10 82

Jonah
3 272

Micah
6:8 7
7:18-19 162

Malachi
2:15 250

Matthew
3:7-8 398
4:19 396
5 . . . . 396, 398
5:14-16 . . . . 210, 366
5:44-47 266
5:48 298

6:19-21 334
6:24 334
6:31, 33 336
9:10-12 136
10:8 337
11:20-24 244
19:4-6 . . . . 235, 250, 259
19:11-12 235
22:34-40 . . . . 279, 290
25:34-35 308
25:34-40 390

Mark
1:17 313
10:14 380

Luke
5:12-13 184
7:36-50 280
10:36-37 398
12:16-21 269
13:1-5 266
15 393
17:1-3 352
17:7-10 298
18:9-14 34
19 280
23:34 22

John
3:8 296
3:17 . . . . 112, 154
4 . . . . 280, 291
4:10 292
8 280
8:10-12 112
9:1-3 279

Acts
7:60 22

Romans
1:18-32 243
1:27 . . . . 234, 236
3:23-24 14
5:12-21 269

6:12-13 162
8:20-23 269

1 Corinthians
2:9 390
4:12-13 266
6:9-11 . . . . 228, 234, 236, 244
6:18-20 162
6:18 . . . . 243, 260
7:8 260
13 263
13:1-2 14
13:4-7 294
15:54 370
15:55 20

2 Corinthians
1:3-5 112
9:6 336

Galatians
3:28 261
5:13-14 316
5:19-21 243
6:7-8 270

Ephesians
2:8-10 210
5:1-2 266
5:21-25,28 . . . . 262, 316

Philippians
2:3 316

Colossians
1:28 298
2:9-10 261
3:12 352

1 Timothy
1:8 228

Titus
2:1 352

Hebrews
1:3 294
2:14-15 370
4:12 290
13:4 250

James
1 346
1:27 379
2:13 309
2:20 308
3:1 352

1 Peter
2:9 286
2:12 210
3:9 22
3:15 237
5:1-5 316

2 Peter
3:9 34

1 John
1:8-10 269
4:8 280

Revelation
1:17-18 136
6:7-8 82
20:10-15 374
22:17 390

Subject Index

Abortion, 378-79, 384
    women activists against, 64
    World Health Organization
        against, 64
Abstinence, 17, 168, 358-59, 361
Achan, 272, 386
Acquired immunodeficiency
    syndrome (AIDS),
    in Africa. *See* Africa and
        AIDS
    in Asia, 103
    in Australia, 103
    baptismal basins and spread
        of, 24
    bathrooms and spread of, 24
    in Caribbean, 104
    celebrity disease, 382
    challenging society's
        cherished myths, 383-84
    children, 150-51
    comparison with mortality of
        other illnesses, 217
    context of AIDS in society, 18
    definition of, 25
    Europe, cases in, 97, 103
    first report, 16
    incubation period of, 25, 85,
        94, 177
    infant spread of, 27, 91, 125-
        27
    infectiousness variability, 167
    minorities over-represented
        in, 126, 150
    most devastating illness of all
        time?, 25, 216
    number of cases, 86, 90, 92,
        95, 97, 99, 216
    origin of, 85
    politics and, 25
    scenarios of, 29-31
    in South America, 104
    stages of infection, 142-44
    Third world problems and,
        26
    tourism and, 26, 103, 104
    unidentified cause in some
        patients with, 127, 219
    urban predominance of, 28
    variety of secondary diseases
        of, 85
    weight loss and, 140
Acute retroviral syndrome, 142

Adultery, 212, 280, 289, 305
Advertisements, 253-54, 358, 385
Africa and AIDS, 88, 94, 97, 100-101
  breast-feeding in, 171
  heterosexual spread, 102, 276
  inflated estimates of AIDS cases, 101
  limited medical funds, 102
  mosquito-infested areas, 195
  "slim disease," 102
  social changes increasing spread, 101
Agape love, 235, 257, 263, 293
Age of first menses, 65
AIDS Related Complex (ARC), 26, 92, 94, 143
Aloneness, 258, 261
American Bar Association and abortion, 64
American Civil Liberties Union, 312, 342
American Family Association, 299
American Medical Association, 63, 64
American Psychiatric Association, 73, 240
Amoeba, 147, 230
Amsterdam, 169
Amyl nitrates ("poppers"), 88
Anal intercourse, 123, 147, 230, 239
Andrea Doria, 52
Anthrax, 199
Antiviral drugs, 152-53, 214
Aquinas, Thomas, 54
Artificial insemination, 171, 172, 240
Assault and battery, 175
Augustine, 54
Autologous transfusions. *See* Transfusions, donor directed
AZT, 100, 152, 153, 323, 330, 339, 362

Bacterial infections, 148, 151
Bailey, Derrick, 75, 236
Bats spreading fungal infection, 147
Bathhouses, 86, 87, 90, 92, 93, 96
Bathsheba, 272, 278
Bell and Weinberg study of homosexuals, 245
Beethoven, Ludwig, 58
Bennett, Michael, 100
Bettelheim, 364
Birds spreading fungal infection, 147
Birth control. *See* Contraception
Bisexual, 317
Bishop in Houston with AIDS, 128
Bites by humans, 197-98, 200
Blindness, 149, 281
Blood banks, 91, 95, 327, 385
Blood donors,
  in Africa, 188
  directed, 95, 99, 124, 169-70
  reduced numbers due to AIDS, 170
Blood ingestion by infants and transmission of HIV, 126
Blood supply safety, 215-16, 347
Botulism, 199
Brain infection by HIV, 150
Breast-feeding and spread of HIV, 126, 171
Brown, Governor Jerry, 86
Buber, Martin, 292-93
Bubonic plague, 175, 216, 217, 381, 382, 385

Calling of God, the, 322
Calvin, John, 336
Campylobacter, 148
Camus, Albert, 279, 373
Canaanites, 272, 277, 386
Cancer, 144, 145, 149
Capitalism, 56, 337
Casual transmission, 95, 175, 186, 216, 325, 357

evidence against, 187, 190, 191, 193, 197, 198, 201
  summary, 202-3
Catholic church, 75, 63-64, 382
Cats, 146, 213
Celibacy, 54, 235
Centers for Disease Control, the, 16, 90, 93, 94, 96, 97, 171, 190, 192, 195, 198, 216, 340
Chanchroid, 123
Chemotherapy, 145, 149, 150
Chesterton, G.K., 51, 255
Chickenpox, 144, 151, 175, 201
Childhood innocence, 385
Children, 74, 187
Chimpanzee as carrier of HIV, 214
Chlamydia, 88
Cholera, 322
Christ, his life and principles, 20, 128-29, 177, 178, 201, 211, 212, 221-24, 233, 236, 246-48, 257, 260, 268, 277, 279, 280, 281, 282, 288, 289, 291, 292, 294, 302-3, 308, 313, 320, 329, 332, 339, 340, 342, 343, 349-50, 366, 374, 376, 380, 387, 388, 395, 401
Christians and the comfortable life, 201, 400
Christians and sexual sin, 75, 234, 256, 260, 305, 384
Chronic illnesses and HIV disease, 153
Church, the, 54, 71, 139, 234, 236, 246, 247, 256-59, 261, 401
"City on a hill, " 263
Cleaning agents and the destruction of HIV, 199, 214
Coccidioides, 147
Cohabitation, 256
Cohn, Roy, 100
Colson, Charles, 288, 402
Coming of Age in Samoa, 60

Community, 386
Compassion, 280-81, 291, 309, 328, 340, 379
Complementariness of men and women, 258, 262
Computerized tomography (CT scan), 146
Comstock laws, 63
Condoms, 63, 165-67, 233, 358-60
Confidentiality, 173, 322, 324-25, 327
Contraception, 58, 63, 64
Cosmetics, 67
Coughing, 197, 219
Covenant House, 311
Cryptococcus, 147
Cryptosporidium, 146
Cystic fibrosis, 330
Cytomegalovirus (CMV), 149

Dancing, changes from the nineteenth century, 66-67
Daniel, 386
Darwin, Charles, 55-56
Date rape, 166
Dating, 306
David, King, 272, 278
Day, Doris, 98
Day-care center, 340
Death,
  in AIDS, 138, 222, 375
  description of, 371-73
  final adversary, 388
  of God, 15
  in the hospital, 375
  of Lazarus, 374
  proximity of, 376
  stages of, 379-80
  wish of homosexual men and IV drug users, 376-77
De Beavoir, Simone, 71-72
Democratic National Convention (1980), 86
Demographics of HIV disease, 190

Dentists, risk for HIV disease, 190, 197
Depression, the Great, 68-69
Desperation therapies, 98
Developmental delay, 151
Dewey, John, 68
Diabetes, 330
Dilemmas,
    of the AIDS epidemic, 164, 212
    "horns of," 288
Dionysius of Alexandria, 36
Discrimination, 324, 339, 343
Disease, inappropriate label to social sins, 386
Divorce, no-fault, 73
Dobson, James, 317
Dolan, Terry, 100
Dominican Republic, 194
Dostoevsky, Fydor, 19
Dressing changes, 189
Drug treatment centers, 329, 361, 377
Drug use, 241, 311
Dugas, Gaetan, 90, 318
Durant, Will, 58-59

Eagle, 287-88, 296
Ecclesiastes, 224, 233
Economics and the AIDS epidemic, 218, 223, 344
Education, 311, 355-56, 360, 361
Ehrlich, Paul, 62
Either-or choices, 288
Elderly, reduction of immune system strength in, 191
Elijah, 273
ELISA test for HIV, 140, 172, 325
Elkind, Lawrence, 364
Ellis, Havelock, 59, 60
Ellis, Perry, 100
Ellul, Jacques, 337
Employers, Christian, 340-41
Encephalitis, 146
Eros, 257, 337

Essex, Max, 215-16
Ethicist, 353
Expertise, fallacy of dependency, 17

Factor VIII, 91, 95, 169
False-positive, 140
Feminine Mystique, The, 72
Feminism and feminists, 72, 261
Financial assistance,
    to cities, 338
    to families of AIDS patients, 345-46
    in housing, 341
    to individuals, 338-39
    nationally, 338
    in nonpayment of rent, 343
Fishers of men, 289, 304-5, 310, 398, 402
Fletcher, Joseph, 75, 235
Florida, question of mosquito spread, 195
"Focus on the Family" radio program, 317
Ford, Henry, 66
Forgiveness, 280-81, 288, 291
Foster, Richard, 295
Foucoult, Michel, 100, 237
Fragmentation of knowledge, 18, 57
Francis, Saint, 261
"Free love," 233, 235, 254, 257, 312
Freedom, 319, 377
Freeman, Derek, 60
Freud, Sigmund, 56-57, 60, 67, 375
Friedan, Betty, 72
Funding problems, 94, 98

Gallo Robert, 94, 96, 100, 196, 215
Gamma globulin, 152, 169
Gandhi, 357
Gangrene, 199
Gay Bowel Syndrome, 230

Gay Freedom Day parade, 86, 229
Genital ulcers, and the spread of HIV, 102, 167
Genocides of the twentieth century, 57
Giardiasis, 147, 230
Ginsberg, Alan, 72
"Global village," 67
Good Shepherd, 154
Gonorrhea, 62-63, 188
Gottlieb, Michael, 87
Great Physician, 19, 178, 224
Greeks, ancient, 375
Groups within the AIDS epidemic, 320-22
Guinness, Os, 400
Gum disease, 144

Hairy leukoplakia, 144
Haiti and Haitians, 91, 104, 147, 194
Health care workers, close contact with HIV, 189, 198, 322
Hebrews and their writings, 253, 290
Heckler, Margaret, 96
Hemingway, Ernest, 58, 290, 319
Hemophiliacs, 28, 91, 95, 124
Hepatitis B, 88, 89, 91, 124, 126, 170, 192, 230, 276
Herpes, 63, 92, 123, 144, 145, 151, 188, 199-201
Histoplasmosis, 145, 147
Homosexuality in the Western Christian Tradition, 236
Homosexuals
  activists, 267-68, 329
  barriers to escaping addiction, 393-94
  behavior as evidence of change, 239
  books written about, 69, 72
  cures by various method-

ologies, 238, 241
denial early in the epidemic, 89, 90, 92, 94
diversity of, 229-30
during World War II, 70
forgiven, 244
former, 239
Freudian psychotherapy and, 237
gay bars, 70, 342
genetic determination of questioned, 238
hormonal determination questioned, 238
identical twins, 139, 238
immoral actions rather than orientation, 237, 342
in preindustrial societies, 237
judgment of God on, 96, 222, 268-69, 275-76
legalization, 242
"liberation" of, 73, 245
lifestyle of, 23, 24, 92, 328
married "closeted," 139
needs, basic, 328
New Testament condemnation of, 235
offensive sexual practices, 218
Old Testament condemnation of, 235, 342
other sins associated with, 243
pastors, 139
political power of, 86
promiscuity of, 86-87, 166, 240, 246
promotion of, 342
segregated culture of, 245
sinfulness of acts, 218, 221, 241, 243, 273
transience of lifestyle, 238
within the church, 23, 24
worst sin, the, 243
Honest to God, 235
Hooker, Evelyn, 238, 240

Hope, 379, 388
Hospices, 378
Hospitals, 218, 387
Hospitality, 236
Housing, 324
"Howl," 72
Hudson, Rock, 98, 326, 341, 385
Human immunodeficiency
    virus, 116, 117, 121, 172
  asymptomatic stage, 139-40
  antibody test for, 140-41
  biochemistry of, 215
  culture of, 127
  drying of, 198
  fetal tissues contain, 126
  fragility, 198-99, 214
  invasion of the cell, 117-18
  mutation into casually
    transmitted virus, 200-201
  numbers floating in the
    blood, 145
  people infected without
    knowing, 140
  reproduction within the cell,
    120
  spread of, 122, 166
  structure of, 215
  test for, 96, 98, 173
  type 2, 102, 200, 215
  vaccine for, 169, 176, 177
  wasting syndrome, 144
Humanism, 400

"I-It" relationship, 292-93
"I-Thou" relationship, 292-94
Ideals of maleness, 244-45
Idols of society, 19
Image of God, 18, 128, 154, 213,
    246, 263, 341, 375, 376, 395
Immunizations in patients with
    AIDS, 152
Imprisonment, for spreading
    HIV, 175, 326
Incest, 232, 251
Independence and individ-
    ualism, 258-59, 319, 386

Industrialization, 66
Infants with AIDS, support of,
    171
Influenza, 199
Insurance, 218, 277, 343-45, 385
Intimacy, 253, 257, 258
Intravenous drug users, 16, 27,
    88-90, 93, 125, 142, 168-69,
    170, 276, 398

James, Henry, 242
Jeremiah, 386
Jesus Christ. *See* Christ
John, the apostle, 279
John, the Baptist, 212, 398
John Paul II, 75
Jones, Stanton, 237
Joshua, 272, 273, 278
Judah, 273, 277
Jude, 236
Judging sources of information
    on AIDS, 220
Judgment of God, 268-69, 289,
    309, 400
  against the United States, 277
  cause-and effect, 270, 275,
    277, 279, 280-81
  definition, 269, 275
  final, 274, 398
  specific divine, 272, 275, 277-
    79
  universal, 269, 278

Kaposi's sarcoma, 86, 87, 149-
    50, 347
Kennedy, Edward, 86
Kingdoms in Conflict, 402
Kinsey, Alfred, 60, 61, 72, 238
Kinsey reports, the, 71, 236
Kissing, 198
Koch, Robert, 62
Koop, C. Everett, 100, 358, 362
Korah, 272, 278
Kramer, Larry, 93, 98

Lab technicians and risk of HIV

disease, 189
"Lancet," 94
Lawsuits, 326-27, 385
Legal restraints on carriers of venereal disease in Europe, 97
Legion of Decency, 69
Legionnaire's disease, 85-86, 346
Leisure, 66, 67, 260
Lenin, Nikolai, 290
Lepers and leprosy, 128-29, 302, 387
Lesbians, 171, 239-40, 276
Levy, Jay, 94
Lewis, C.S., 261, 288, 400
Liberace, 100
Light for the world, 305, 329, 401
Limitations of science, 384
Lister, Joseph, 62
Look magazine, 60
Los Angeles, 27, 96, 311
Love, 235, 281, 288-89, 293-95, 303-4, 320, 329
Luther, Martin, 54
Lying about probable method of acquisition of AIDS, 128
Lymph node enlargement, 143
Lymphoma, 150

Macrophage, 117, 143, 176
Malaria, 102, 196
Marx, Karl, 56, 290
Masters, William and Johnson, Virginia, 61, 238
Materialism, 234, 339, 349, 400
Maternal spread to infant, 126, 151, 170
May, Rollo, 71
McLuhan, Marshall, 69
McNeill, William H., 186
"Me generation," 72, 319
Mead, Margaret, 55, 60
Media, the mass, 92, 94, 306, 311, 365

in education, 356, 358
liberal bias, 356-57
sensationalist stories, 356-57
Medical schools, drop in applicants, 385
Meningitis, 147, 151
Metropolitan church, 235
Middle Ages, 54
Ministering, 199, 305, 307-11, 339
Miriam, sister of Moses, 128
Missionaries, 103, 387
Mistakes in the AIDS epidemic medical, 213-20
theological, 221-24
Monasticism, 54
Money, 336-38
Money, John, 238
Monkeys as host for HIV, 213
Monogamy, 17, 168, 245, 312, 359
Mononucleosis, 144
Montagnier, Luc, 93
Moral relativism, 18, 20
Moses, 278, 359
Mosquitoes, 194-97, 215, 357
Mother Teresa, 261, 312
Movies, 66, 68, 305-6, 364
Muggeridge, Malcolm, on education, 354
Muscular dystrophy, 330

Napoleon Bonaparte, 211-12
National Cancer Institute, 94, 215
National Enquirer, 220
National Gay and Lesbian Task Force, 241
Needle sticks, accidental, 125, 142, 170, 173, 192, 322
Needles, clean, 360-61
Needs of AIDS patients, 302
New Age spirituality, 362, 400
New Deal, 69
New England Journal of Medicine, 89, 220

New Jersey, 93
New York City, 27, 93, 96, 98,
    311, 338
"New morality," 52
Newsweek, 89
Niebuhr, H. Richard, 75
Nietzsche, Friedrich, 15, 19, 57
Ninevah, 272
Noah, 278
"The Normal Heart," 98
Nurses, infected by contact
    with blood, 189

Occupational spread of HIV,
    125, 170, 188
Old Testament, 293
Old woman/young woman
    drawing, 163-64
Opportunities, 398-401
Organ transplants, 171
Orphanages, 387

Parables, 291, 304
Paradigm shift, 164
Parasites, 144
Partner notification, 322-23,
    325-27
The Pasteur Institute, 93, 215
Pasteur, Louis, 62
"Patient Zero," 90, 318
Patients without identified risk
    factor, 193, 194
Paul, the apostle, 54, 235, 243,
    257, 260
Pediatrician, exposed as being
    HIV-positive, 340
Peer pressure, 306, 365
Penicillin, 52, 62
Pentamidine, 84, 146
Peter, the apostle, 235
Phagocytosis, 117
Pharisees, 222, 281, 289-90, 295, 398
Pilate, 386
The Pill, 52, 53, 63-64, 72, 166
Plague, and AIDS compared,
    322, 381-82

The Plague, 93, 279, 282, 373
Planned Parenthood, 74, 168,
    362-65
Playboy, 71, 263, 305
Pneumocystis carinii pneumonia,
    84-87, 145-46, 152, 317, 347
Pneumonia, 151
Political arena, 311, 312
Pornography, 66, 70, 73, 241,
    254, 328, 364
Possessions, 336, 344, 358
Post-Christian era, 245, 258, 328
Presley, Elvis, 72
Pre-teens, 172
Prisoners,
    mandatory HIV testing of,
        331
    medical care of, 332
    ministries to, 332
    rape of, 331
    rights of, 331
    solitary confinement of AIDS
        patients, 332
Prostitutes, 54, 70, 188, 254, 295,
    311, 330-31, 340, 398
Pseudo-scientists, 59-62
Psychologists, think
    homosexuality aberrant,
    241
Psychology, self-actualizing, 67,
    71
Public health authorities, 323
Public schools, dangers to AIDS
    patients, 330
Puritans, 54, 253

Quakers, and liberal sexual
    morality, 75
Quarantine, problems with,
    175, 176, 324

Rainbow coalition, 329
Rationalism, 289-90
Reagan, President, 96
Rebellion, 243-44, 271
Receptors on cells, 117

Redfield, Robert, 17
The Reformation, 54
Refusal to treat AIDS patients
    by health care workers, 322
Rekers, George Alan, 238
Relapse of previous infections
    in HIV disease, 145
Relationship, 293, 307, 329, 361,
    366, 377-78, 387
Rental property, 341
Repression, sexual, 59
Research, 85, 193, 346-48
Responsibility, 175, 321
    (diagram), 327
Restaurant workers, 340
Retinal infection, 149
Retrovirologists, 346
Retroviruses, 86, 94, 101, 116,
    214, 347
Reverse transcriptase, 152
Ribonucleic acid (RNA) viral
    vaccines, 214
Rights, personal, 319, 320
Robinson, Bishop, 235
Robinson, Max, 100
Rogers, Carl, 71
Romance novels, 70
Roosevelt, Franklin, 69
Rural society, 65
Russell, Bertrand, 55, 57-58, 60,
    290

Sadomasochism, 254
"Safe sex," 140, 164-66, 178, 233,
    312, 323, 356, 361
Saliva, 197-98
Salmonella, 148, 325
Salvation Army, 387
Samaritan, the good, 396-98
Samaritan woman, 280, 291-92
San Francisco, 27, 93, 96, 230,
    338
Sanger, Margaret, 58, 63
Sartre, Jean Paul, 376
Schaeffer, Francis, 396
Schlossberg, Herbert, 288

Science magazine, 94
Science and morality, 312
Secularization, 19, 322, 355
Self-centered, 303, 318, 319-20
Self-condemnation, 378
Self-esteem, 292, 306
Self-righteousness, 212, 223,
    231, 234, 279, 281, 290, 304,
    313, 396, 400
Semen, 123, 171
Sermon on the Mount, 201, 243,
    303
Servanthood, 262, 320
Sex education, 74, 311, 353-54,
    362-66
Sex manuals, 59
Sexologists, 61
Sexual addiction, 167, 233, 239,
    247, 255, 307, 318, 359, 377,
    384, 395
*Sexual Behavior in the Human
    Male*, 60
Sexual identity crisis in
    children, 242
Sexual immorality, 231, 233,
    290, 302, 359-60
Sexual promiscuity, cause of the
    AIDS epidemic, 18, 52, 86,
    88, 90, 101, 123, 255
Sexual revolution, 247, 253, 263,
    305, 307, 385
Sexual roles of males and
    females, 65, 262
Sexually transmitted diseases,
    63, 70, 242, 399
Sheep as host for HIV, 213
Shelley, Percy, 290
Shigella, 148
Shingles, 144
Simian immunodeficiency virus
    (SIV), 214
Single mothers, 232, 234
Singles, 256-57
Situation Ethics, 75, 235
Sleeping sickness in Africa, 102,
    196

Smallpox, 217
Soap operas, 254, 364
Social changes leading to the
	sexual revolution, 17, 67-76
Sodom and Gomorrah, 236, 243,
	272-73, 277, 278, 400
Sontag, Susan, 385
Sovereignty of God, 187, 277-78,
	310
Sperm as possible cause of
	AIDS, 88
Spinal cord, 150
Spouses, transmission of HIV,
	174
Statistics misused, 188, 219
Stein, Gertrude, 242
Sterility due to gonorrhea, 62
Steroids and immune
	suppression, 145
Stonewall Inn riot, 73, 342
Suffering Servant, 295
Suicide, 138, 378-79
Sulfa drugs, 146
Sunlight and HIV destruction,
	199, 214
Swindoll, Charles, 224
Syphilis, 62, 123, 148, 153, 173,
	188
Szanz, Thomas, 61

Taxes, 277, 289, 385
Teenagers, 165, 167, 233, 312,
	359, 364-65
Ten Boom, Corrie, 261
Ten Commandments, 270
Test animals, 177, 214
Testimony, laws as, 342
Testing, HIV,
	controversy, 324
	financial considerations, 173
	general, 172
	in insurance, 343-45
	mandated, 325-26
	in marriage, 172
	open reporting of, 173, 174
	prisoners, 173

in rape and incest, 173, 327
selective reporting, and, 174
syphilis, 173
voluntary notification, 174
T-cell leukemia, 94, 116
T-helper cell, 91, 95, 117, 120,
	121, 137, 142, 143, 145, 152,
	176, 356
Tetanus, 199, 382
Thoreau, Henry David, 362
Thrush, 143-44
Time magazine, 89, 92, 319
Time with children, 306
Timothy, 260
Tolerance, 319
Tolstoy, Leo, 305
Toxic shock syndrome, 86, 346
Toxoplasmosis, 146
Transcendent value, 319
Transfusions,
	donor-directed, 169, 170
	transmission of AIDS, 89,
	124, 142
Treatment, 143, 147, 148, 149,
	150, 151, 152, 153, 361-62
Treatment, withholding due to
	sin, 153
Trinity, the, 290
True Spirituality, 396
Tuberculosis, 144, 148, 197, 199-
	200, 219
Tuberculosis-like infections, 148

Unclean, ceremonially, 128-29,
	289
Unconscious, the, 56
"Understanding AIDS," 100

Value judgments, 168
Venereal diseases. *See* Sexually
	transmitted diseases
Victorians, 54
Vietnam war, 72
Virus, description of, 115
Warnings, 399-401
Weaver, Mark, 299-300, 304